Spinal Injury
and
Stroke
Rehabilitation

Spinal Injury and Stroke Rehabilitation

Editor

Mouli Madhab Ghatak MD (PMR)
Incharge and Chief Consultant
Department of Physical Medicine and Rehabilitation (PMR)
Medical Rehabilitation Center
TRA General Hospital
Formerly, Assistant Professor, Nopany College of Physiotherapy
Formerly, Visiting Consultant, KPC Medical College and Hospital
AMRI Hospital, Kolkata, West Bengal, India

Assistant Editors

Souvik Sen MD MS MPH FAHA
Director
UNC Hospital Stroke Center
Associate Professor
Department of Neurology
University of North Carolina, USA

Milind Deogaonkar MD MS MCh
Neurosurgeon and Fellow
Neural Transplantation and
Gene Therapy Program
Department of Neurosciences
Cleveland Clinic Foundation
Cleveland, OH, 44195, USA

Foreword

AK Mukherjee

JAYPEE **The Health Sciences Publisher**
New Delhi | London | Philadelphia | Panama

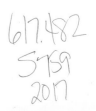

Jaypee Brothers Medical Publishers (P) Ltd.

Headquarters
Jaypee Brothers Medical Publishers (P) Ltd.
4838/24, Ansari Road, Daryaganj
New Delhi 110 002, India
Phone: +91-11-43574357
Fax: +91-11-43574314
E-mail: jaypee@jaypeebrothers.com

Overseas Offices
J.P. Medical Ltd.
83, Victoria Street, London
SW1H 0HW (UK)
Phone: +44-20 3170 8910
Fax: +44(0) 20 3008 6180
E-mail: info@jpmedpub.com

Jaypee Medical Inc.
325, Chestnut Street
Suite 412, Philadelphia, PA 19106, USA
Phone: +1 267-519-9789
E-mail: support@jpmedus.com

Jaypee-Highlights Medical Publishers Inc.
City of Knowledge, Building 235, 2nd Floor
Clayton, Panama City, Panama
Phone: +1 507-301-0496
Fax: +1 507-301-0499
E-mail: cservice@jphmedical.com

Jaypee Brothers Medical Publishers (P) Ltd.
17/1-B, Babar Road, Block-B
Shaymali, Mohammadpur
Dhaka-1207, Bangladesh
Mobile: +08801912003485
E-mail: jaypeedhaka@gmail.com

Jaypee Brothers Medical Publishers (P) Ltd.
Bhotahity, Kathmandu, Nepal
Phone: +977-9741283608
E-mail: kathmandu@jaypeebrothers.com

Website: www.jaypeebrothers.com
Website: www.jaypeedigital.com

Inquiries for bulk sales may be solicited at: jaypee@jaypeebrothers.com

Spinal Injury and Stroke Rehabilitation

First Edition: **2017**
ISBN: 978-93-80704-89-0
Printed at Rajkamal Electric Press, Plot No. 2, Phase-IV, Kundli, Haryana.

Dedicated to

*My late father
the beacon
light of my path*

Contributors

Amit Pathak BOT (NIOH, Kolkata)
Occupational Therapist
Department of Occupational Therapy
Howrah Orthopedic Hospital
Howrah, West Bengal, India

Arun B Taly MD DM (Neurology)
Professor and Head
Department of Neurology
National Institute of Mental Health
and Neurosciences
Bengaluru, Karnataka, India

Bhabani Kumar Chowdhury MD (PMR)
Diploma in Sports Medicine
Professor and Head
Department of Physical Medicine
and Rehabilitation (PMR)
Calcutta Medical College
Kolkata, West Bengal, India

HS Chhabra MS (Ortho)
Consultant Orthopedic Surgeon
Department of Orthopedic
Spine Surgery
Chief of Spine Service and
Medical Director
Indian Spinal Injuries Center
New Delhi, India

Indrajit Roy MS MCh
Senior Consultant Neurosurgeon
Department of Neurosurgery
Calcutta Medical Research Institute
Kolkata, West Bengal, India

Indu Marium Jacob
BSLH (Manipal) BSc (Speech Therapy with Honors)
Australia
Speech Therapist
Department of Physical Medicine
and Rehabilitation (PMR)
Christian Medical College (CMC)
and Hospital
Vellore, Tamil Nadu, India

K Venugopal DNB (PMR)
Ex-Senior Lecturer
Department of Physical Medicine
and Rehabilitation (PMR)
Christian Medical College
and Hospital (CMC)
Vellore, Tamil Nadu, India

KPS Nair MD DM (Neurology)
Assistant Professor
Department of Psychiatric and
Neurological Rehabilitation
National Institute of Mental Health
and Neurosciences
Bengaluru, Karnataka, India

Mahima Agarwal MBBS MD DNB
MNAMS (PMR)
Assistant Professor
Department of PMR
Jawaharlal Nehru Medical College and
Attached Hospitals
Ajmer, Rajasthan, India

Milind Deogaonkar MD MS MCh
Neurosurgeon and Fellow
Neural Transplantation and
Gene Therapy Program
Department of Neurosciences
Cleveland Clinic Foundation
Cleveland, OH, 44195, USA

Mouli Madhab Ghatak MD (PMR)
Incharge and Chief Consultant
Department of Physical Medicine and
Rehabilitation (PMR)
Medical Rehabilitation Center
TRA General Hospital
Formerly, Assistant Professor
Nopany College of Physiotherapy
Formerly, Visiting Consultant, KPC
Medical College and Hospital
AMRI Hospital
Kolkata, West Bengal, India

Mrinal Joshi MBBS MD DNB MNAMS (PMR)
Professor
Department of Physical Medicine and
Rehabilitation (PMR)
Rehabilitation Research and
State Spinal Injury Center
SMS Medical College and Attached
Hospitals
Jaipur, Rajasthan, India

Partha Pratim Pan MD (PMR)
Assistant Professor and Head
Department of Physical Medicine
and Rehabilitation (PMR)
North Bengal Medical College
Kolkata, West Bengal, India

Parthasarathi Bhattacharya MD DNB DM
Pulmonologist and Director
Department of Pulmonary Medicine
Institute of Pulmocare and Research
Kolkata, West Bengal, India

Ranen Kumar Ghatak MD (PMR)
Associate Professor
Department of Physical Medicine
Burdwan Medical College
Kolkata, West Bengal, India

Rupam Sinha MPT (Ortho)
Physiotherapy Officer
Department of Physiotherapy
Technical and Academics
GM Rehabilitation of Research Services
Kolkata, West Bengal, India

Rupnarayan Bhattacharya MS DNB MCh
Assistant Professor and Head
Department of Plastic Surgery
RG Kar Medical College
Kolkata, West Bengal, India

S Srinivas Rau Dip PT
Assistant Professor (Physiotherapy)
Department of Physiotherapy
National Institute for the
Orthopaedically Handicapped (NIOH)
Kolkata, West Bengal, India

S Ziauddin BPT (NIOH, Kolkata)
Physiotherapist
Department of Physiotherapy
Indian Railways

Shobini L Rao PhD (Psychology)
Former Professor and Head
Department of Clinical Psychology
National Institute of Mental Health
and Neurosciences
Bengaluru, Karnataka, India

Shrabani Sanyal Bhattacharya
BSc Clinical Nutrition and Dietetics (Hon)
Chief Nutritionist
Department of Nutrition and
Clinical Dietetics
Medical Rehabilitation Center
Kolkata, West Bengal, India

Souvik Sen MD MS MPH FAHA
Director
UNC Hospital Stroke Center
Associate Professor
Department of Neurology
University of North Carolina, USA

Srilekha Biswas
DPM (Eng) MRC Psych (London) MRCP (UK)
Ex-Professor and Head
Department of Psychiatry
RG Kar Medical College
Kolkata, West Bengal, India

Syed Ali Asad MS (Surgery) MS (Anatomy)
Extramural Teacher
Department of Anatomy
Vivekananda Institute
of Medical Sciences
Kolkata, West Bengal, India

Tanmay Sengupta BPO
Orthotist and Prosthetist
Medical Rehabilitation Center
Kolkata, West Bengal, India

West E Ray MS LTR/CTRS
Formerly Incharge
Department of Recreational Therapy
UNC Medical Center, USA
Chair
ATRA Higher Education Task
Force, USA

Dr. A.K. Mukherjee
MS (Orth.), D. Phil (Oxford), F.A.M.S.
Member Board of Governors
&
Director General

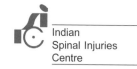

**Indian
Spinal Injuries
Centre**

Sector-C, Vasant Kunj, New Delhi-110070
Ph. : +91-11-4225 5225 (30 Lines) 4225 5213
(Direct) Fax : +91-11-2689 8810
E-mail : directorgeneral@isiconline.org
Web : www.isiconline.org

NABH, NABL, ISO 9001, ISO 14001 & OHSAS 18001

Foreword

It is a privilege to write the foreword of this book.

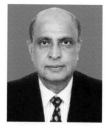

The global community today is passing through an exciting phase of development. The achievements in scientific fields have improved the quality of life of the human race. As a byproduct of this, the disability burden is on the increase. It is well known that disability is a human condition and disability load can be minimized in society.

Spinal injuries and strokes are important causes of disabilities leading to devastating disorders arising suddenly in life. Both are partially preventable and can be minimized with timely comprehensive rehabilitation intervention.

During the last decade, awareness about the need of rehabilitation program and the rights of persons with disabilities are strengthened through various global and regional instruments such as the UN Convention on the Rights of Persons with Disabilities (UNCRPD) and Incheon Strategy of the United Nations Economic and Social Commission for Asia and the Pacific (UNESCAP). It is mandatory for countries to make an inclusive developmental program of societies with a focus on disabilities. Thus, there is a need for an effective rehabilitation program to prevent and minimize disability burden in society. The contributors have presented the chapters in lucid form and added the recent scientific approaches to address various disability related issues.

The book will be valuable to professionals and to others who are involved with disability movements.

Dr AK Mukherjee
Member-Working Group (Disability), UNESCAP

Preface

The complex nature of the neurological and musculoskeletal disabilities is a real challenge in modern days. The 50 years back concept of "Not to move" after spinal injury and stroke, has gradually been changed by the grace of the great science—The Rehabilitation Medicine. With the spirit of this quickly progressing science, at least the disability of medical science is recovered up to a great extent and the huge load of stroke patients has obtained an option to avail rehabilitation treatment. In reality, conquering disability is not an easy job, and it demands proper application of rehabilitation science with a hearty and sympathetic care system.

Stroke and spinal injury are two major medical issues, where rehabilitation may be the pathfinder to get back to a productive life. It helps regain the lost function of the involved body parts and enhances the performance of the residual sound parts up to an above normal state to compensate the malfunctions of the impaired body parts. Moreover, the various medical hazards and complications arising out of stroke and spinal cord injury (SCI) need a continuous medical intervention with phases and monitored rehabilitation measures, which justifies the integrated and multidisciplinary approach of stroke and SCI rehabilitation.

The number of living stroke and SCI patients is only increasing because of the number of attacks (due to fast and pressurized life style) and highly improved emergency management (resulting in the number of survivors). Such an increased load of disabled persons should be properly dealt with integrated rehabilitation process, to reduce the social and family burden. This book has been planned to guide medical professionals towards an updated rehabilitation management, which I hope, will eventually contribute a lot to have a newer orientation on this subject.

Though this book had been assigned for providing information regarding only the rehabilitation stroke and spinal cord injury, but eventually, it is furnished with the complete science of stroke and SCI. The basic anatomy, pathology and all aspects of management with a deliberate focus on rehabilitation have been covered in different chapters of the book. Such a complete book, I hope will be helpful for not only a student or a doctor of physical medicine, but also to the neurologists, neurosurgeons, orthopedicians, other specialties and subspecialties who are working on stroke and SCI patients.

The book will provide advanced and multifocal management procedures for stroke and SCI patients. The scientific discussion and descriptions emphasized in the book are free for criticism and further opinion. I extend my thanks to Shrabani Sanyal Bhattacharya, Sanchita Ghatak and Rupam Sinha for their unstinting help and support.

Mouli Madhab Ghatak

Acknowledgments

I am grateful to all contributors and sub-editors for their contribution and support towards the publication of the book.

I also appreciate the support of some of my associates such as Dr Ranen Kumar Ghatak, Dr KM Das, Dr Sanchita Ghatak, etc.

I would remain grateful to Shri Jitendar P Vij (Group Chairman), Mr Ankit Vij (Group President), Mr Tarun Duneja (Director-Publishing) and associates of M/s Jaypee Brothers Medical Publishers (P) Ltd, New Delhi, India, especially Mr Sabyasachi Hazra (Commissioning Editor) and Ms Samina Khan (Executive Assistant to Director-Publishing) who always monitored the situations of the process very nicely.

Lastly, I thank my Associate and Nutritionist Mrs Shrabani Sanyal Bhattacharya, whose constant efforts and assistance have helped a lot for completing the whole process.

I acknowledge to all others who have directly or indirectly helped me to make the journey a success.

Contents

SECTION 1: Stroke Rehabilitation

1. Blood Supply of Brain and its Disorders   3
Syed Ali Asad

• Supply of Cerebrum *3* • Vascular Supply of Midbrain *6*
• Effects of Lesion *7* • Summary of the Principal Cortical
Areas of Cerebrum and their Lesions *12*

2. Clinical Presentation of Stroke Syndromes   14
Souvik Sen

• Clinical Diagnosis of Acute Ischemic and Hemorrhagic
Stroke *16* • Clinical Syndromes and Arterial Distribution
of Stroke *17* • Clinical Stroke Scales *25*

3. Evaluation of Stroke   28
Ranen Kumar Ghatak, Mouli Madhab Ghatak

• Stroke *28* • History *29* • Clinical Examination of
Stroke Patient *31* • Investigation *34* • Activity of Daily
Living *35* • Scales Used for Outcome Assessment *35*

4. Acute Stroke Management   40
Souvik Sen

• Mechanisms of Ischemic Stroke *43*
• Mortality/Morbidity *44* • Clinical History and
Symptomatology *45* • Physical Examination *45*
• Common Stroke Mimics (Differential Diagnosis) *47*
• Blood Tests in Acute Stroke *47* • Neuroimaging Studies
in Acute Stroke *48* • Other Tests that Might Assist in
Acute Stroke Management *51* • Stroke Medical Care *51*
• Surgical Care *53* • Consultations *54* • Diet *54*
• Physical Activity *55* • Further Inpatient Care *55*
• Outpatient Care/Rehabilitation *55* • In/Outpatient
Measures in Secondary Prevention *56* • Transfer to a
Stroke Capable Hospital *56* • Complications *57*
• Patient and Health Personnel Education *57*
• Palliative Care *58*

5. **Concepts in Stroke Rehabilitation**   **60**

Mouli Madhab Ghatak

- Neural Plasticity: The Light in Rehabilitation *60*
- The Learning: Plasticity Duet *61* • Basic Factors
in Stroke Rehabilitation *62* • Goal of Stroke
Rehabilitation Programs *62* • Stroke Recovery
Predictors (SRP) *62* • When Rehabilitation? *63*
- Where and Whom to Rehabilitate? *63*
- Phases of Poststroke Rehabilitation *64*
- Long-term Rehabilitation *72*

6. **Management of Complications and Deconditioning
Hazards of Stroke and Spinal Cord Injury Patients**   **78**

Partha Pratim Pan, Mouli Madhab Ghatak

- Musculoskeletal Changes *79* • Cardiovascular
Hazards *89* • Deep Vein Thrombosis and Pulmonary
Embolism *89* • Pulmonary Complications *91*
- Integumentary System *92*

7. **Therapeutic Exercise Program for Stroke Patients**   **97**

S Srinivas Rau

- Goals of Exercises during the Early Stage *97*
- Positioning the Patient *97* • Choice of Positioning *98*
- Reflex Inhibiting Movement Patterns *100* • Selective
Movements of the Upper Extremity *102* • The Lower
Extremity *102* • Trunk Mobilization in Hemiplegia *104*
- The Pelvis in Hemiplegia *106* • Gait and Gait
Training *106* • Some Useful Methods to Facilitate
Walking *107*

8. **Speech and Language Dysfunction in Stroke:
Diagnosis and Management**   **109**

K Venugopal, Indu Marium Jacob

- General Characteristics of Aphasia *110*
- Types of Aphasia *111* • Differential Diagnosis *111*
- Evaluation of Aphasia *114* • Assessment Instruments *115*
- Independent Test of Specific Skills *116* • Treatment of
Aphasia *117* • Variables that affect Treatment Outcome *117*
- Principles of Treatment of Aphasic Patients *118*
- Therapy Approaches *119* • New Therapeutic Approaches
for Teaching Aphasia *122* • Alternative Augmentative
Communication in Aphasia *122*

9. **Pressure Sore and Skin Care in Stroke and Spinal Cord Injuries** 128
   Rupnarayan Bhattacharya
   - Etiology of Pressure Sore *128* • Pathology *129*
   - Pressure Sore Grading *130* • Distribution of Pressure Sore *131* • Management of Pressure Sore *132*

10. **Swallowing Problems in Stroke and Brain Injury** 138
    K Venugopal, Indu Marium Jacob
    - Oral Preparatory Phase *139* • Oral Transport Stage *139*
    - Central Control of Swallowing *141* • Role of the Cerebral Cortex *141* • Characteristics of Swallowing Disorders in the Brain Injury *142* • Impaired Cognition *143*
    - Assessment of Swallowing *145* • Management of Dysphagia *147* • Alternatives to Rehabilitation of Oral Feeding *149*

11. **Psychiatric Rehabilitation in Stroke** 152
    Srilekha Biswas
    - Psychological Consequences of Stroke and their Management *152*

12. **Nature, Impact and Retraining of Cognitive Deficits in Stroke** 158
    Shobini L Rao
    - Nature of Cognitive Deficits in Stroke *158*
    - Prevalence of Cognitive Deficits *159*
    - Assessment of Cognitive Deficits *159*
    - Impact of Cognitive Deficits on Stroke Outcome *161*

13. **Nutritional Management of Stroke** 172
    Shrabani Sanyal Bhattacharya
    - Nutrition-related Risks and Preventive Diets for Stroke *175*
    - Dietary Management *176* • Hypocholesterolemic Agents *178*

SECTION 2: Spinal Cord Injury Rehabilitation

14. **Anatomy of Spinal Cord** 183
    Syed Ali Asad
    - Laminar Concept of Spinal Gray Matter *184*
    - White Matter of Spinal Cord *185* • Pain Control Mechanism *193* • Blood Supply of Spinal Cord *194*

15. Pathophysiology of Spinal Injury 202
Milind Deogaonkar

- *Spinal Column Injury:* Traumatic Forces *202*
- *Spinal Column Injury:* Mechanism of Injury *203*
- *Spinal Cord Injury:* Pathophysiology *205*

16. Evaluation of Spinal Cord Injury 207
HS Chhabra

- History *208* • Impairment, Disability and Handicap *208*
- Neurological Assessment *209* • Asia Scoring *210*
- Steps in Assigning an Asia Level *212* • Functional
Outcome Scales *214* • Assessment/Evaluation for
Complications *218* • Psychological Assessment *218*
- Evaluation for Requirement of Equipment, Aids
and Appliances *220* • Evaluation of Home, Workplace
and Environment *220*

17. Role of Electrodiagnostics in Spinal Cord Injury
and Stroke Rehabilitation 222
Arun B Taly, KPS Nair

- Evoked Potentials *223* • Electromyography *224*
- Nerve Conduction Studies *226* • Evaluation of
Autonomic Function *226* • Muscle Strength Testing *227*
- Evaluation of Fatigue *228* • Posturography *228*
- Gait Analysis *228* • Quantification of Spasticity *229*
- Pudendal Nerve Latency *235* • Assessment of
Residual Function *235*

18. Acute Care and Surgical Aspects of Spinal Injuries 239
Milind Deogaonkar

- Historical Aspects *239* • Epidemiology *240*
- Prehospital Management *242* • Acute in-hospital
Care *242* • Surgery for Spinal Cord Injury *245*

19. Concepts in Spinal Cord Injury Rehabilitation 248
Mouli Madhab Ghatak

- A Comprehensive SCI Rehabilitation *249*
- The Predischarge Preparation *251*
- Long-term Care for Quadriplegics *252*
- Modern Technologies in Spinal Cord Injury
Rehabilitation *254* • Management of Chronic
Pain in SCI Patients *254* • Assistive Technology
for People with Spinal Cord Injuries *258*

- Rehabilitation of Spinal Cord Injury Patients *264*
- Reintegration of a Spinal Cord Injury: Person *264*

20. **Therapeutic Rehabilitation and Medical Management of Spasticity**   **268**
   Rupam Sinha, S Ziauddin, Mouli Madhab Ghatak

   - Pathophysiology *268* • Factors Related to Movement Dysfunction after Stroke *269* • Positive and Negative Roles of Spasticity *269* • Movement Problems Associated with Spasticity *270* • Spasticity Treatment Planning *272* • Therapeutic Approaches in the Treatment of Spasticity *272* • Medical Management of Spasticity *276* • Intrathecal Baclofen Pump for Treatment of Spasticity *277*

21. **Therapeutic Exercises for Spinal Cord Injuries**   **285**
   S Srinivas Rau

   - Physiotherapy Assessment during the Acute Phase *286* • Physiotherapy Treatment during Acute Phase *287* • Passive or Active Movements *288* • Physiotherapy Treatment in the Subacute Phase *291*

22. **Surgical Management of Spasticity**   **297**
   Milind Deogaonkar

   - Surgical Strategies for Management of Spasticity *297*

23. **Functional Restoration of Spinal Cord Injury Patients**   **303**
   Amit Pathak

   - Basic Principles *303* • Preliminary Training for Functional Activities *304*

24. **Management of Neurogenic Bladder, Sexual and Bowel Dysfunction in Spinal Cord Injuries**   **309**
   Mahima Agarwal, Mrinal Joshi

   - Classification of Neurogenic Bladder *309* • Evaluation of Voiding Dysfunction *311* • Management of Voiding Dysfunctions *311* • Bladder Management Techniques *312* • Pharmacological Management *313* • Enhancing Bladder Emptying Pharmacologically *314* • Other Pharmaceutical Treatments for Bladder Emptying *314* • Surgical Treatment Options *314* • Pathophysiology and Clinical Features *315* • Aims of Neurogenic Bowel Management *316* • Neurogenic Bowel Management *316*

25. **Respiratory Care in Spinal Cord Injury**   319
Parthasarathi Bhattacharya

• Respiratory Problems in Spinal Cord Injury *320*
• Assessment of Pulmonary Function in Spinal
Cord Injury *323* • Others Issues: Prevention and
Treatment of Complications *328*

26. **Nutritional Management in Spinal Cord Injuries**   336
Shrabani Sanyal Bhattacharya

• Metabolic and Endocrine Changes after Spinal
Cord Injury *336* • Weight Management *337*
• Understanding Calories, Grams and Nutrients *338*
• Bowel Management *339* • Strategies for the
Prevention of Osteoporosis *340* • Skin Care *341*

27. **Wheelchair Selection and Training in Spinal
Cord Injury Patients**   342
Amit Pathak

• Evaluation *342* • Wheelchair Types (On the Basis
of Mobility) *343* • Ergonomic Consideration in
Wheelchair Selection *344* • Wheelchair Maneuvers
by Tetraplegic Patient without a Grip *346*
• Wheelchair Maneuvers by Paraplegic Patient *347*
• Wheelchair Prescription on the Basis of Level
of Injury *348*

28. **Orthotic Management in Stroke and
Spinal Cord Injury**   349
Mouli Madhab Ghatak, Tanmay Sengupta

• Types of Splints *349* • Lower Extremity *352*
• Levelwise Orthotic Management of Spinal
Cord Injury *353* • Advanced Orthosis *355*

SECTION 3: Brain Injury Rehabilitation

29. **Consequences of Traumatic Brain Injury**   361
Indrajit Roy

• Neurophysical Sequelae *362* • Neurobehavioral
Sequelae *364* • Case Reports *365*

30. **An Outline of Brain Injury Rehabilitation** 372

Bhabani Kumar Chowdhury

- Rehabilitation of Cases with Traumatic Brain Injury *373*
- Assessment Scale *373* • Diaschisis *373*
- Active Rehabilitation *375* • Cognitive Rehabilitation *377*
- Sexuality Rehabilitation *377* • Outcome of Brain Injured *377*

SECTION 4: Integration and Extension

31. **Models of Rehabilitation in Spinal Cord Injury and Stroke** 381

Mouli Madhab Ghatak

- Systems of Rehabilitation in Stroke and Spinal Cord Injuries *387*

32. **Recreational Therapy in Rehabilitation** 392

West E Ray

- Introduction to Recreational Therapy *392*
- Definition of Recreational Therapy *393*

33. **Epilogue: Regeneration Research—A Hope for Future** 416

Milind Deogaonkar

- Nature of Spinal Cord Injury *416* • Spinal Cord Repair Research *417* • Electrostimulus Devices: Paraplegics Walk Again *419*

Appendix 421

K Venugopal, Indu Marium Jacob

- Clinical Bedside Swallowing Assessment *421*

Index *423*

Plate 1

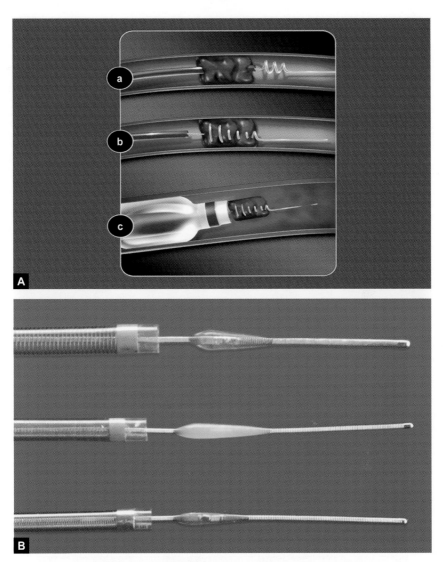

Figs 4.1A and B: (A) The MERCI system; (B) The Penumbra system

Plate 2

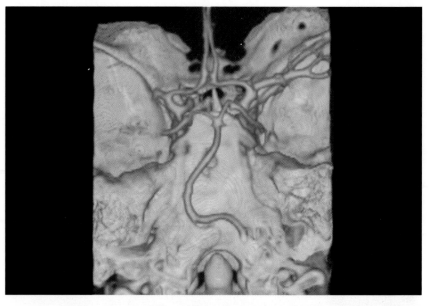

Fig. 4.4: Right middle cerebral artery occlusion

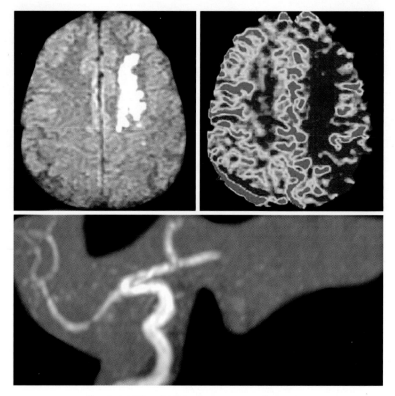

Fig. 4.5: MRI and MRA of an acute stroke patient

Plate 3

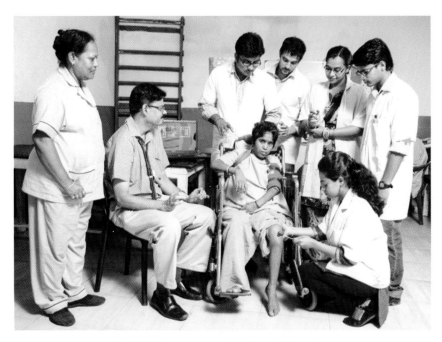

Fig. 5.1: The group examination and discussion

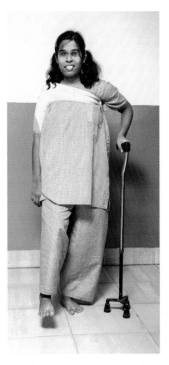

Fig. 5.2: Functional (gait) training in a stroke patient having
Bobath cuff in shoulder to prevent shoulder subluxation

Plate 4

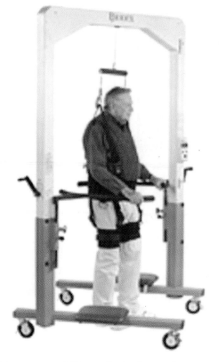

Fig. 5.3: Body weight supported (Harness) standing and gait training (on Treadmill) allows vertical shift of center of gravity and functional pelvic rotation
Courtesy: Hospimedica International

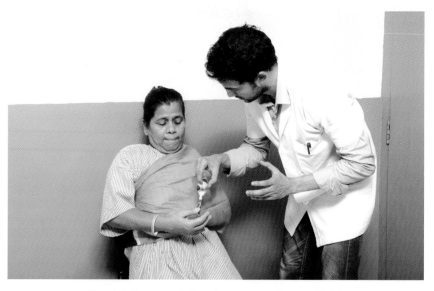

Fig. 5.4: Constraint-induced movement therapy (CIMT)

Plate 5

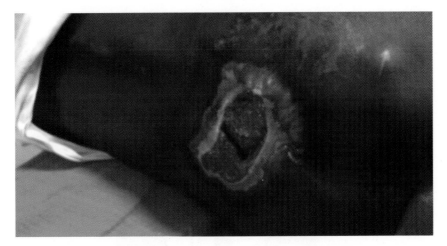

Fig. 9.1: Grade III pressure sore (sacral) in a paraplegic

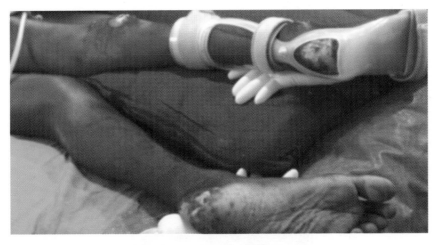

Fig. 9.2: Pressure sores at different sites

Plate 6

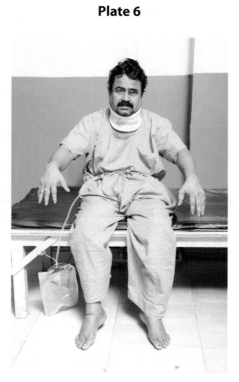

Fig. 19.1: A quadriplegic on acute care rehabilitation

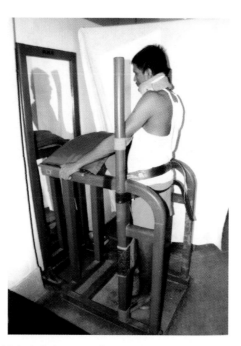

Fig. 19.2: A quadriplegic being trained to stand in a specially made "stand-in-frame"

Plate 7

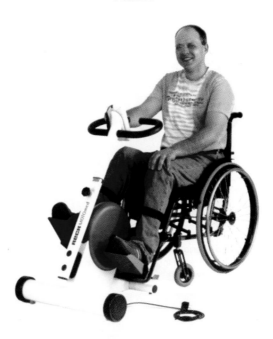

Fig. 19.3: MMT I—Motor-driven, software-controlled movement therapy system for passive, active and antispastic muscle training for paraplegics, quadriplegics and hemiplegics

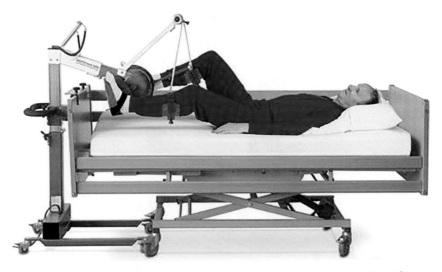

Fig. 19.4: MMT II—Patients confined to bed are trained with bed attached unit far remobilization and preventing contracture, pressure sore, thrombosis, etc.
Courtesy: Hospimedica International

Plate 8

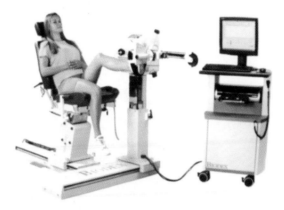

Fig. 19.5: Computerized strength and muscle function evaluation system (BIODEX)
Courtesy: Hospimedica International

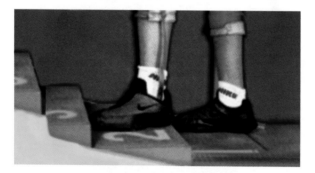

Fig. 19.6: Adjustable step height with push button control for SCI and stroke patients

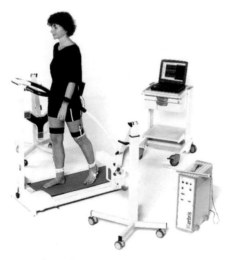

Fig. 19.7: Three-dimensional motion analysis system

Plate 9

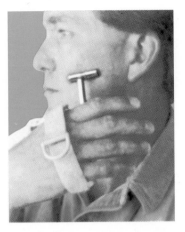

Fig. 19.8A: Adaptive hand device for ADL

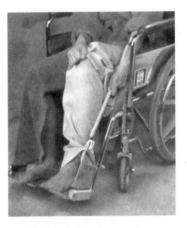

Fig. 19.8D: Assistive devices for self-care

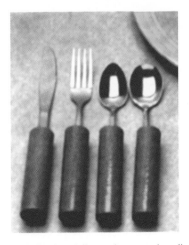

Fig. 19.8H: Specially made spoon handles

Plate 10

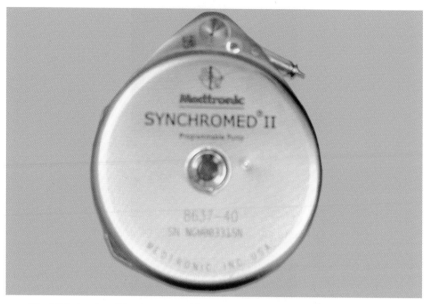

Fig. 20.1: Implantable, programmable Medtronic SynchroMed® Infusion System
(Medtronics, Minniapolis, MN) pump

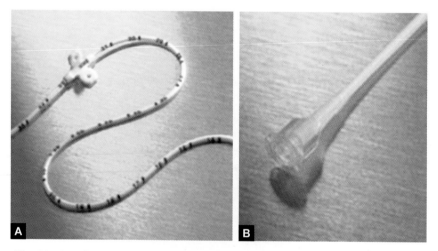

Figs 20.2A and B: Implantable, programmable Medtronic SynchroMed® Infusion System
(Medtronics, Minniapolis, MN) pump catheter (A) and connection (B)

Plate 11

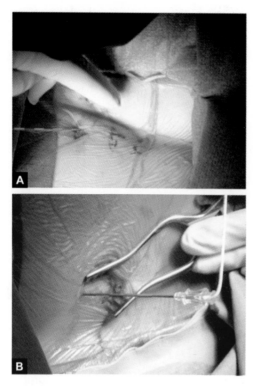

Figs 20.3A and B: Technique of implantation of intrathecal catheter

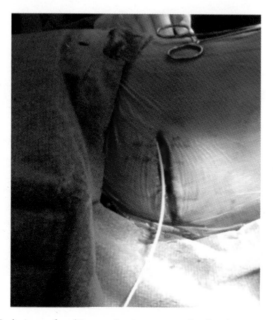

Fig. 20.4: Technique of making a subcutaneous pocket for the pump placement

Plate 12

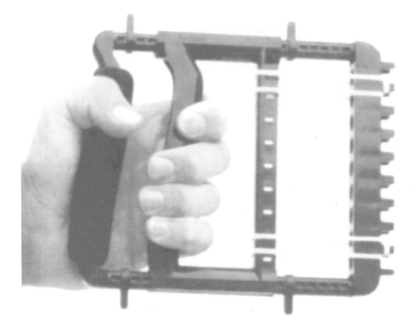

Fig. 21.1: Grip strength training

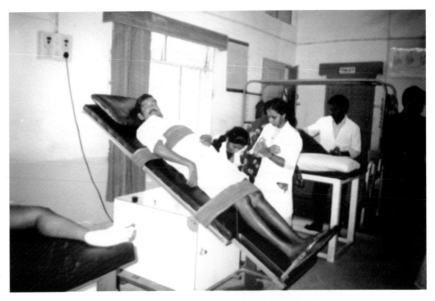

Fig. 21.2: Physical therapy sessions

Plate 13

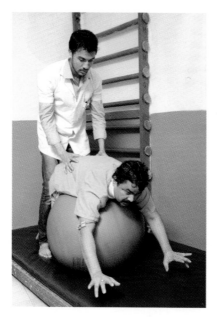

Fig. 21.3: Mat and ball activities in spinal cord injury patient

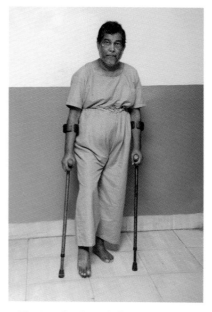

Fig. 21.4C: Bilateral elbow crutch gait

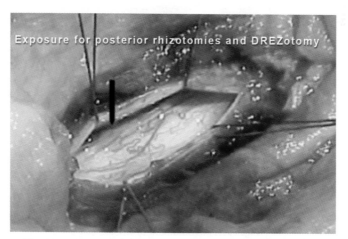

Fig. 22.2: Approach for the DREZotomy and posterior rhizotomy

Plate 14

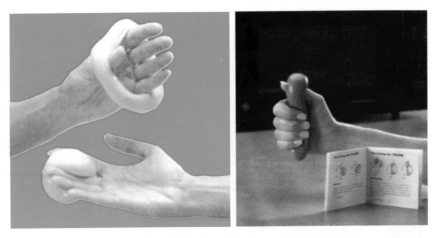

Fig. 23.1: Training of hand (coordination, manipulation, etc.)

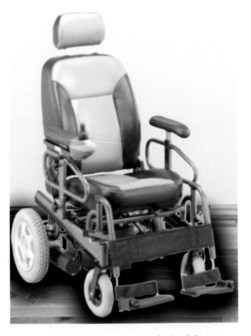

Fig. 27.1: Measurement of wheelchair

Plate 15

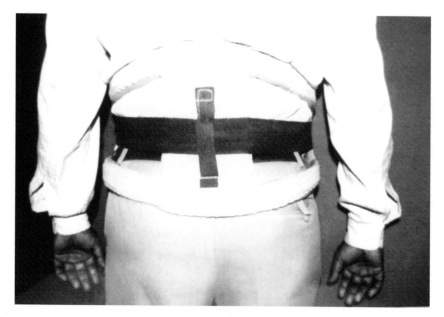

Fig. 28.1: Lumbosacral brace

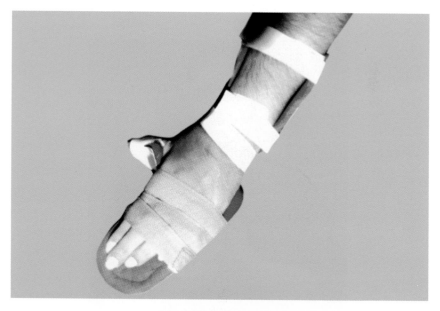

Fig. 28.2: Cock up splint

Plate 16

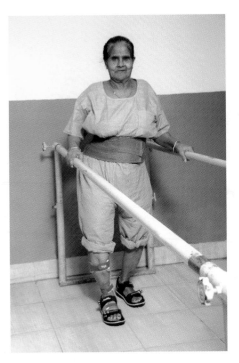

Fig. 28.3: Knee-ankle-foot orthosis

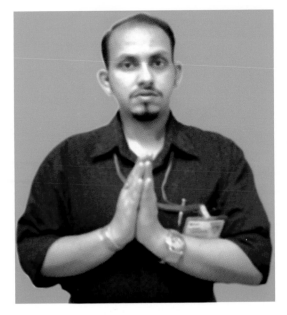

Fig. 29.3: RM January, 2005

Plate 17

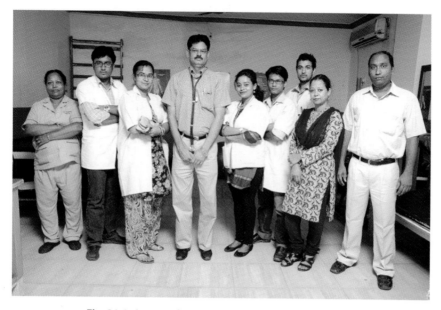

Fig. 31.1: A group discussion session with a stroke patient
at Medical Rehabilitation Center, Kolkata

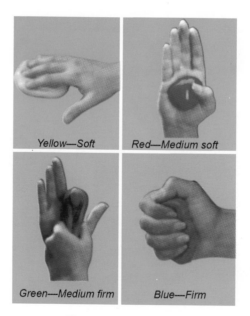

Fig. 31.2: Hand exercises

Plate 18

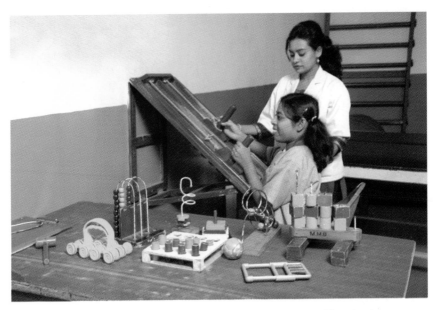

Fig. 31.3: The occupational therapy unit operating functional hand training

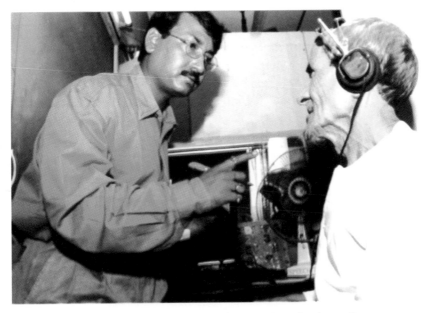

Fig. 31.4: A speech communication therapy unit performing audiogram

Plate 19

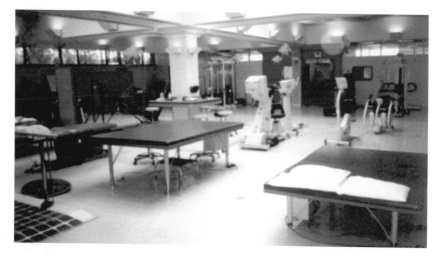

Fig. 31.5: Part of a rehabilitation gym

Section 1

Stroke Rehabilitation

Stroke rehabilitation is a continuous process of medical management of a stroke-affected patient having a minor to multifactorial problems to restore or regain the maximum functional capability, with the aim of reinstituting the patient to a normal or near normal physical, mental, social, familial and professional health status.

1

Blood Supply of Brain and its Disorders

Syed Ali Asad

The nervous system is of prime importance in our day-to-day life activities. It requires copious and profuse supply of oxygen through blood circulation and as such two systems of arteries are put to service for its proper functioning. Interruption of the supply of blood even for a period of ten seconds can produce unconsciousness and results in damage to nervous tissue.

The two sets of arteries that are destined to supply the brain form a polygonal anastomosis, the *Circle of Willis*, at the base of the brain around interpeduncular fossa. They are the carotid and the vertebral systems.

Internal carotid arteries supply frontal, parietal and a portion of temporal lobes. Two vertebral arteries unite to form basilar artery which supplies through its branches the occipital and rest part of temporal lobes, along with brainstem and the cerebellum. Without going into the details of branching mode of the parent arteries, only the branches supplying the functional areas of the brain including the brainstem and spinal cord will be dealt with.

Supply of Cerebrum

Superolateral Surface

It is supplied by the following arteries **(Fig. 1.1)**:
  a. Middle cerebral artery—it is a larger branch of internal carotid artery.
  b. Anterior cerebral artery—it is a smaller branch of internal carotid artery.

Middle cerebral artery runs in the stem of lateral sulcus and on the surface of the insula. Its branches supply almost two-thirds of this surface including temporal pole. Parts supplied by the cortical branches by this artery are:
  i. Greater parts of the primary motor and primary sensory areas of the cortex including the frontal eyefield.

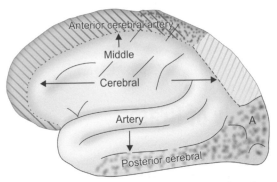

Fig. 1.1: Arterial supply of superolateral surface of cerebrum

ii. Broca's (area 44 and 45) and Wernicke's (area 22) areas of speech in dominant hemisphere.
iii. Lateral part of orbital surface.

Occlusion of this Artery Produces

- Contralateral paralysis affecting face and upper limb mostly.
- Sensory loss for position sense and discriminating touch of the opposite side.
- Severe aphasia (loss of speech) when dominant hemisphere is affected.

Anterior Cerebral Artery (Cortical Branches) Supply

- Medial part of orbital surface.
- Corpus callosum.
- Medial parts of frontal and parietal lobes extending upto parieto-occipital sulcus.
- Strip of cortex 2.5 cm on superolateral surface parallel to the superomedial border of the hemisphere.

Occlusion of this Artery Produces

- Paralysis of the lower limb (leg area) of the opposite side.
- Mild sensory deficit affecting contralateral lower limb. Two sets of capillary plexuses are formed by few branches of anterior cerebral artery while going to supply lamina terminalis. One set superficial to pia mater and the other in the substance of lamina terminalis. The plexuses form sinusoidal plexuses ultimately drain into the hypothalamic veins. Such portal system of vessels is known as *Organum Vasculosum lamina terminalis:* possibly they convey neurochemical substances to the hypothalamic neurons.

Posterior Cerebral Artery

It is the paired terminal branches of basilar artery.

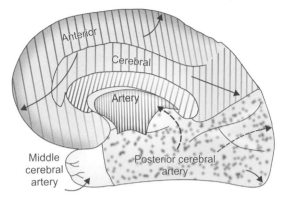

Fig. 1.2: Arterial supply of medial surface of cerebrum

Supplies: Having three Sets of Branches

Cortical, posterior choroidal and posterolateral striate branches—they supply the following:

- A narrow strip along lower border of the lateral aspect of the temporal lobe and lateral aspect of occipital lobe—i.e. primary visual cortex (area 17 through calcarine branch).
- Occlusion of this branch leads to homonymus hemianopia of opposite side vision.

Macular vision: Macula is spared due to presence of anastomosis of the cortical branches between the posterior and middle cerebral arteries close to the occipital pole.

Medial Surface of Cerebrum (Fig. 1.2)

- The anterior cerebral artery supplies anterior two-thirds of the medial surface that includes paracentral lobule also.
  So the areas are:
  Motor and sensory cortical areas, which are related to the perineum and opposite leg and foot areas.
- The middle cerebral artery supplies temporal pole.
- The posterior cerebral artery medial surface of occipital lobe. Its calcarine branch supplies the visual cortex.

Inferior Surface of Cerebrum (Fig. 1.3)

- *The posterior cerebral artery:* Inferomedial surface of temporal and occipital lobes except temporal pole (including visual area).
- *The middle cerebral artery:* Lateral part of the orbital surface of frontal lobe and temporal pole.
- *The anterior cerebral artery:* Medial part of the orbital surface of the frontal lobe.

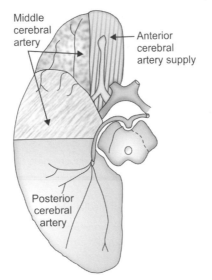

Middle cerebral artery

Anterior cerebral artery supply

Posterior cerebral artery

Fig. 1.3: Arterial supply of inferior surface of cerebrum

Thalamus

Supplied by the branches of the posterior cerebral, posterior communicating and anterior choroidal arteries.

- *Severe lesion of the thalamus:* Impairment of all forms of sensibility on opposite side of the body, as a result of damage to the ventral nuclei.
- *Korsakoff's syndrome:* It is due to injury to the mediodorsal nucleus of thalamus, characterized by difficulty in remembering new incidents and with loss of recent memory.
- Due to lesion of posterior choroidal artery (branch of posterior cerebral artery), the threshold for pain, touch and temperature is raised on opposite side of the body and sensations become exaggerated. This is known as thalamic syndrome **(Fig. 1.4)**.

Vascular Supply of Midbrain (Fig. 1.4)

Prelude: The branches derived from the vertebral system supply the brain stem in three arterial territories:

1. The *paramedian branches* penetrate the brainstem near the median plane and supply the *medial zone* on each side of the midsagittal plane.
2. The short circumferential branches supply the *anterolateral zone.*
3. The *long circumferential* branches (represented by posterior inferior cerebral arteries) supply the *posterolateral zone* and the cerebellum.

   So, the neurological signs following vascular lesion depend on the location and size of the affected area.

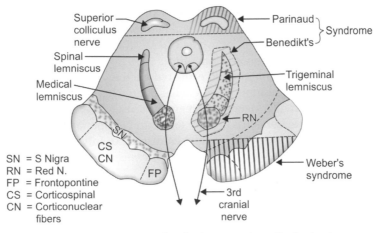

Fig. 1.4: Cross-section of midbrain at superior colliculus level

The arteries supplying the midbrain area are as follows:
- Central branches of posterior cerebral artery.
- Posterior communicating.
- Basilar (direct branches).
- Anterior choroidal.
  (Quadrigeminal artery emerging from circumferential branches supply mainly the colliculi).

Effects of Lesion

1. Lesion at mid tectum—by pressure from pineal tumor produces (due to involvement of superior colliculi nucleus).
   Paralysis of upward gaze, which may first be manifested as nystagmus in a vertical plane. Other eye movements are normal. *This area may contain a "centre for upward movement of the eyes."*
   Anatomical cause is not certain.
   It is known as *Parinaud's syndrome.*
2. Lesion affecting oculomotor nucleus and basis pedunculi with the involvement of pyramidal tract due to occlusion of posterior cerebral artery features are:
   a. Ipsilateral paralysis of the eye muscles supplied by 3rd cranial nerve (lower motor neuron).
   b. Producing ptosis (paralysis of levator palpebrae superioris).
   c. External strabismus—eyeball moves laterally because of medial rectus paralysis and pulled by lateral rectus (supplied by VIth cranial nerve).
   d. Loss of accommodation due to loss of ciliaris muscle and due to paralysis of sphincter pupillae, pupil dilates.

    e. Contralateral paralysis of the lower part of the face, the tongue and the arm and leg, i.e. contralateral hemiplegia.

      The whole episode is known as *Weber's syndrome.*

3. Lesion affecting midbrain tegmentum:
   a. It involves oculomotor nerve, the red nucleus, medial lemniscus and the fibers of the superior cerebellar peduncle.
   b. Causes (Vascular necrosis of tegmentum):
      i. Contralateral loss of pain, touch and temperature and vibratory and proprioceptive senses due to involvement of medial lemniscus—*which joins in the lateral spinothalamic tract at this level.*
      ii. Ipsilateral oculomotor palsy—*lateral squint and ptosis of same side.*
      iii. Tremor, chorea and athetosis due to involvement of the red nucleus and superior cerebellar peduncle.
      iv. Involuntary movements of the opposite limbs.
          All these signs and symptoms are together known as Benedikt's syndrome.

4. Ventral tegmental area contains (between red nucleus and substantia nigra) similar neurons like substantia nigra (dopaminergic). These neurons enter the mesolimbic pathway, which supplies the limbic structures of the forebrain. Excess activity in this pathway is thought to be related to the onset of *schizophrenia* exhibited by thought disturbances and delusions.

5. Internal squint and diplopia on looking down (superior oblique muscle of eyeball by trochlear nerve).

6. Involuntary movements and rigidity (red N, substantia nigra and reticular formation) due to affecting extrapyramidal system, produces Parkinson's disease, it is associated with tremor, rigidity and bradykinesis.

Lesions in the Pons (Fig. 1.5)

1. *Lesions in the medial and ventral part of the caudal pons:*
   a. Paramedian area is affected by the occlusion of paramedian and short circumferential branches of the basilar artery. This involves abducent nerve, facial nerve and pyramidal tract.

       This lesion produces alternating abducent hemiplegia (Raymond's syndrome), characterized by ipsilateral paralysis of lateral rectus muscle, producing internal squint with horizontal diplopia and contralateral hemiplegia.
   b. When facial nerve and pyramidal tract are involved—alternating facial hemiplegia results—manifested as paralysis of same side muscles of facial expression and contralateral hemiplegia.

       This is known as Millard—Gubler syndrome.

2. *Lesions in the lateral part of the midpons:*
   a. The lesion may involve the trigeminal nerve and the pyramidal tract resulting in alternating trigeminal hemiplegia.

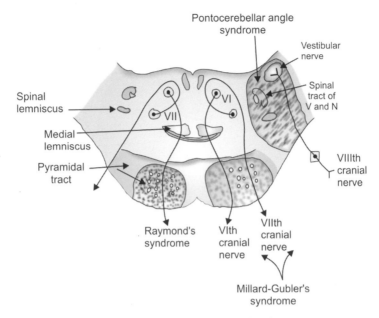

Fig. 1.5: Different parts of pons and its lesions

Features
- Paralysis (LMN) of the muscles of mastication on the same side of the lesion (spinal nucleus and tract of trigeminal nerve involvement) and anesthesia of face (same side of the lesion).
- Contralateral hemiplegia.
- Impaired sensation on the contralateral side of the body (spinothalamic tract involvement).

b. *Pontine hemorrhage:* The hemorrhage when occurs, produces extensive damage bilaterally.

Effects are:
i. Pin point pupil due to involvement of pontine sympathetic fibers for eye.
ii. Bilateral paralysis of face and limbs due to involvement of facial nerve nuclei and corticospinal tracts.
iii. Hyperpyrexia as the injury to the pons severs the connection with heat regulating center in hypothalamus.
iv. Deep coma due to involvement of reticular formation in pons.
v. Ataxic nystagmus is observed while attempting a lateral gaze (may be due to posterior internuclear ophthalmoplegia) in an abducted eye.

The Effects of Lesion in Internal Capsule (Fig. 1.6)

Internal capsule is a compact bundle of afferent and efferent cortical fibers, which connect the cerebral cortex to the brainstem and spinal cord.

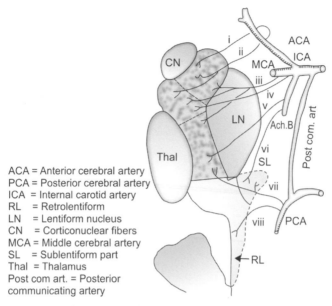

ACA = Anterior cerebral artery
PCA = Posterior cerebral artery
ICA = Internal carotid artery
RL   = Retrolentiform
LN   = Lentiform nucleus
CN   = Corticonuclear fibers
MCA = Middle cerebral artery
SL   = Sublentiform part
Thal = Thalamus
Post com art. = Posterior
communicating artery

Fig. 1.6: Internal capsule with blood supply

- Lesions at genu—lead to paralysis of face and upper limb of the opposite side, due to involvement of corticonuclear fibers for head and neck and corticospinal fibers for upper limb.
- Lesions at anterior 2/3rds of posterior limb—lead to contralateral hemiplegia due to involvement of corticospinal fibers for lower and upper limbs and corticorubral fibers.
- Lesions at posterior 1/3rd of posterior limb—lead to loss of sensation on the opposite side.
- Lesions of sublentiform and retrolentiforms—cause visual and auditory loss due to involvement of optic and auditory fibers respectively.

Internal capsule is supplied by **(Fig. 1.6)**:
- *Anterior limb:*
    i.   Striate branch of anterior cerebral artery (ACA),
    ii. Recurrent branch of Heubner of ACA,
    iii. Striate branch of middle cerebral artery (MCA) (Charcol's artery of cerebral hemorrhage)
- *Genu:* Recurrent branch of ACA (ii)
          Striate branch of MCA (iii)
          Direct branch from internal carotid artery (ICA) (iv)
- *Posterior limb:* Striate branch of MCA (iii)
                    Anterior choroidal artery (A.Ch.A) (v)
                    Branch from posterior cerebral artery (PCA) (vii)
- *Sublentiform part (SL):* Anterior choroidal artery (vi)
                            Posterior cerebral artery (vii)
- *Retrolentiform part (RL):* Branch from PCA (viii)

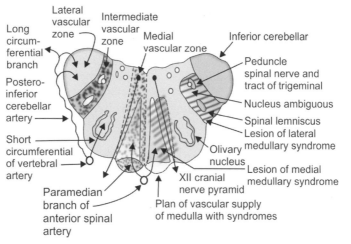

Fig. 1.7: Plan of vascular supply of medulla with syndromes

Lesions in the Medulla Oblongata (Fig. 1.7)

Its ventromedial part is supplied by medullary branches of vertebral artery and dorsolateral part by medullary branches of the posterior inferior cerebellar artery.

1. Lesion (occlusion) of a paramedian artery and anterior spinal artery that supply medially situated structures will lead to contralateral hemiplegia (UMN paralysis) (pyramidal tract involvement), loss of position sense and vibration sense in the limbs (medial lemniscus involvement) and ipsilateral paralysis of the tongue (hypoglossal nerve involvement) (LMN paralysis). The tongue when protruded the tip will be deviated to the affected side due to unopposed action of contralateral genioglossus muscle. *This is known as medial medullary syndrome (Dejerine's anterior bulbar syndrome).*
   This is also known as alternating hypoglossal hemiplegia.

   • If the lesion is further extended posteriorly involves inferior cerebellar peduncle and vestibular nuclei, produces hypotonia and ataxia of ipsilateral limbs (inferior cerebellar peduncle involved) and cerebellar asynergia and nystagmus (vestibular nuclei irritation) and giddiness.

   • Spinal lemniscus (lateral spinothalamic tract) lesion leads to loss of pain and temperature on the opposite half of body down the neck. Lesion of spinal nucleus and tract of trigeminal nerve leads to ipsilateral loss of pain and temperature from the face and forehead.

   • Nucleus ambiguous lesion leads to paralysis of the muscles of the soft palate, pharynx and larynx on the side of the lesion. This condition of ipsi-and contralateral sensory loss is known as *alternating hemianesthesia.*

   The whole episode is known as *lateral medullary syndrome* (Wallenberg's syndrome). It is also known as syndrome of the posterior inferior cerebellar artery as the lateral medullary arteries usually take origin from the proximal part of this artery.

Summary of the Principal Cortical Areas of Cerebrum and their Lesions

1. Lesion of *sensory area (areas 3, 1, 2)*—produces contralateral paraesthesia, e.g. numbness, "pins and needles" feelings on the opposite side of the body.
2. Lesion of *motor area (area 4)* convulsive seizure, start as focal twitchings on the opposite side of the body. Destructive lesions—contralateral paresis or paralysis.
3. Lesions of *promotor area (area 6)*—similar to area 4, when lesion includes area 4 along with area 6, irritation produces stereotyped movements along with head turning and torsion of the body. In premotor area involvement there will be impairment of learned movements (apraxia) execution occurs. This area mainly concerns with successful voluntary motor activities through extrapyramidal fibers, which arise from this area. So, the patient has hesitancy in performing complex, skilled and learned movements.
4. Lesion of *area of smell (area 28)*—anosmia—loss of sense of smell.
5. Lesions of the *auditory area—(areas 41 and 42)*—unilateral injury—mild deafness, bilateral injury—cortical deafness, stimulation of this area—buzzing and roaring sensations perceived.
6. Lesions of frontal eye field *(area 8)* affect conjugate movements of the eyeball (deviation of the eyes to the ipsilateral side).
7. Lesions of *ascending reticular activating system (ARAS)*—loss of consciousness or disruption in the arousal mechanism. Hypnotic drugs selectively block transmission of impulses in ARAS.
8. When *sensory speech area (area 22) of Wernicke* is involved, the patient suffers from receptive or sensory aphasia; he cannot understand spoken words although his hearing is normal (Area 22 is responsible for interpretation of sounds and comprehension of spoken language).
9. When there is damage to *"motor speech area of Broca" (areas 44 and 45)*: (left hemisphere of right handed person)—these areas control production of speech. Damage to these areas produce inability to articulate the sounds i.e., motor aphasia without *paralysis* of muscles of lips, tongue and rocal cord, when one speaks, his whole brain speaks.
10. Formation of *aneurysm*—the arteries forming the *circle of Willis* are prone to formation of aneurysm. When these aneurysms rupture they may produce *subarachnoid hemorrhage*. The anterior communicating artery aneurysm cause *bitemporal lower quadrantanopia* due to pressure effect on optic chiasma.
11. *Areas 39-40 (angular and supramarginal gyri)* are center for the process of learning, e.g. reading, writing and computing. So, lesions of these areas result in wide range of aphasic disorders, e.g. alexia (difficulty in reading), acalculia (computing disorder), agraphia (writing disorder) and anomia (disorder in recognizing names of objects).

12. *Prefrontal area (areas 9 to 12) lesion*—the patient with tumors of frontal lobe of prefrontal cortex shows symptoms of lack of sense of responsibility, vulgarity in speech and feeling of euphoria.
13. Unilateral lesion of *area 17* due to thrombosis of the posterior cerebral artery produces homonymous hemianopia since it receives visual impulses from the temporal half of the retina of same side and nasal half of the retina of the opposite side.
14. Unilateral lesions of *visuopsychic areas (areas 18 and 19)* lead to impairment of the identification of objects and its distance since these areas are responsible for association of the visual impressions with the past experience.

Bibliography

1. Alexander MP. Mild traumatic brain injury: pathophysiology, natural history and clinical management. Neurology. 1995;45(7):1253-60.
2. Belooseky, et al. The importance of brain infarct size and location in predicting outcome after stroke. Age and Ageing. 1995;24(6):515-8.
3. Bouma, et al. Cerebral circulation and metabolism after severe traumatic brain injury: the elusive role of ischaemia. J Neurosurg. 1991;75:685-93.
4. Chen, et al. Brain lesion, size and location: effects on motor recovery and functional outcome in stroke patients. Archive of Physical Medicine and Rehabilitation. 2000;81(4):447-52.
5. Dettmers, et al. Relations between cerebral activity and force in the motor areas of human brain. J Neurophysiol. 1995;74(2):802-15.
6. Halsband, et al. The role of premotor cortex and the supplementary motor area in the temporal control of movement in man. Brain. 1993;116:243-66.
7. Hardy, et al. Microsurgical anatomy of the superior cerebellar artery. Neurosurgery. 1980;6(11):1-120.
8. Henri MD. Surface, blood supply and three-dimensional section anatomy. The Human Brain, 2nd edn. Spinger, 1999.
9. J. De Reuck. The human periventricular arterial blood supply and anatomy of cerebral infraction. European Neurology. 1971;5(6):321-34.
10. Lammie. Pathology of small vessel stroke. British Medical Bulletin. 2000;56(2):296-306.
11. Stein, et al. Delayed and progressive brain injury in closed-head trauma: radiological demonstration. Neurosurgery. 1993;32(1):25-31.
12. Tatu, et al. Arterial territories of the human brain: cerebral hemispheres. Neurology. 1998;50(6):1699-708.
13. Zeal, Rhoton. Microsurgical anatomy of the posterior cerebral artery. Journal of Neurosurgery. 1978;48(4):534-59.

2

Clinical Presentation of Stroke Syndromes

Souvik Sen

Introduction

Stroke is the sudden onset neurological deficit of vascular origin. It is broadly classified into ischemic and hemorrhagic type, and the clinical presentation depends on the type of stroke and the territory of the brain affected. Physicians involved in management of acute stroke are generally interested in distinguishing between these two categories of stroke, as well as differentiating the etiological and prognostic subtypes, as the management may differ based on them. Although sometimes it is possible to distinguish clinically between ischemic and hemorrhagic stroke, the method is often not reliable and frequently need the assistance of imaging assessment such as non-contrast computed tomography (CT) scan or magnetic resonance imaging (MRI).

In order to distinguish clinically between ischemic and hemorrhagic stroke at the bedside, scoring systems have been designed and validated such as the Allen score, the Siriraj stroke score and the Besson score. However since 80% of strokes are ischemic and only 20% hemorrhagic, it is hard to find a score that is reliable greater than 90%. Determination of the cause of ischemic stroke in patients is important for the clinical management. The diagnostic test pursued and the stroke prevention strategy advocated is often dependent on the suspected cause of ischemic stroke. Ischemic stroke etiology may be classified using the Trial of Org 10172 in acute stroke treatment (TOAST) criteria. Cardioembolic etiology was considered in patients, with a major brain artery or a branch of cortical artery occlusion, who had at least one cardiac source identified, according to the TOAST criteria (example-atrial fibrillation). Potential large-artery atherosclerosis the source of thrombosis or embolism was assessed by carotid ultrasound and/or MRA. Small vessel occlusive disease is a consideration when a patient present with one of the lacunar stroke syndrome, with a corresponding lacunar infarct on CT/MRI and absence of any identified cardioembolic or large artery atherosclerosis. Uncommon causes of stroke identified on testing include CNS vasculitis, a hypercoagulable state, and "watershed infarct" from a hypoperfusion state or a traumatic dissection of a cerebral blood vessel. Stroke may be classified according to their clinical presentation, using the Oxfordshire community stroke project (OCSP) criteria. In brief: Lacunar infarcts (LACI) are diagnosed if patients present clinically with pure motor, sensorimotor or ataxic hemiparetic findings, confirmed with an appropriate CT/MRI lesion; total anterior circulation infarcts (TACI) are diagnosed if patients present with a cortical disorder (such as dysphasia, dyscalculia) and/or homonymous hemianopsia and/or ipsilateral sensory or motor findings involving at least two regions (with CT/MRI confirmation); posterior circulation infarct (POCI) are diagnosed in the presence of cranial nerve palsies and contralateral motor or sensory deficits, or bilateral motor or sensory findings or disorders of eye movement or cerebellar dysfunction. Partial anterior circulation infarct (PACI) is diagnosed if patients present with only two of the three components of the TACI syndrome and CT/MRI confirmation of an appropriate lesion.

Substantial progress has been made in recent times in stroke prevention strategies and treatment of acute ischemic stroke. Most of the stroke prevention strategies can be advocated after an initial assessment and may be instituted at a small cost, such as antithrombotic therapy, management of stroke risk factors such as hypertension, diabetes, smoking and hypercholesterolemia. These strategies may be implemented with minimal resources available in the setting of primary care. The more advance strategies such as carotid endarterectomy, carotid angioplasty and stenting may only be accomplished in the setting of an advanced tertiary referral center with infrastructure for vascular surgery and interventional neuroradiology. The treatment of acute ischemic stroke includes strategies to promote recanalization of an occluded artery such as thrombolysis and mechanical revascularization and ancillary management of cardiac and pulmonary comorbidities, blood pressure management, management of cerebral edema, anticoagulation and antiplatelet therapy and prevention of complications such as deep venous thrombosis, bedsore, stress ulcers nutritional care. The approach requires a massive multidisciplinary team approach and infrastructure that is often expensive and unaffordable. It is feasible that these strategies may be partly or wholly implemented and with adequate rehabilitation may achieve modest to good stroke outcome. Stroke outcome measures have been reliably assessed utilizing clinically based stroke scales such as the NIH stroke scale (NIHSS), the Canadian Neurological Scale (CNS), the Scandinavian Neurological stroke scale (SCNSS) and European stroke scale (ESS). These scales have the greatest utility in assessing severity of the stroke, monitoring stroke outcome and possibly prognosticating stroke outcome.

In this chapter, we shall emphasize specifically three aspects of the clinical assessment of stroke syndromes. Early clinical diagnosis of acute ischemic and hemorrhagic stroke, clinical stroke syndromes and stroke scales used to assess and prognosticate stroke at the time of presentation.

Clinical Diagnosis of Acute Ischemic and Hemorrhagic Stroke

The management of ischemic and hemorrhagic strokes is significantly different which makes it important to distinguish the two types of stroke in the acute setting. The typical symptoms of a hemorrhagic stroke are related to acute increase in intracranial pressure such as headache, vomiting, decrease in level of consciousness and occasionally signs of meningeal irritation. Lacunar stroke syndromes and resolution of stroke symptoms do not necessarily point towards an ischemic or hemorrhagic stroke.

Neuroimaging modalities such as a non-contrast CT or MRI can reliably distinguish between ischemic and hemorrhagic stroke. However, access to such diagnostic test are not available in a timely fashion to clinicians stressing the importance of clinical scoring system. In such a setting, there is need for a scoring system that is easy, reproducible and performed immediately after a stroke. The lack of a scoring system that is accurate and reliable, is a major setback to clinical scoring system. Nevertheless, such scoring systems have roles in assessment of the acute stroke. The three scoring systems those have used, are briefly summarized in **Table 2.1**.

Table 2.1: Clinical scores for differentiation of ischemic compared with hemorrhagic stroke		
Allen score	*Siriraj stroke score*	*Besson score*
1. Apoplectic onset	1. Level of consciousness	1. History of hypertension
2. Level of consciousness	2. Vomiting	2. History of TIA
3. Plantar responses	3. Headache	3. History of hyperlipidemia
4. Diastolic blood pressure	4. Diastolic blood pressure	4. Alcohol consumption
5. Atheroma markers	5. Atheroma markers	5. Headache
6. History of hypertension		6. Peripheral arterial disease
7. Previous TIA or stroke		7. Atrial fibrillation on admission
8. Heart disease		8. Plantar response

The Allen score is a validated, weighted, linear, clinical score that was developed from a multivariate analysis of the clinical data in large groups of patients. It was developed to help clinicians without immediate access to CT or MRI. A score greater than 6 is more likely to be secondary to ischemic stroke than a score of less than 6. The Siriraj stroke score was developed and validated in Thailand. It uses five elements and is easier to use than the Allen score. The Besson score is a simple validated score with a high positive predictive value. Factors such as history of transient neurological deficit, peripheral arterial disease, hyperlipidemia and atrial fibrillation lead to the diagnosis of ischemic stroke. Alcohol consumption, extensor plantar response, a history of hypertension and headache lead to 'uncertain' diagnosis. The score is computed using the formula (2 × alcohol consumption) + (1.5 × plantar response) + (3 × headache) + (3 × hypertension) – (5 × transient neurological deficit) – (peripheral arterial disease) – (1.5 × hyperlipidemia) – (2.5 × atrial fibrillation) <1 translates to a likely diagnosis of nonhemorrhagic stroke. The three scores have not been validated in the same patient group. The scores have their best utility in prioritizing patients for neuroimaging study such as CT scan or MRI scan and is best used to conjunction with such imaging. CT scan remains the test of choice for early exclusion of hemorrhagic.

Clinical Syndromes and Arterial Distribution of Stroke

Stroke is defined as a sudden onset of focal neurological deficit that is vascular in origin and typically the symptoms last more than 24 hours. Traditionally symptoms lasting less than 24 hours have been referred to as Transient Ischemic Attack or TIA. With the advent of advanced neuroimaging modalities such as Magnetic Resonance Diffusion Weighted Imaging (MR-DWI) the traditional definition has been muddied by the "DWI-positive TIA". Independent of the definition the sudden onset of focal neurological signs such as hemianopsia, hemiparesis and aphasia should tip off towards a possibility of a cerebrovascular syndrome. Although the focus is on the suddenness in onset, it must be pointed out that occasionally it may be rapidly progressive or even fluctuating and stuttering in onset. Ischemic stroke typically manifests itself as a syndrome that relates to its localization in terms of the part of the brain it affects and its arterial supply. In the following section, we will describe some of the traditional stroke syndromes those are based on a particular arterial supply.

Middle Cerebral Artery Stroke Syndrome

Physical findings in patients with middle cerebral artery (MCA) stroke syndrome depend on the location of middle cerebral artery occlusion and dominant versus nondominant hemisphere involvement. In most of the persons, the left MCA territory controls speech and language function.

Proximal MCA occlusion leads to contralateral hemiplegia, eye deviation away from the side of the weakness, contralateral hemianopsia, and contralateral hemisensory loss. Proximal MCA occlusion of the dominant hemisphere causes global aphasia, whereas in the nondominant hemisphere causes impaired perception of deficits (anosognosia) resulting from the stroke. Superior division of MCA strokes lead to contralateral deficits with weakness of the upper extremity and face greater than the lower extremity. Inferior division of MCA stroke on either side can result in a superior quadrantanopsia or homonymous hemianopsia. In the dominant hemisphere, it can lead to Wernicke's aphasia. In the nondominant side, it may lead to a visual neglect. MCA stroke syndrome rarely cause decrease in level of consciousness at onset of symptoms, which if present should raise suspicion for other reasons such as seizures, swelling from edema or hemorrhagic transformation leading to herniation and brainstem compression, or brainstem ischemia from vertebrobasilar ischemia.

The pattern of weakness sometimes provides a clue to a MCA territory stroke. Typically MCA stroke weakness produces weakness in the face and arm greater than in leg, with facial weakness of the upper motor neuron type (affecting lower half of stroke only). The face, arm and leg weakness are all on the same side. Occasionally, the face arm and leg are densely paralyzed suggestive of internal capsular involvement supplied by the lenticulostriate branches of the proximal MCA. Uncommonly the presentation is of faciobrachial paresis (the weakness of the lower face) and the upper extremity distal hand affected greater than the proximal forearm. Such deficits result from stroke in the insula and operculum.

Unilateral movement disorders such as hemiathetosis, hemichorea, and hemidystonia are rarely seen MCA stroke syndromes and reflect, involvement of the basal ganglia.

Visual deficits: Field cut or hemianopsia can occur with MCA stroke syndromes. Quadrantanopsia can be attributed to a parietal infarct affecting a division of the MCA (superior or inferior) supplying the deep fibers of the upper or lower optic radiation respectively.

Neglect or inattention is MCA stroke syndrome reflecting ischemic injury to the parietal lobe. Two types of neglect are commonly tested. Visual and sensory neglect are tested by double simultaneous stimulation of the visual and sensory modalities. Patients with visual neglect will frequently ignore objects or person approaching the patient from that side. They may have difficulty in naming objects presented on the affected side. Motor neglect with underutilization of the side contralateral to cerebral insult appears much like a hemiparesis. Special efforts must be made by the examiner to encourage the patient to demonstrate strength. Typically, the patient has delayed withdrawal to noxious stimuli, fails to place the affected hand in the lap when seated, and falls heavily to the affected side with no apparent effort to minimize impact.

Left-MCA (dominant) stroke syndrome: The left cerebral hemisphere is dominant for speech and language in vast majority of right-handed individuals. Defining cerebral dominance for left-handed and ambidextrous individuals is more difficult.

Aphasia or language disturbance is typically seen in strokes resulting from the dominant MCA (left MCA in a right-handed person). They are broadly classified as global, expressive or nonfluent, receptive or fluent and conduction aphasias.

Global aphasia, refers to a large entire MCA territory stroke affecting both expressive and receptive components of speech. Typically, these patients are mute. Global aphasia needs to distinguish from anarthhria resulting from paralysis of the oropharyngeal muscles. Although the patients appear mute their comprehension is spared.

Broca's or expressive or motor aphasia, results in difficulty in expression of either spoken or written language. Comprehension of written and spoken language is spared. Typically, such form of aphasia is seen with strokes affecting the insula and frontoparietal operculum.

Wernicke's or receptive or sensory aphasia, results in difficulty in comprehension of written and spoken language. Expression of either spoken or written language is spared resulting in a fluent speech with few understandable words and frequent paraphasic errors. It is caused most often by stroke affecting the lower division of the MCA bifurcation or one of its branches. The Wernicke's aphasia, localizes to a stroke affecting the dominant posterior temporal, inferior parietal, and lateral temporo-occipital areas.

Conduction aphasia results from stroke affecting the arcuate fasciculus connecting the motor and sensory area of speech. This hard to elucidate syndrome, both receptive and expressive component of speech are preserved. It is the inability to put the written or spoken language into action. They have difficulty in repetition of spoken sentences and often try to correct the misspoken words.

Specific Aphasia Syndromes

Alexia: It is the inability to recognize or comprehend written language. It is associated with lesion in the left occipitotemporal cortex.

Agraphia: It is inability to write, is associated with left occipital lesion.

Apraxia of speech: Results from inability to use the oropharyngeal and respiratory muscles necessary for speech resulting in a hesitant and telegraphic speech output. This syndrome is associated with lesion in the rolandic area.

Agrammatism is described when the individual uses fewer words to communicate an idea. This is associated with lesion in the Broca's area.

Transcortical aphasia: It is characterized by inability to repeat, may be motor, sensory or mixed, resulting from isolation of the individual speech areas in the cortex.

Apraxia refers to the inability to perform a previously learned tasks despite preserved strength, vision, and coordination. The condition is due to an insult to the dominant hemisphere.

The most common form of apraxia is ideomotor apraxia. On verbal command, the patient is unable to perform simple tasks, such as imitating the use of a common object such as combing the hair. Apraxia results from a stroke resulting in disconnection between the cortex containing plans for movement and the cortex responsible for execution.

Ideational apraxia results in inability to complete an idea and is tested by examining the ability to complete complex multistep tasks, such as taking a piece of paper, folding it into two and leaving it on the table.

Besides ideomotor and ideational apraxia, few specific form of apraxias have been described. Limb-kinetic apraxia results in impaired clumsy manipulation of objects in such tasks as combing one's hair. Oral-buccal-lingual apraxia results in ability to perform complex movements involving the described muscles.

In addition to the above-mentioned symptomatology, it is important to recognize that the dominant hemispheric strokes more common than the nondominant hemisphere strokes are associated with depression. This often bears impact on the overall prognosis as well as prognosis for rehabilitation.

Right MCA (nondominant) stroke: Strokes of the nondominant hemisphere can lead to behavioral abnormalities. The patients are confused, agitated and disoriented. General confusion and delirium often are more appreciated in patients with nondominant hemisphere stroke. The right hemisphere is responsible for attention, vigilance, and distinguishing stimuli. Such stroke presentations are predictive of an unfavorable long-term outcome after rehabilitation.

Extinction describes inattention to one stimulus when double simultaneous stimuli are applied. Generally, the ignored stimulus is on the left side. The stimulus may be visual or auditory or tactile.

Impersistence is used to describe an inability to persist in performing motor tasks and often is accompanied with visuomotor and visuospatial deficits. This indicates an unfavorable rehabilitation outcome.

Dressing apraxia is seen with right-hemispheric stroke and results in difficulty distinguishing right from left and up from down. The patient is unable to dress without assistance despite having no apparent weakness or coordination difficulties that would prevent performing this task.

Memory deficit, which occurs when individuals become lost in familiar surroundings, often accompanies nondominant hemisphere stroke. Confabulation of information is due largely to inability to recognize errors, disinhibition, and memory deficits.

Constructional apraxia defines difficulty in manipulating objects in space. This kind of apraxia can be appreciated by having affected patients copy designs or build-3 dimensional models.

Aprosody, lack of intonation in speech, and affective agnosia refer to the inability to comprehend emotional intonation of speech. The two deficits correlate with stroke in the right temporoparietal region.

Lacunar Stroke Syndrome

The five classical lacunar syndromes have symptoms that are relatively specific to it. Occasionally, cortical infarcts and intracranial hemorrhages can mimic a lacunar syndrome. Cortical signs and symptoms (e.g. hemianopsia, aphasia, neglect) are absent.

Pure motor stroke/hemiparesis: This is the most common of all the lacunar syndromes. It consists of hemiparesis or hemiplegia that typically affects the face, arm, and leg equally. Sensory symptoms, dysarthria and dysphagia may also be present. The lacunar stroke is usually present in the posterior limb of the internal capsule or the basis pontis.

Ataxic hemiparesis syndrome: This is the next most common lacunar syndrome, consisting of weakness and clumsiness on one side of the body. The onset of symptoms may stutter over hours or days. The most frequent site of infarction is the posterior limb of the internal capsule, basis pontis, and corona radiate.

Dysarthria clumsy hand syndrome: The main symptoms are dysarthria and clumsiness of the hand, which often is most prominent when the patient is writing. It results from a small infarct in the dorsal basis pontis just below the medial lemniscus.

Pure sensory stroke: This syndrome consists of persistent or transient numbness and/or paresthesias (pins and needles) on one side of the body. Occasionally, it is associated with pain, burning, or other unpleasant sensation. The stroke is usually in the thalamus (VPL and VPM nuclei).

Mixed sensorimotor stroke: This syndrome consists of a combination of hemiparesis and sensory impairment on one side of the body.

The stroke is usually in the thalamus and adjacent posterior limb of the internal capsule.

Anterior Cerebral Artery Syndromes

Stroke in the anterior cerebral artery (ACA) territory is uncommon, commonly resulting from atherothrombosis of the proximal segment of the ACA. The ACA supplies the whole of the medial surfaces of the frontal and parietal lobes, majority of the corpus callosum, the frontobasal cerebral cortex, the anterior diencephalons, and the deep structures including the head of the caudate nucleus. ACA strokes often go unrecognized because of paucity of detectable signs and symptoms. ACA strokes can lead to weakness in the legs typically out of proportion to leg weakness, apathy and abulia. It can cause personality changes and urinary incontinence in bilateral ACA infarcts. It is not uncommon to have an anatomical variation where a single ACA supplies both sides of the brain. In such a case, ACA stroke can result in paraparesis.

Anterior choroidal artery (AChA) is a branch of the ACA. It supplies the lateral thalamus and posterior limb of the internal capsule. AChA stroke is rare and can result in hemiparesis and hemisensory loss. It also supplies the lateral geniculate body resulting in certain unusual homonymous field abnormalities.

The "recurrent artery of Heubner" is a branch of the ACA that supplies the head of the caudate nucleus and the adjacent internal capsule. Stroke in this specific distribution can result in hemiparesis.

Internal Carotid Artery Syndromes

The internal carotid artery (ICA) supplies the MCA, ACA and less commonly a fetal posterior cerebral artery (PCA). Occlusion of ICA commonly results from atherothrombosis, less commonly from dissection, embolism and other causes. This commonly results in a combination of MCA syndrome and ACA syndrome with homonymous hemianopsia.

Ophthalmic artery is a branch of the ICA. Ischemia in the distribution of the ophthalmic artery is transient in the setting of symptomatic internal carotid artery occlusion (i.e. transient monocular blindness) is common, but central retinal artery ischemia is relatively uncommon, presumably because of the efficient collateral supply.

Vertebrobasilar Insufficiency Syndromes

Patients with vertebrobasilar artery thrombosis typically have a waxing and waning course of symptoms. When caused by atherothrombosis, it is frequently preceded by prodrome that includes TIAs and rarely a "herald hemiparesis". In contrast, embolic events are sudden, without prodrome or warning, with acute and dramatic presentation. Commonly reported symptoms associated with the vertebrobasilar insufficiency (VBI) include vertigo, nausea, vomiting decrease in the level of consciousness, oculomotor signs, dysarthria, dysphagia, dysphonia, lower motor neuron pattern (both upper and lower halves) weakness of facial muscles and tongue, sensory loss, ataxia, crossed motor weakness and sensory loss, bladder or bowel incontinence and visual-field defects. Common clinical findings observed in patients include abnormal level of consciousness and hemiparesis or quadriparesis, which is usually asymmetric. Papillary abnormalities and oculomotor signs are common, and bulbar manifestations, such as facial weakness, dysphonia, dysarthria, and dysphagia, occur less commonly.

Oculomotor signs are usually reflex involvement of the abducens nucleus, the horizontal gaze center located in the pontine paramedian reticular formation (PPRF), contiguous to the abducens nucleus, and/or the medial longitudinal fasciculus (MLF). Lesions to these structures result in ipsilateral lateral gaze or conjugate gaze palsy. Ocular bobbing is described as a brisk downward movement of the eyeball with a subsequent return to the primary position. This deficit localizes the lesion to the pons. Other reported signs of pontine ischemia include ataxia and tremor associated with mild hemiparesis. The signs described can occur in different combinations presenting a diagnostic challenge in lesion localization.

Certain constellations of findings may serve as clues for narrowing down the search, including the following examples. Midbrain syndromes (Coarse tremor on one side of the body, cranial nerve III lesion or vertical gaze palsy), Pontine syndrome (Clue-Cranial nerve VI lesion, horizontal gaze palsy, or VII nerve palsy), medullary syndrome (crossed pain and temperature loss, Horner syndrome, ataxia, paralysis of the tongue, soft palate, vocal cord or sternocleidomastoid muscle), posterior cerebral artery (macular sparing hemianopsia).

A variety of specific neurologic syndromes have been described based on constellations of findings. Some examples are listed below:

Wallenberg (lateral medullary) syndrome: It is the most common of all the posterior circulation syndromes and is due to vertebral artery occlusion. Patients present with nausea, vomiting, vertigo, dysarthria and gait unsteadiness. Ipsilateral clinical features include ataxia and dysmetria, due to damage of the inferior cerebellar peduncle and cerebellum; Horner syndrome (including ptosis, miosis, hypohidrosis or anhidrosis, enophthalmos), due to the damage to descending sympathetic fibers; facial pain and temperature loss; reduced corneal reflex from damage to the descending spinal tract and trochlear nerve nucleus resulting in nystagmus, hypoacusis (cochlear nucleus), dysarthria, dysphagia, paralysis of the pharynx, palate, and vocal cord; and loss of taste from the posterior third of the tongue (nuclei or fibers of glossopharyngeal and vagus nerves). The prognosis of patients with the lateral medullary syndrome is usually benign with good functional outcome. However, patients may die in the acute phase from aspiration pneumonia, and death has been reported from sleep apnea in a number of cases.

Dejerine (medial medullary) syndrome: This syndrome is due to occlusion of anterior spinal branches of the vertebral artery and it involves the pyramid, the medial lemniscus, and the hypoglossal nerve.

The clinical features include ipsilateral paresis of the tongue with deviation towards the lesion (lower motor neuron lesion of the hypoglossal nerve), contralateral hemiplegia with sparing of the face (corticospinal tract), and loss of ipsilateral vibration and proprioception (medial lemniscus).

Cerebellar infarction: A stroke involving the cerebellum may result in a lack of coordination, clumsiness, intention tremor, ataxia, dysarthria, scanning speech, and occasionally difficulties with memory and motor planning. Early diagnosis of cerebellar infarctions is important since swelling may cause brainstem compression or hydrocephalus.

Locked-in syndrome: This dramatic clinical syndrome occurs when there is an infarction of the upper ventral pons. Locked-in syndrome results from occlusion of the proximal and middle segments of the basilar artery, or hemorrhage involving that region, and also may be caused by trauma, central pontine myelinolysis, encephalitis, or tremor. Bilateral ventral pontine involving both corticospinal and corticobulbar tracts lead to quadriplegia. The patient is unable to speak, or produce facial movement (damage to the corticobulbar tracts) as well as look to either side (horizontal eye movement is impaired due to a lesion of bilateral abducens nerve nuclei). Because the tegmentum of the pons is spared, the patient's consciousness is preserved, with the patients fully awake, sensate, and aware. The only movements preserved are vertical eye movements and blinking. The patient is paralyzed completely and communicates only by blinking. Some recovery of facial muscle movement and horizontal gaze may occur with time or in an incomplete form of this syndrome.

Top of the basilar syndrome: This syndrome is the manifestation of upper brainstem and diencephalic ischemia caused by occlusion of the rostral basilar artery, usually due to an embolism. The syndrome is characterized by visual, oculomotor, and behavioral abnormalities, often without significant motor dysfunction. Rostral brainstem infarction produces oculomotor and pupillary signs that are identical to those in thalamic hemorrhage. Somnolence, vivid hallucinations and dreamlike behavior may also accompany rostral brainstem infarction. Temporal and occipital infarctions are frequently accompanied by hemianopia with distinctive characteristics, fragments of the Balint syndrome, amnestic dysfunction, and agitated behavior.

Internuclear ophthalmoplegia: Clinically, internuclear ophthalmoplegia (INO) is a horizontal gaze palsy resulting from a brainstem lesion affecting the MLF between the nuclei of abducens and oculomotor nerves, most commonly in the pons. When a patient with a lesion in the right MLF attempts to look to his/her left (i.e. away from the involved side), he/she shows no adduction of the right eye and full abduction of the left eye with the end-point abduction nystagmus. By the same logic, in the case of bilateral INO, there is no adduction to either side with nystagmus of the abducting eye in both directions. Convergence is preserved since both nuclei of oculomotor nerve and peripheral innervation of the medial recti muscles are intact. Since horizontal gaze requires coordinated activity of the ipsilateral oculomotor nerve and communication pathway (i.e. MLF) between the nuclei of oculomotor nerve (in the midbrain) and abducens nerve (in the pons) results in the inability of the eye ipsilateral to the lesion to adduct and contralateral eye to exhibit abduction nystagmus when looking away from the involved side. In elderly patients, INO is caused most often by occlusion of the basilar artery or its paramedian branches. In younger adults, it may occur due to multiple sclerosis, commonly with bilateral involvement and occasionally partial INO.

One-and-a-half syndrome: This syndrome is caused by a lesion affecting the PPRF and MLF simultaneously, resulting in ipsilateral conjugate gaze palsy and INO. The patient with a lesion in the ipsilateral PPRF or abducens nucleus and MLF connecting to the contralateral abducens nerve exhibits horizontal gaze palsy when looking towards the side of the lesion (one), and INO when looking away from the side of the lesion (half). Associated features may include vertical nystagmus, exotopia of the contralateral eye, and skew deviation. Vertical gaze and convergence generally are preserved. A patient with this syndrome is completely unable to move the ipsilateral eye, and he/she is able only to abduct the contralateral eye, with resulting nystagmus.

Millard-Gubler (Ventral pontine) syndrome: This syndrome occurs after paramedian infarction in the pons and results in ipsilateral lateral rectus palsy (abducens nerve) with diplopia, complete facial paresis (unilateral facial nerve palsy), and contralateral hemiparesis/hemiplegia (corticospinal tract involvement). It is also referred to as "crossed hemiplegia".

Raymond-Céstan (Upper dorsal pontine) syndrome: This syndrome is due to obstruction of flow in the long circumferential branches of the basilar artery. This occlusion results in ipsilateral ataxia and coarse intention tremor (indicating involvement of the superior and middle cerebellar peduncles), weakness of mastication and sensory loss in the face (suggesting sensory and motor trigeminal nuclei and tracts), and contralateral loss of all sensory modalities due to damage to medial lemniscus and spinothalamic tract) with or without facial weakness and hemiparesis (corticospinal tract). Horizontal gaze palsy also may occur.

Foville (Lower dorsal pontine) syndrome: This syndrome may result from lesions to the dorsal tegmentum of the lower pons. The patient exhibits ipsilateral paresis of the whole face (nucleus and fibers of facial nerve), horizontal gaze palsy on the ipsilateral side (PPRF ± abducens nucleus), and contralateral hemiplegia (corticospinal tract) and sensory loss.

Weber (Ventral midbrain) syndrome: Weber syndrome occurs with an occlusion of the median and/or paramedian perforating branches of the basilar artery. Typical clinical findings include ipsilateral oculomotor nerve palsy, ptosis, and mydriasis with contralateral hemiplegia.

Benedikt (Dorsal midbrain) syndrome: This syndrome is due to lesion in the midbrain tegmentum from occlusion of paramedian branches of either the basilar artery, PCA, or both. The patient demonstrates ipsilateral oculomotor palsy, ptosis and mydriasis (like in Weber syndrome), along with the contralateral involuntary movements, such as intention tremor, ataxia, or chorea (due to the involvement of the red nucleus).

Posterior cerebral artery infarct: The most common finding in occipital lobe infarction leading to contralateral hemianopsia with macular sparing. Clinical symptoms associated with occlusion of the PCA vary depending on the location of the occlusion and may include the thalamic syndrome, thalamic perforate syndrome, Weber syndrome, cortical blindness, and color blindness, failure to see to-and-for movements, verbal dyslexia, and hallucinations.

Clinical Stroke Scales

The introduction of specific modalities of treatment for acute stroke has emphasized the interest in the clinical measurement of stroke severity. A number of quantitative stroke scores have been devised to enable outcome measurement in clinical trials, prognosis stratification and assess quantitative changes in neurological status of stroke patients. The commonly used stroke scales are listed in **Table 2.2**.

Table 2.2: Clinical stroke scale			
CNS	*SNSS*	*ESS*	*NIHSS*
1. Level of consciousness	1. Level of consciousness	1. Level of consciousness	1. Level of consciousness
2. Orientation	2. Eye movement	2. Comprehension	2. Orientation
3. Speech	3. Arm power	3. Speech	3. Comprehension
4. Motor weakness	4. Hand power	4. Visual field	4. Gaze
5. Motor response	5. Leg power	5. Gaze	5. Visual field
	6. Orientation	6. Facial movement	6. Facial palsy
	7. Speech	7. Arm position	7. Limb weakness
	8. Facial palsy	8. Leg raising	8. Ataxia
	9. Gait	9. Wrist extension	9. Sensory
		10. Finger strength	10. Language
			11. Neglect

Bibliography

1. Adams, et al. Guidelines for the early management of adults with ischemic stroke: A guideline from the American heart association/American Stroke Association Stroke Council, Clinical Cardiology Council, Cardiovascular Radiology and

Intervention Council, and the Atherosclerotic Peripheral Vascular Disease and Quality of Care Outcomes in Research Interdisciplinary Working Groups. Circulation. 2007;115(20):e478-e534.

2. Celani, et al. Comparability and validity of two clinical scores in the early differential diagnosis of acute stroke. British Medical Journal. 1994;308(6945): 1674-6.

3. Chalela, et al. Magnetic resonance perfusion imaging in acute ischemic stroke using continuous arterial spin labeling. Stroke. 2000;31(3):680-87.

4. Coull, et al. Nderestimation of the early risk of recurrent stroke: evidence of the need for a standard definition. Stroke. 2004;35(8):1925-9.

5. Edwards, et al. Unified neurological stroke scale is valid in ischemic and hemorrhagic stroke. Stroke. 1995;26(10):1852-8.

6. Flossmann, et al. Reliability of clinical diagnosis of the symptomatic vascular territory in patients with recent transient ischemic attack or minor stroke. Stroke. 2008;39(9):2457-60.

7. Gérard Besson. Is it clinically possible to distinguish nonhemorrhagic infarct from hemorrhagic stroke? Stroke. 1995;26:1205-09.

8. Goldstein, et al. Improving the clinical diagnosis of stroke. Stroke. 2006;37(3): 754-5.

9. Goldstein, et al. Improving the reliability of stroke subgroup classification using the trial of org 10172 in acute stroke treatment (TOAST) criteria. Stroke. 2001;32(5):1091-7.

10. Hideaki, et al. Deteriorating ischemic stroke in 4 clinical categories classified by the Oxfordshire community stroke project. Stroke. 2000;31(9):2049-54.

11. Higashida, et al. Should interventional radiologists be involved in acute stroke intervention? Re: Emergency interventional stroke therapy: A statement from the American Society of Interventional and Therapeutic Neuroradiology and the Society of Cardiovascular and Interventional Radiology. Journal of Vascular and Interventional Radiology. 2001;12(2):145-6.

12. J Bogousslavsky, et al. The Lausanne stroke registry: Analysis of 1,000 consecutive patients with first stroke. Stroke. 1988;19:1083-92.

13. Jager HR. Diagnosis of stroke with advanced CT and MR imaging. British Medical Bulletin. 2000;56(2):318-33.

14. Kobayashi, et al. Oxfordshire community stroke project clinical stroke syndrome and appearances of tissue and vascular lesions on pretreatment CT in hyperacute ischemic stroke among the first 510 patients in the third international stroke trial (ist-3). Stroke. 2009;40(3):743-8.

15. Mallen C. Predicting the outcome of acute stroke: A prognostic score. Journal of Neurology, Neurosurgery, and Psychiatry. 1984;47:475-80.

16. MG Celani. Comparability and validity of two clinical scores in the early differential diagnosis of acute stroke. British Medical Journal. 1994;308:1674-6.

17. Pelz, et al. Stroke review: Advances in interventional Neuroradiology 2004. Stroke. 2005;36(2):211-4.

18. Peter D Schellinger. A standardized MRI stroke protocol comparison with CT in hyperacute intracerebral hemorrhage. Stroke. 1999;30:765-8.

19. Phillips, et al. Clinical diagnosis of lacunar stroke in the first 6 hours after symptom onset: Analysis of data from the glycine antagonist in neuroprotection (gain) Americas Trial. Stroke. 2007;38(10):2706-11.

20. Qureshi, et al. New grading system for angiographic evaluation of arterial occlusions and recanalization response to intra-arterial thrombolysis in acute ischemic stroke. Neurosurgery. 2002;50(6):1405-15.

21. Sato, et al. Baseline NIH stroke scale score predicting outcome in anterior and posterior circulation strokes symbol. Neurology. 2008;(70):2371-7.
22. Thanvi, et al. Early neurological deterioration in acute ischaemic stroke: predictors, mechanisms and management. Postgraduate Medical Journal. 2008;84(994):412-7.
23. Toni, et al. Pure motor hemiparesis and sensorimotor stroke: Accuracy of very early clinical diagnosis of lacunar strokes. Stroke. 1994;25(1):92-6.
24. Wilterdink, et al. Effect of prior aspirin use on stroke severity in the trial of org 10172 in acute stroke treatment (TOAST). Stroke. 2001;32(12):2836-40.

3

Evaluation of Stroke

Ranen Kumar Ghatak, Mouli Madhab Ghatak

Stroke

Stroke or cerebrovascular accident (CVA) is an acute neurologic dysfunction of vascular origin, with relatively rapid onset, causing focal or sometimes global signs of disturbed cerebral function lasting more than 24 hours. Clinically there will be affection of higher function as well as motor and sensory systems of the patient.

Stroke Affects the Patients at three Different Levels

1. Biological level which includes the cardiovascular system, respiratory system, gastrointestinal system and genitourinary system.
2. Practical level of ADL (activity of daily living) which includes feeding, bathing, dressing, communication, and ambulation.
3. Social level which includes their work, their enjoyment and their family. The loss of neurological function directly or indirectly affects the psychological state of the individual.

Caring for stroke patients presents a great challenge to our present day society. This challenge becomes even more formidable when one takes into consideration that the life expectancy of stroke patients continues to increase with the advances in modern medical care. As resources are limited in rehabilitating these patients, particularly in a developing country, they must be used in a judicious manner to get maximum benefit for the patients.

To formulate a plan of treatment for stroke patients, data are collected by proper evaluation. For evaluation of stroke patients, proper history taking, clinical examination and investigations are important. In addition, different assessment tools are used to find different deficits. Finally, results of all assessment procedures are combined to ascertain present status of the patients so that planning of treatment and rehabilitation can be done.

Evaluation of a stroke patient varies with the stage of involvement of an attending physician who first comes in contact with him.

In the initial stage of the disease process, the main concern is survival of the patient. Here assessment of certain neurological signs is important. But in the later stage when the condition of the patient is stable and the main concern is physical and social function, different sets of tools should be used. Thus choice or selection of assessment tools differs for different patients.

The aim of use of the assessment tools is to identify as well as measure lost and preserved function of the stroke patient. Ideal assessment tools should be *valid, reliable, sensitive, simple and generate easily communicable data.*

Valid: The assessment tool should measure the particular deficit for which it is used.

Reliable: The assessment tool must give the same result on repeated application.

Sensitive: The assessment tool should be able to detect genuine change in the patient's ability.

Simplicity: The assessment tool must be simple so that it can be used without much difficulty. Complex tests, even if valid, reliable and sensitive, are not widely accepted. Simplicity is important for both patient and examiner. Some tests require active participation of the patient. A complex test, where patient cannot participate fully due to complexity, does not give good result.

Communicability: The ultimate aim of the assessment tools in rehabilitation set up is to generate data, which are easily communicable to other members of the rehabilitation team. Numerical data, when generated by the assessment tools, is good in communicable quality but the interpreter must be familiar with the test.

The treatment of stroke requires synchronized team effort where members of the team would be able to communicate with each other to understand deficits detected in the patient by each of them. The whole team must meet soon after the first contact with the patient so that they can appreciate the full extent of the patient's deficit and plan to assist him in overcoming the deficits.

With this preliminary idea regarding evaluation, let us consider the detailed evaluation of a stroke patient.

Components of Evaluation of the Stroke Patient

1. History.
2. Clinical examination.
3. Investigation.

History

Taking history of a stroke patient is an art of knowing the patient entirely which is never limited to the event of attack but from the premorbid health status to the downfall of it in all aspects. The history of a stroke rehabilitation process should always elaborate the lost function compared to the disease-free healthy life of the individual before attack. It varies from individual to individual and there is no distinct universal relationship between the disease and the amount of residual disability. The complex variability of physiological, psychological, metabolic and pathological adaptability of different individuals affected by stroke always demands a vivid and detail premorbid and morbid history, which also needs a scientific eye to assess and explain the changing nature of different incapacitating factors at different time.

A poststroke patient may be received in a rehabilitation setup any time from the day one up to after a long time from the attack. But as because stroke rehabilitation should be started from the very 1st day, the general history taking in the earlier days are mostly concentrated towards the acute events and functional losses present at that time along with premorbid data recording. A rehabilitation specialist should keep proper predictive assumption in mind regarding the aim, goal and possible outcome of a particular patient while taking the history. The patient himself may be able to answer the queries asked by the doctor but very frequently a near relative or friend accompanying the patient is the best individual to enlighten the full spectrum of premorbid and morbid events.

The stroke patient should be evaluated with a general norm of medical history taking, like recording the chief complains, family history, history of present and past illness, etc. But a specialized rehabilitation history should always focus the exact nature of illness, its intensity, the neuromusculo-psychocognitive and metabolic impairments arising out of the attack and the exact residual functional capability restored along with the history and exact nature of other associated complicating factors like DM, HTN, IHD, CRF, etc. A good assessment for the rehabilitation of a stroke patient always focuses each and every disability factors and the factors complicating or delaying the rehabilitation process and outcome.

Such a History should include the following points:
1. *Premorbid:*
   a. Physical activity status.
   b. Life style.
   c. Occupation and job involvement.
   d. Mental performance and psychological adaptabilities.
   e. Body weight and obesity or malnutrition.
   f. Habits and interest.
   g. Social attachments and stabilities.
   h. Financial status and stability.
   i. Pre-existing illness, which can restrict the rehabilitation outcome.
   j. Addiction like smoking, alcohol intake, etc.
2. *History of and after the event of stroke:*
   a. Onset.
   b. Progression.
   c. Level of consciousness.
   d. Cognition and higher motor function.

    e. Speech and communication affection.

    f. Nature of paralysis.

    g. Associated events like cardiac instability, hypertension, respiratory insufficiency, stress bleeds, infections, diselectrolytemia, renal compromise, etc.

    h. Bladder and bowel status (? catheterized).

    i. Feeding and nutrition (? nasogastric intubation).

    j. Development of any pressure sore or skin complications.

    k. Psychological complication.

    l. *Functional history including the:*

        i. Ambulation.

        ii. Assistance (total, partial or stand by).

        iii. Capacity of transfer.

        iv. Dressing history.

        v. Eating and personal hygiene activity status.

    m. Social and family support system.

The records of this detailed history is reconfirmed and scientifically justified by a thorough clinical examination of the involved systems and formulated and organized with proper calculative measures of different scaling systems and instruments.

The specified evaluation procedures are elaborately discussed in different chapters dealing with various domain of disability in this book. However, the basic assessment protocol emphasizing the neuromuscular disability parts are covered here in this chapter.

Clinical Examination of Stroke Patient

Level of consciousness of the patient is important. In an unconscious patient, rehabilitation process cannot be started effectively as the patient cannot follow simple commands and comprehend the instruction of basic exercises.

A commonly used scale for measuring depth of coma is The Glasgow coma scale. The scale has three components, e.g. eye opening, verbal response and motor response and has a score ranging from minimum of 3 to a maximum 15.

Cognition and memory: Consciousness, cognition and memory are all related to higher function of neurological examination. Cognitive changes in stroke patient may be due to the affect of CVA on the brain or due to old age. When there is gross affection of cognition or memory, patient cannot cooperate fully with the rehabilitation team. Rehabilitation is teamwork where active participation of the patient with his relatives is important. Patient with cognitive changes cannot also set a realistic goal. A tool frequently used is Mini-Mental Status Examination (MMSE). Component of the scale are questionnaires that assesses a patient's orientation, memory, attention, language and construction functions. Maximum score possible is 30. Neurobehavioral Cognitive Status Examination (NCSE) is another tool where impairment in consciousness, orientation, memory, language, and reasoning are considered.

Language and Communication

Speech is an important means of communication. Loss of speech is also a cause of frustration and anger on the part of the patient. Disturbance in language or dysphasia may be exhibited by disturbances in comprehension, naming, repetition, fluency, reading or writing. Commonly used tools are American speech-language-hearing association, functional assessment of communication skills for adults and Boston diagnostic aphasia examination.

Vision

Vision is another area, which is usually overlooked. Impaired vision is an important factor for failure of rehabilitation process. In stroke there may be monocular visual loss, homonymous hemianopia, or cortical blindness.

Hearing Impairment

Impairment of hearing may be present in some stroke patient and should be examined in every stroke patient.

Depression

Depression may be primary due to CVA or secondary reaction to significant neurological loss in the patient.

Two important assessment scales are the Geriatric Depression Scale (GDS) and Center for Epidemiologic Studies Depression (CES-D).

Motor Examination

Stroke is considered mainly as a cause of loss of muscle power of some part of the body. Actually, loss of power in stroke patient may not be responsible for the disability of the patient. The main problem may be that patient cannot use his affected limb either due to spasticity or involuntary movement.

Commonly used muscle power assessment tool like Medical Research Council (MRC) scale which grades muscle power from 0 to 5 may not be helpful in a stroke patient due to presence of spasticity, exaggerated reflexes and synergy dominance. By observing the functional task of upper extremity (shoulder flexion, elbow flexion and prehension) and lower extremity (hip flexion, knee extension, ankle dorsiflexion) of stroke patients, 'Motricity Index' score can be calculated which ranges from 0 (total paralysis) to 100 (normal).

Brunnstrome used a different approach to ascertain muscle power in hemiplegic patients. Movement patterns are observed and motor function is rated according to stages of motor recovery. Presence of flexor and extensor synergy as well as selective muscle activation from synergy pattern are also considered.

Other important scales are Fugl-Meyer Assessment of Physical Performance (FMA) and Motor Assessment Scale (MAS).

Muscle Tone

Spasticity is increased tone of muscle to passive movement. Increased tone or spasticity of muscle is one of the cause of disability. Spasticity can be measured by modified Ashworth Scale.

Sensory Examination

Sensory affection, when present, affects total rehabilitation process. Stroke patient with good muscle power and less spasticity may be a bad subject for rehabilitation when there is sensory deficiency. Pain, touch, temperature, vibration sensation, position and joint sense, stereognosis, should be examined routinely.

Balance, Coordination

Impairment of balance may be due to abnormalities in motor, sensory, cerebellar and vestibular functions. Clinical tests like finger-nose test, rapid alternating movement are done. In addition ataxia from sensory impairment must be differentiated from ataxia of cerebellar dysfunction.

Other Systems

The morbid factors which complicates, delays and restricts the rehabilitation outcome are to be properly evaluated and monitored and treated during an active rehabilitation process and also during the residual future life of such a patient.

As because stroke is predominantly a disease of elderly, coexistance of CVS abnormalities are very frequent. Rehab team should be aware and a thorough cardiovascular evaluation is mandatory before starting the rehabilitation programs and in some persons, a continuous monitoring or even a midterm assessment is necessary.

1. *Pulse:* To look for any sinus tachycardia or sinus bradycardia or any other rhythmic disturbances.

   Testing the nature of pulse with mild to moderate exercises or training is also important to see the reflection of cardiac response to exercises and activities.

2. *Blood pressure:* To look for any hypertension or hypotension before and during and after exercises. Postural hypotension is to be assessed and monitored in a prolonged bed ridden patient.

   The cardiovascular response of patient from lying to sitting, sitting to standing, standing to walking and in stair climbing, performing other activities are clinically evaluated in a rehabilitation gym usually by the pulse rate, blood pressure, presence of sweating, shortness of breath, chest pain, palpitation, etc.

3. *ECG, TMT, echocardiography:* While the resting ECG demarked commonly found ischemia, arrhythmia, infarction, etc. TMT is important to record

the exercise tolerance and the metabolic equivalent (METS) reflecting any provocable ischemia on exercise. Specially made treadmills are now available for hemiplegic patients. Ergometric evaluation of exercise tolerance and stress test is a useful tool.

Any wall motion abnormality, the left ventricular ejection fraction (LVEF) or detection of valvular problems, etc. are clearly recorded by echocardiogram which reflects the capacity of heart to sustain and tolerate the rehabilitation training programs. A patient with less than 40% of ejection fraction or gross wall motion abnormality is a poorer case for a successful rehabilitation.

4. *Evaluation of other metabolic and risk factors:* Diabetes, renal impairments, arthritis (RA or OA), hypothyroid state or any other metabolic or systemic illness should be properly evaluated and monitored with proper clinical examination and investigation to treat such ailments meticulously as these diseases retard the rehabilitation process.

Investigation

In addition to history and clinical examination, diagnostic procedures help in better understanding of the condition of the patient of stroke. Diagnostic procedures used are as follows:

1. *Imaging of the brain*
   Computerized tomography scan (CT scan): Produces cross-sectional horizontal and vertical images of the brain. CT scan is able to identify type as well as location of lesion.
   Magnetic resonance imaging (MRI): Uses magnetic fields to locate site of lesion in the brain.
   Radionuclide angiography: Can detect diminished blood flow and damage of tissue of brain and gives an idea about the functions of the brain.
2. *Electrical activity of brain*
   Electroencephalography (EEG): Records electrical activity of the brain by means of electrodes placed on the scalp.
   Evoked potential: Records brain's response to visual, auditory and sensory stimuli.
3. *Tests to measure cerebral blood flow*
   Carotid phonoangiography: Microphone placed over carotid artery picks up sound of blood flow.
   Doppler sonography: Evaluates blood flow through a vessel by sound wave.
   Ocular plethysmography: Measures pressure on the eye.
   Cerebral blood flow test (inhalational method): Measures amount of oxygen in blood in different parts of the brain.
   Digital substraction angiography (DSA): Images of blood vessels of brain, taken after administering contrast dye, helps to detect problem of blood flow in brain.

Evaluation of Stroke patient should be done during initial contact with the patient and then subsequently during several visits. Initial assessment gives a clue to the present status of the patient and also helps in planning of proper utilization of resources available for the fullest benefit of the patient. Subsequent assessments are important for following the patient and to assess result of treatment given to the patient. If interpretation of the result showed no improvement in a particular patient, alteration of treatment planning can be done.

Activity of Daily Living

This is very much important as it exposes actual disability of the stroke patient. Patient should actively participate in activity of daily living (ADL) tests. When active participation of the patient is not possible due to some cause, physician should not interpret what the patient can do but should depend on the information from relatives of the patient about the actual performance of the patient.

Basic activities of daily living (BADL) is assessed by Barthel Index and Functional Independence Measure (FIM)

The Barthel Index can be used both for initial assessment and for outcome measure. It measures ten different activities like feeding, bathing, grooming, dressing, bladder control, bowel control, toileting, transfer (chair/bed), mobility and stair climbing and total score ranges from 0 (totally dependant) to 100 (independent).

Functional Independence Measure (FIM) instrument have 18 items and evaluate self-care, sphincter control, transfer, locomotion, communication, and social cognition. Score ranges from 1(total assistance) to 7 (completely independant).

Instrumental activities of daily living scales (IADL) consider activities related to living environment of stroke patients and include items like use of telephone, shopping, food preparation, housekeeping, laundry, public transportation and managing money. Important scales are Functional Health Status, Older Americans Resources and Services Multidimensional Functional Assessment Questionnaire (OARS MFAQ) and Philadelphia Geriatric Center (PGC) Instrumental Activities of Daily Living, and Frenchay Activities Index.

Scales Used for Outcome Assessment

These scales are used in gauging success of various interventions for acute stroke patients, e.g. American Heart Association Stroke Outcome Classification (AHASOC), National Institute of Health Stroke Scale (NIHSS), and Health Survey SF-36 and SF-12.

AHASOC: Components are number of domain affected, severity of stroke and functional classification level.

NIH Stroke scale: Considers level of consciousness, gaze, visual, facial palsy, motor involvement of arm and leg, ataxia, sensory, dysarthria, etc.

SF-36: The 36-item short-term questionnaire has 8 domain like physical problem, general health, social functioning, emotional problem, mental health and body pain, etc.

Some other scales used in stroke patients are Hemispheric Stroke Scale (HSS), Mathew Stroke Scale, Canadian Neurological Scale, Orgogozo Stroke Scale, Cincinnati Stroke Scale, Modified Rankin Scale, Hunt and Hess Scale.

Mini-Mental Status Examination (MMSE): It deals with testing some higher motor functions like orientation, registration, attention and calculation, recall, language, etc. and scoring the specific points.

Barthel index: It deals with functional capability assessment in regards to feeding, bathing, grooming, dressing, bladder, toilet use, transfer, mobility, stairs. A score ranging from 0 to 100 is available to assess the patients' capability.

Glasgow Coma Scale

Test	Score	Response
Eye opening (E)	4	Eyes open spontaneously
	3	Opens eyes to verbal stimulus
	2	Opens eyes to painful stimulus
	1	Eyes do not open
Best verbal response (V)	5	Fully alert and oriented
	4	Converses but disoriented
	3	Inappropriate words
	2	Incomprehensible sounds
	1	Nil
Best motor response (M)	6	Follows command
	5	Localized movement to painful stimulus
	4	Makes withdrawal movement to pain
	3	Flexor (decorticate) posturing to pain
	2	Extensor (decerebrate) posturing to pain
	1	No motor response to pain

Coma score = E+V+M. Maximum score = 15. Minimum score = 3.

MRC Muscle Grading (Medical Research Council, 1976)

Grade	Strength
0	No movement or contraction whatsoever
1	A palpable contraction, but no movement observed
2	Movement seen at the appropriate joint, with gravity eliminated
3	Able to move the joint against gravity
4	Able to move the joint against resistance, but less than normal side.
5	Fully normal power

(Reprinted from Stroke–A critical approach to diagnosis treatment and management. D.T. Wade, R. Langton Hewer, C.E. Skilbeck and R. M. David. Pub. Chapman and Hall Medical. 1985. Page 138.)

Brunnstrom Stages of Motor Recovery

Stage	Characteristic
Stage 1	No activation of the limb.
Stage 2	Spasticity appears, and weak basic flexor and extensor synergies are Present.
Stage 3	Spasticity is prominent; the patient voluntarily moves the limb, but muscle activation is all within the synergy patterns.
Stage 4	The patient begins to activate muscles selectively outside the flexor and extensor synergies.
Stage 5	Spasticity decreases; most muscle activation is selective and independent from limb synergies.
Stage 6	Isolated movements are performed in a smooth, phasic, well-coordinated manner.

(Reprinted from Rehabilitation Medicine – Principles and Practice. 3rd Ed. Joei A. Delisa and Bruce M. Gans. Lippincott, Ravan Publishers. Page 1179)

Modified Ashworth Scale

0	No increase in tone.
1	Slight increase in muscle tone, manifested by a catch and release or by minimal resistance at the end of their range of motion when the affected part(s) is moved in flexion or extension.
1+	Slight increase in muscle tone, manifested by a catch, followed by minimal resistance throughout the remainder (less than half) of the range of motion.
2	More marked increase in muscle tone through most of the range of motion, but affected part(s) easily moved.
3	Considerable increase in muscle tone, passive movement difficult.
4	Affected part(s) rigid in flexion or extension.

(From Bohannon RW, Smith MB: Interrater reliability on a modified Ashworth scale of muscle spasticity. Phys Therapy. 1989;67:206-7.)

Functional Independence Measure (FIM)

Self-care	Admission	Discharge	Follow-up
A. Eating			
B. Grooming			
C. Bathing			
D. Dressing-Upper Body			
E. Dressing-Lower Body			
F. Toileting			
Sphincter-Control			
G. Bladder Management			
H. Bowel Management			

Contd…

Contd...

Self-care	Admission	Discharge	Follow-up
Transfers			
I. Bed, Chair, Wheelchair			
J. Toilet			
K. Tub, Shower			
Locomotion			
L. Walk/Wheelchair			
M. Stairs			
Motor Subtotal Score			
Communication			
N. Comprehension			
O. Expression			
Social Cognition			
P. Social Interaction			
Q. Problem Solving			
R. Memory			
Cognitive Subtotal Score			
TOTAL FIM SCORE			

Bibliography

1. Andrew, et al. Quantitative cerebral blood flow determinations in acute ischemic stroke: Relationship to computed tomography and angiography. Stroke. 1997;28:2208-13.
2. Arboix, et al. Clinical study of 222 patients with pure motor stroke. Journal of Neurology, Neurosurgery, and Psychiatry. 2001;71:239-42.
3. Banks and Marotta. Outcomes validity and reliability of the modified rankin scale: Implications for stroke clinical trials: A Literature review and synthesis. Stroke. 2007;38:1091-6.
4. Benaim, et al. Validation of a standardized assessment of postural control in stroke patients: The postural assessment scale for stroke patients (PASS). Stroke. 1999;30:1862-8.
5. Blackburn, et al. Reliability of measurements obtained with the modified ashworth scale in the lower extremities of people with stroke. Physical Therapy. 2002;82(1):25-34.
6. Blanco, et al. Predictive model of functional independence in stroke patients admitted to a rehabilitation programme. Clinical Rehabilitation. 1999;13:464-75.
7. Camargo, et al. Acute brain infarct: Detection and delineation with CT angiographic source images versus nonenhanced Ct scans. Radiology. 2007;244:541-8.
8. Christensen, et al. Insular lesions, ECG abnormalities, and outcome in acute stroke. Journal of Neurology, Neurosurgery, and Psychiatry. 2005;76:269-71.
9. Donkervoort, et al. The course of apraxia and ADL functioning in left hemisphere stroke patients treated in rehabilitation centres and nursing homes. Clinical Rehabilitation. 2006;20:1085-93.

10. Ferraro, et al. Assessing the motor status score: A scale for the evaluation of upper limb motor outcomes in patients after stroke. Neurorehabilitation and Neural Repair. 2002;16:283-9.

11. Gladman, et al. Use of the extended ADL scale with stroke patients. Age ageing. 1993;22:419-24.

12. Goldstein, et al. Is this patient having a stroke? Journal of American Medical Association. 2005;293:2391-402.

13. Haan, et al. A comparison of five stroke scales with measures of disability, handicap, and quality of life. Stroke. 1993;24(8):1178-81.

14. Hsueh, et al. Analysis of combining two indices to assess comprehensive ADL function in stroke patients. Stroke. 2004;35(3):721-6.

15. Janet H Carr, et al. Investigation of a new motor assessment scale for stroke patients. Physical therapy. 1985;65(2):175-80.

16. Linda, et al. Development of a stroke-specific quality of life scale. Stroke. 1999;30:1362-9.

17. Litchman, et al. Clinical examination is more predictive of ambulation recovery than CT lesion location following subcortical ischemic stroke. Neurorehabilitation and Neural Repair. 1994;8:55-61.

18. Meyer, et al. The post-stroke hemiplegic patient. 1. A method for evaluation of physical performances. Scandinavian Journal of Rehabilitation Medicine. 1975;7(1):13-31.

19. Muir, et al. Comparison of neurological scales and scoring systems for acute stroke prognosis. Stroke. 1996;27(10):1817-20.

20. Muir, et al. Interconversion of stroke scales: Implications for therapeutic trials. Stroke. 1994;25(7):1366-70.

21. Olivares, et al. Risk factors in stroke: A clinical study in Mexican patients. Stroke. 1973;4:773-81.

22. Palle Moller. The impact of aphasia on ADL and social activities after stroke: The Copenhagen stroke study. Neurorehabilitation and Neural Repair. 1996;10:91-6.

23. Prescott, RJ et al. Predicting functional outcome following acute stroke using a standard clinical examination. Stroke. 1982;13:641-7.

24. Salter, et al. Health-related qualit of life after stroke: What are we measuring? International Journal of Rehabilitation Research. 2008;31(2):111-7.

25. Santus, G et al. Social and family integration of hemiplegic elderly patients 1 year after stroke. Stroke. 1990;21:1019-22.

26. Schellinger, et al. A standardized MRI stroke protocol comparison with CT in hyperacute intracerebral hemorrhage. Stroke. 1999;30:765-8.

27. Silliman, RA. The social and functional consequences of stroke for elderly patients. Stroke. 1987;18:200-3.

28. Simondson, et al. The mobility scale for acute stroke patients: Concurrent validity. Clinical Rehabilitation. 2003;17:558-64.

29. Thomas, et al. Progression in acute stroke: Value of the initial NIH stroke scale score on patient stratification in future trials. Stroke. 1999;30:1208-12.

30. Wade DT, Collin C. The Barthel ADL index: A standard measure of physical disability? Disability and Rehabilitation. 1988;10(2):64-67,1464-5165.

31. Wade DT, Hewer RL. Functional abilities after stroke: measurement, natural history and prognosis. Journal of Neurology. Neurosurgery, and Psychiatry. 1987;50:177-82.

32. Wolfe, et al. Assessment of scales of disability and handicap for stroke patients. Stroke. 1991;22(10):1242-4.

4

Acute Stroke Management

Souvik Sen

Introduction

Background

Stroke is the third leading cause of death and the leading cause for adult disability, worldwide. It is defined as the sudden onset focal neurological dysfunction that results from loss of circulation to an area of the brain. It manifests with the sudden onset of focal neurologic deficits, such as weakness, unsteadiness, sensory deficit, or difficulties with vision or language, or headache. Strokes are broadly classified as either as ischemic or hemorrhagic strokes. Ischemic strokes are further subclassified based on causes, into thrombosis, embolism, small vessel occlusive disease and others, whereas hemorrhagic strokes can be subclassified based on location as either intracerebral or subarachnoid.

Recent advances have enabled physicians to significantly improve the outcome of this disabling disease. A new era in acute stroke treatment began in 1996, when the FDA, based on the National Institute of Neurologic Disorders and Stroke (NINDS) tissue plasminogen activator (t-PA) Stroke Study Group approved the early administration (less than 3 hours) of t-PA in patients with acute ischemic stroke. More recently as in 2008, the European Cooperative Acute Stroke Study (ECASS) 3 trial showed the effectiveness of IV t-PA 3-4.5 hours from symptom onset. Also recently, in 2004, the FDA has approved the use of a mechanical embolus retrieval device ("cork-screw") and in 2008 the FDA has approved a microaspiration device referred to as the Penumbra system in acute ischemic stroke patients with major vessel embolic occlusion and contraindication to use of IV t-PA. The devices may be used up to 8 hours from symptom onset. These devices are yet to be made widely available in India. The mechanical embolus removal in cerebral ischemia (MERCI) and the Penumbra system are depicted in **Figures 4.1A and B**.

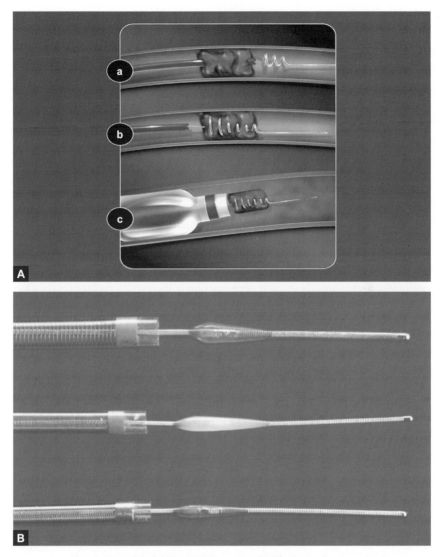

Figs 4.1A and B: (A) The MERCI system; (B) The Penumbra system
(For color version, see Plate 1)

Pathophysiology

The average normal cerebral blood flow in healthy young adults is approximately 50 mL/100 g/min. It is four times higher in the gray matter (80 mL/100 g/min) compared with the white matter (20 mL/100 g/min). The brain is the most metabolically active tissue in the body. It consumes approximately one third of the oxygen and one tenth of the glucose delivered by blood. Ischemic strokes result from events that limit or stop blood flow. As blood flow decreases, neurons cease functioning, and irreversible neuronal ischemia and injury begin at blood flow rates of less than 20 mL/100 mg/min. The gray matter in general is more susceptible to ischemic injury in comparison with the white matter.

As a result of decreased blood flow the nerve cell suffers from injury. The neuronal injury at the cellular level is referred to as the ischemic cascade. Within seconds to minutes of the loss of glucose and oxygen delivery to neurons, the cellular ischemic cascade begins. This is a complex process that begins with cessation of the electrical function of the cells. The resultant neuronal and glial injury produces edema in the ensuing hours to days after stroke, causing further injury to the surrounding neuronal tissues. The quantity of local blood flow is comprised of any residual flow in the major arterial source and the collateral supply, if any. Regions of the brain without significant flow are referred to collectively as the core, and these cells are presumed to die within minutes of stroke onset. Zones of decreased or marginal perfusion are collectively called the ischemic penumbra. Tissue in the penumbra can remain viable for several hours because of marginal tissue perfusion, and currently studied pharmacologic interventions for preservation of neuronal tissue target this penumbra. The natural history of infarction core and ischemic penumbra in absence of intervention is depicted in **Figure 4.2**.

Administration of t-PA to the patient with an acute stroke allows attempts to establish revascularization, so that cells in the penumbra can be rescued before irreversible injury occurs. Restoring blood flow can mitigate the effects of ischemia only if performed quickly. Neuroprotective strategies are intended to preserve the penumbral tissues and attempt to extend the time window for revascularization techniques, but none have shown broad benefit in clinical trials as of this writing.

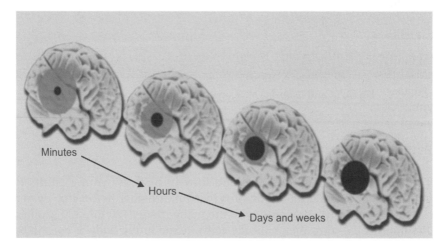

Fig. 4.2: Ischemic penumbra

Mechanisms of Ischemic Stroke

Atherothrombotic Strokes

Atherothrombosis is implicated in the pathophysiology of large-vessel strokes (70%) and small-vessel strokes (30%). In large vessel strokes they are due to *in situ* occlusions, characteristically on atherosclerotic lesions in the carotid, vertebrobasilar, and cerebral arteries, typically proximal to major branches. Thrombogenic factors include injury to and loss of endothelial cells exposing the subendothelium and platelet activation by the subendothelium, activation of the clotting cascade, inhibition of fibrinolysis, and blood stasis. Thrombotic strokes are thought to originate from rupture of unstable atherosclerotic plaques, similar to that known to result in myocardial infarction. Among the Indian, other Asian and African-American population, intracranial atherosclerosis is a common cause of stroke. Among the Caucasian population, extracranial atherosclerosis affecting the internal carotid artery and vertebral artery at its origin is more common.

Lacunar Stroke

Lacunar stroke is the common name for strokes resulting from small vessel atherothrombosis and it represents approximately 20% of all ischemic strokes. They occur when the penetrating branches of the middle cerebral artery (MCA), the lenticulostriate arteries, or the penetrating branches of the circle of Willis, vertebral artery, or basilar artery become occluded. Causes of lacunar infarcts include microatheroma, lipohyalinosis, fibrinoid necrosis secondary to hypertension or vasculitis, hyaline arteriosclerosis, and amyloid angiopathy. The great majority are related to hypertension. Of all stroke types, lacunar strokes have the best prognosis. It is a common type of stroke noted among Indian, other Asian and African-American population.

Cardio- and Atheroembolic Strokes

Emboli may either be of cardiac or arterial origin. Cardiac sources include atrial fibrillation, recent myocardial infarction, prosthetic valves, native valvular disease, endocarditis, mural thrombi, dilated cardiomyopathy, and others. Arterial sources are atherothrombolic or cholesterol emboli that develop in the arch of the aorta and in the extracranial arteries (i.e. origin of internal carotid and vertebral arteries). Embolic strokes tend to have a sudden onset, and neuroimaging may demonstrate previous infarcts in several vascular territories.

Other Known Causes of Stroke

In younger patients, other causes should be considered, including coagulation disorders, sickle cell disease, fibromuscular dysplasia, arterial dissections, vasculitis and vasoconstriction associated with substance abuse. In patients of all age group low blood pressure and hypoperfusion can lead to watershed infarcts. These infarcts, also known as border zone infarcts, develop from relative hypoperfusion in the most distal arterial territories and can produce bilateral symptoms. Frequently, these are associated with surgical procedures as a result of severe hypotension.

Cryptogenic Stroke

In approximately 15% of all strokes, an identifiable cause is not detected despite an extensive work-up. It is believed that these patients may have an etiology that is only transiently present (example paroxysmal atrial fibrillation or transient vasospasm) or it may be truly unknown.

Stroke Etiology in India

Little is known, about stroke etiology in India. Available data suggest that hemorrhagic stroke is more common in India compared to the west. There is not much data on the stroke subtypes in India. Stroke registry of Nizam's Institute of Medical Sciences, for the past few years reports intracranial large artery atherosclerotic disease seems to be the most common stroke mechanism in India, followed by lacunar, cardioembolic and extracranial carotid disease respectively. Two earlier studies from India, one based on conventional angiography and the other on magnetic resonance angiography (MRA) also reported the high frequency of intracranial lesions. Common risk factors for the development of large and small artery disease are similar and constitute hypertension, diabetes and smoking. No significant differences have been found in the risk factors between extra and intracranial large artery disease. For cardioembolic stroke, rheumatic heart disease , and ischemic heart disease seem to be dominant risk factors in India.

Mortality/Morbidity

Stroke is the third leading cause of death worldwide, following cardiac diseases and cancer-related deaths. Approximately a quarter of patients die within one year following a stroke; this percentage rises in the elderly and those with other comorbidities.

Stroke is the leading cause of adult disability. Approximately a third of stroke survivors need help in taking care of themselves after a stroke, a fifth need some type of assistance for walking. At least one third of stroke survivors have depression.

Stroke adds a huge financial burden to the society. The cost of stroke includes direct costs resulting from medical care and indirect costs arising from inability to return to full-time employment. The exact financial impact of stroke in India is unknown.

Stroke can occur in patients of all ages, including children. Risk of stroke increases with age, especially in patients older than 65 years, in whom majority of all strokes occur. The incidence of stroke is greater in males compared to females. The incidence of stroke among Indian population is greater than the Caucasian population and matches the African-American and Hispanic counterparts in the United States.

Clinical History and Symptomatology

The American Stroke Association advises the public to be aware of the five symptoms of stroke those are easily recognized. These symptoms are:

- Sudden numbness or weakness of face, arm, or leg, especially on one side of the body
- Sudden confusion, difficulty in speaking or understanding
- Sudden deterioration of vision of one or both eyes
- Sudden difficulty in walking, dizziness, and loss of balance or coordination
- Sudden, severe headache with no known cause.

Consider stroke in any patient presenting with acute neurological deficit or any alteration in level of consciousness. Common signs of stroke include hemiparesis or hemiplegia, complete or partial hemianopia, monocular or binocular visual loss, or diplopia, dysarthria or aphasia, ataxia, vertigo, or nystagmus, sudden decrease in consciousness.

Medical history is focused on identifying risk factors for atherosclerotic and cardiac disease, including hypertension, diabetes mellitus, tobacco use, high cholesterol, and a history of coronary artery disease, coronary artery bypass, or atrial fibrillation.

In younger patients, history of trauma, coagulopathies, drug use (especially cocaine), migraines, or use of oral contraceptives or over-the-counter sympathomimetic medications are to be elicited. History also can suggest other causes of the patient's symptoms, such as recent trauma, migraine headaches, oral contraceptive use, recent infections, or seizure activity. Family members, bystanders, and especially prehospital personnel can provide valuable information regarding the time and events surrounding the onset of symptoms.

Establishing time of onset is especially critical when thrombolytic therapy is an option. If the patient awakens with the symptoms, then the time of onset is defined as the time the patient was last seen without symptoms. Family members, coworkers, or bystanders may be required to help establish the exact time of onset, especially in right hemispheric strokes accompanied by neglect or left hemispheric strokes with aphasia.

If the patient is a candidate for thrombolytic therapy, a thorough review of the inclusion and exclusion criteria from the NINDS trial must be performed in the patients presenting <3 hours from symptom onset and exclusion criteria from the ECASS3 trial must be performed in the patients presenting 3–4.5 hours from symptom onset. The exclusion criteria largely focus on identifying risk of hemorrhagic complication associated with thrombolytic use.

Physical Examination

Physical examination is directed towards the following areas: (1) assessing the airway, breathing, and circulation (ABCs), (2) defining the severity of the patient's neurological deficits, (3) identifying potential causes of the stroke (4) identifying potential stroke mimics, and (5) identifying comorbid conditions.

The physical examination must start with the ABCs and the vital signs. Patients with stroke can deteriorate quickly; therefore, constant reassessment is critical. Ischemic strokes, unless very large or affect the posterior circulation, do not tend to cause immediate problems with airway patency, breathing abnormalities, or circulation issues. On the other hand, patients with intracerebral or subarachnoid hemorrhage frequently require intervention with both airway protection and ventilation. Vital signs, while nonspecific, can point to impending clinical deterioration and may assist in narrowing the differential diagnosis. Many patients with stroke are hypertensive at baseline, and their blood pressure can become more elevated after stroke. While hypertension is common, blood pressure decreases spontaneously over time in many patients, and medical intervention is not proven to be beneficial in these patients in the absence of signs and symptoms of associated malignant hypertension, AMI, congestive heart failure (CHF), or aortic dissection.

Systemic Examination

A careful and quick examination of the head and neck is essential. Contusions, lacerations, and deformities may suggest trauma as the etiology for the patient's symptoms. Auscultation of the neck may elicit a bruit, suggesting carotid disease as the cause of the stroke. Cardiac arrhythmias, such as atrial fibrillation, are found commonly in patients with stroke. Similarly, strokes may occur concurrently with other acute conditions, such as AMI and acute CHF. Auscultation for murmurs and gallops is crucial. Thoracic aortic dissections, may cause ischemic stroke. Unequal pulses or blood pressures in the extremities may reflect the presence of aortic dissections.

The Neurological Examination

Must be thorough, and quick. A directed and focused examination can be performed in minutes and not only provides great insight into the potential cause of the patient's deficits, but also helps to determine the intensity of treatment required.

A very useful tool in measuring neurological impairment is the National Institutes of Health Stroke Scale (NIHSS). This scale can be used easily, is reliable and valid, provides insight to the location of vascular lesions, and can be correlated with outcome in patients with ischemic stroke. It focuses on 11 items. The NIHSS is used by most stroke teams and stroke neurologists; it enables the consultant to rapidly determine the severity and possible location of the stroke. A patient's score on the NIHSS is associated strongly with outcome, and it can predict those patients who are likely to respond to thrombolytic therapy and those who are most likely to develop hemorrhagic complications of thrombolytic use. One limitation of the NIHSS is its inability to quantify deficits in posterior circulation strokes.

Stroke Risks and Etiology

Risk factors for ischemic stroke comprise both modifiable and nonmodifiable characteristics. Identification of risk factors in each patient can uncover clues to the cause of the stroke and the most appropriate treatment plan. Nonmodifiable risk factors include age, race, sex, ethnicity, sickle cell disease, fibromuscular dysplasia, and heredity. Modifiable risk factors include hypertension, diabetes, cardiac disease—atrial fibrillation, valvular disease, mitral stenosis, etc. hypercholesterolemia, transient ischemic attacks (TIAs), carotid stenosis, and lifestyle issues—excessive alcohol intake, tobacco use, illicit drug use, obesity, physical inactivity, oral contraceptive use among women.

Common Stroke Mimics (Differential Diagnosis)

Stroke mimic is a term employed for manifestations of nonvascular disease processes when a stroke like clinical picture is produced. The presentation resembles or may even be indistinguishable from a stroke syndrome. The mimics include both processes occurring within the central nervous system and systemic disease processes. Distinguishing these stroke mimics from strokes is increasingly important in this era of stroke therapies with potential adverse effects. Broadly stroke mimics may be grouped into those that are likely to and those less likely to have focal neurological findings. Those that are likely to present with focal neurological findings are seizure, complicated migraine, structural brain lesions, hypoglycemia, rare manifestation of multiple sclerosis and functional hemiparesis.

Blood Tests in Acute Stroke

Blood test evaluation of the patient with ischemic stroke should be driven by comorbid illnesses as well as the potential acute stroke. In the setting of acute stroke when IV t-PA is considered blood glucose, platelet count, prothrombin time (PT) and activated partial thromboplastin time (aPTT) are important for eliminating hypoglycemia and bleeding diathesis that may exclude a patient from such treatment.

Glucose and electrolyte tests: Hypoglycemia is the most common blood abnormality that produces stroke like symptoms. It is corrected easily, and correction leads to rapid resolution of symptoms. Electrolyte disorders, hyperglycemia, hypoglycemia, and uremia should be considered carefully as the cause of ongoing mental and physical deficits while pursuing the diagnosis of stroke.

Complete blood count: CBC provides key information regarding hemoglobin and hematocrit, thus evaluating for anemia and possible deficiencies in oxygen-carrying capacity. Additionally, sickle cell disease, polycythemia, and thrombocytosis increase the risk for stroke.

PT and aPTT tests: Many patients with acute stroke are on anticoagulants, such as heparin or warfarin. Treatment decisions, such as thrombolytic use, require data on coagulation status. An elevated international normalized ratio (INR) may preclude patients from receiving thrombolytics.

Cardiac enzymes and arterial blood gas (ABG) analysis: Not infrequently, patients with acute stroke also experience acute myocardial ischemia. In addition to ECG findings, increased cardiac enzymes might suggest concomitant cardiac injury. In patients with suspected hypoxemia, ABG will define the severity of hypoxemia and may detect acid-base disturbances. It must be borne in mind that arterial puncture in a noncompressible site is a contraindication to IV t-PA.

Neuroimaging Studies in Acute Stroke

CT is, and probably will likely remain for the next decade, the most commonly used form of neuroimaging in the evaluation of patients with apparent acute stroke. Noncontrast CT is very sensitive in detecting intracerebral and subarachnoid hemorrhage, as well as subdural hematomas. Treatment algorithms are dichotomous for the presence of intracranial blood, and most interventions for ischemic stroke require the absence of blood on CT scan.

Although CT is not very sensitive for early ischemia (<24 hours), several findings can suggest ischemic changes relatively early in the time course of stroke. Loss of the gray-white matter interface, loss of sulci, and loss of the insular ribbon are subtle signs of early ischemia. Early mass effect and areas of hypodensity suggest irreversible injury and identify patients at higher risk of hemorrhage if given thrombolytics. Significant hypodensity on the baseline scan should prompt the physician to question the time of onset. Hypodensity in an area greater than one third of the MCA distribution is considered by some a relative contraindication for thrombolytics.

A hyperdense MCA sign suggests a clot in the MCA. These patients are at risk for strokes with significant deficit, poor outcome and occasionally poorer response to intravenous t-PA. Some authorities believe that these patients may benefit most from aggressive thrombolytic therapy, including intra-arterial therapies, but this has not been specifically proven in double-blind randomized trials. An illustrative example has been depicted in **Figure 4.3**. CT scan can also demonstrate other causes of the patient's symptoms, including neoplasm, epidural and subdural hemorrhage, aneurysm, abscess, arteriovenous malformation, and hydrocephalus.

Xenon CT is a relatively new technique that complements noncontrast head CT and provides quantitative measurement of regional blood flow. Like *MRI*, it is being studied for its contributions to patient selection for thrombolytic therapy and to management of medical therapies in patients with increased intracranial pressure (ICP).

CT angiography can demonstrate the vascular occlusion and areas of perfusion deficits. CT perfusion studies are capable of producing perfusion images similar to xenon CT and together with CT angiography may become more available and utilized in the acute evaluation of stroke patients. A patient with right middle cerebral artery (RMCA) occlusion is depicted in **Figure 4.4**.

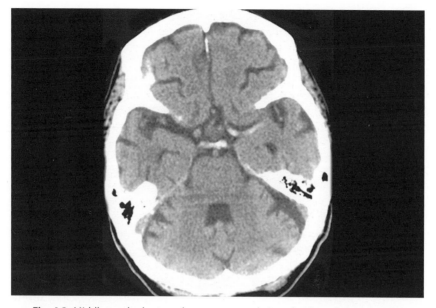

Fig. 4.3: Middle cerebral artery clot—recommendations for thrombolytic therapy

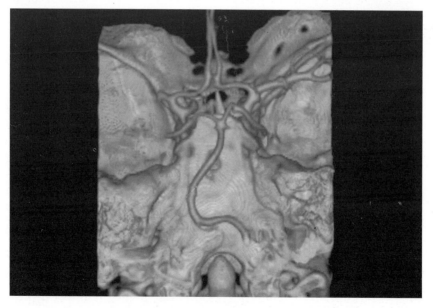

Fig. 4.4: Right middle cerebral artery occlusion
(For color version, see Plate 2)

MRI with magnetic resonance angiography (MRA) is a major advance in the neuroimaging of stroke. MRI not only provides great structural detail but also can demonstrate stroke within minutes of onset of symptoms. A major limitation of MRI in acute stroke is the fact that it is time consuming

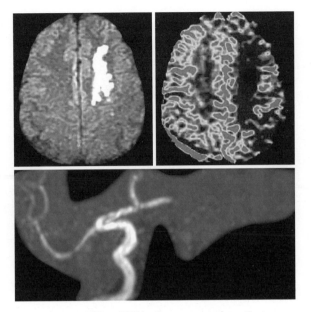

Fig. 4.5: MRI and MRA of an acute stroke patient
(For color version, see Plate 2)

and requires the cooperation of the stroke patient to obtain reliable images. Diffusion-weighted MRI (DWI) can detect areas of ischemic brain injury more quickly than standard MRI or CT scan by detecting changes in water molecule mobility. Perfusion MRI (PWI) uses injected contrast material (usually Gadolinium) to demonstrate areas of decreased perfusion. Recent advances use the technology of arterial spin labeling (ASL) to produce CBF maps without the use of contrast agents. DWI-PWI mismatch, theoretically identifying potentially salvageable tissues. *MRA:* This noninvasive technique demonstrates vascular anatomy and occlusive disease of the head and neck without the need for contrast material. An illustrative example of MRI and MRA of an acute stroke patient is depicted in **Figure 4.5**.

Digital subtraction angiography is considered the definitive method for demonstrating vascular abnormalities, including occlusion, stenosis, dissections, and aneurysms. Cerebral angiography not only provides useful information on the extracranial and intracranial vasculature, but also allows for intra-arterial therapies, both intra-arterial thrombolytics and catheter devices (MERCI and Penumbra system). Angiography requires special facilities and a skilled operator and it carries a stroke risk of approximately 1%.

Transcranial Doppler (TCD) ultrasonography can assess the location and degree of arterial occlusions in the extracranial carotid and large intracranial vessels, including the middle cerebral and vertebrobasilar arteries. It can also be used to detect restoration of flow after thrombolytic therapy, and the recent Combined Lysis of Thrombus in Brain Ischemia Using Transcranial Ultrasound and Systemic TPA (CLOTBUST) study has suggested that TCD may facilitate recanalization. The use of single-photon emission computed tomography (SPECT) and positron-emission tomography (PET) in stroke is still relatively experimental and available only at select institutions; it can define areas of altered regional blood flow.

Other Tests that Might Assist in Acute Stroke Management

Echocardiography

Transthoracic echocardiography (TTE) and transesophageal echocardiography (TEE) are useful tools in evaluating patients with possible cardiogenic sources of their stroke. TEE is more sensitive than TTE and can evaluate the aortic arch and thoracic aorta for plaques or dissections. TEE is however is semi-invasive test that requires conscious sedation and requires patient cooperation, that may be difficult in the acute stroke patient.

ECG

Stroke and coronary artery disease share many risk factors. ECG may demonstrate cardiac arrhythmias, such as atrial fibrillation, or may indicate acute ischemia. All patients with stroke should have an ECG as part of their initial evaluation. ECG may fail to detect paroxysmal atrial fibrillation, the limitation may be overcome by long-term monitoring. Chest radiography should be performed when clinically indicated.

Lumbar Puncture

A lumbar puncture (LP) is required to rule out meningitis or subarachnoid hemorrhage when the CT scan is negative but the clinical suspicion remains high. Performing an LP on patients with acute stroke will preclude them from receiving thrombolytics.

Stroke Medical Care

Stroke care begins in the prehospital setting and ending at home after discharge. Prehospital care personnel are critical elements in the stroke chain of survival. Emergency medical services (EMS) personnel should begin with the ABCs and, once the patient's condition is stable, should perform a more directed assessment and administer supportive treatment. Prehospital stroke scales, such as the Cincinnati Prehospital Stroke Scale or Los Angeles Prehospital Stroke Scale, can be useful in identifying patients with potential stroke. Providing supplemental oxygen when indicated, establishing intravenous lines, measuring serum glucose, and administering glucose in hypoglycemic patients are elements of prehospital stroke care. Equally important is prehospital notification of emergency room of a potential stroke patient. This allows for early activation of stroke teams and mobilization of necessary resources, such as a stroke team, radiology, and pharmacy. The goal of acute stroke management in the emergency department is rapid and efficient care. Continuing from the assessment of the ABCs, stroke patient evaluation and treatment should be performed within one hour from presentation as shown in **Table 4.1**. Again, general Stroke management is a team effort with the nursing and medical staff working closely together. General stroke care issues are outlined in the **Table 4.2** below.

Hypoglycemia and hyperglycemia need to be identified and treated early in the evaluation. Not only can both produce symptoms that closely mimic ischemic stroke, but both also can aggravate stroke induced neuronal damage. Administration of glucose in hypoglycemia produces profound and prompt improvement, while insulin should be started for patients with stroke and hyperglycemia. Hyperglycemia has also been found to be associated with thrombolysis induced intracerebral hemorrhage. Hyperthermia is infrequently associated with stroke but can increase morbidity. Administration of acetaminophen, by mouth or per rectum, is indicated in the presence of fever.

Supplemental oxygen is needed only when the patient has a documented oxygen requirement. No evidence exists to date suggesting that supernormal oxygenation improves outcome, and some studies suggest it may worsen outcome. Blood pressure management is delicate and controversial. Many

Table 4.1: NINDS recommended stroke evaluation targets for potential thrombolysis candidates	
Time interval	*Time target*
Door to doctor	10 min
Access to neurologic expertise	15 min
Door to CT scan completion	25 min
Door to CT scan interpretation	45 min
Door to treatment	60 min
Admission to monitored bed	3 hours

Table 4.2: General management of patients with acute stroke	
Blood glucose	Treat hypoglycemia with D50 Treat hyperglycemia with insulin if serum glucose >150–200 mg/dL
Blood pressure	See recommendations for thrombolysis candidates and noncandidates (**Table 4.3**)
Cardiac monitor	Continuous monitoring for ischemic changes or atrial fibrillation
Intravenous fluids	Avoid D5W and excessive fluid administration IV isotonic sodium chloride solution at 50 mL/h unless otherwise indicated
Oral intake	NPO initially; aspiration risk is great, avoid oral intake until swallowing assessed
Oxygen	Supplement if indicated (SaO_2 < 90%, hypotensive, etc.)
Temperature	Avoid hyperthermia, oral or rectal acetaminophen as needed

patients are hypertensive on arrival. Recent American Stroke Association guidelines have reinforced the need for caution in lowering blood pressures acutely. **Table 4.3** shows current recommendations for both candidates and noncandidates for thrombolytic therapy. In the small proportion of patients with stroke who are relatively hypotensive, pharmacologically increasing blood pressure may improve flow through critical stenoses.

Surgical Care

Surgical intervention is rarely required urgently in acute stroke; however, current recommendations suggest that neurosurgical care should be available within 2 hours when needed, e.g. to evaluate surgical options in symptomatic hemorrhagic conversion following t-PA or in the management of life-threatening elevations of ICP. Increased ICP is a life-threatening event arising from edema and mass effect; it is more common in large, hemispheric

Table 4.3: Blood pressure management in patients with stroke*		
	Blood Pressure	*Treatment*
Candidates for fibrinolysis	Pretreatment SBP >185 or DBP >110 mm Hg	Labetalol 10–20 mg IVP 1–2 doses or Enalapril 1.25 mg IVP
	Post-treatment DBP >140 mm Hg	Sodium nitroprusside (0.5 mcg/kg/min)
	SBP >230 mm Hg or DBP 121–140 mm Hg	Labetalol 10–20 mg IVP and consider labetalol infusion at 1–2 mg/min or nicardipine 5 mg/h IV infusion and titrate
	SBP 180–230 mm Hg or DBP 105–120 mm Hg	Labetalol 10 mg IVP, may repeat and double every 10 min up to maximum dose of 150 mg
Noncandidates for fibrinolysis	DBP >140 mm Hg	Sodium nitroprusside 0.5 mcg/kg/min; may reduce approximately 10–20%
	SBP >220 or DBP 121–140 mm Hg or MAP >130 mm Hg SBP< 220 mm Hg or DBP 105–120 mm Hg or MAP <130 mm Hg	Labetalol 10–20 mg IVP over 1–2 min; may repeat and double every 10 min up to maximum dose of 150 mg or nicardipine 57 mg/h IV infusion and titrate
		Antihypertensive therapy indicated only if AMI, aortic dissection, severe CHF, or hypertensive encephalopathy present

* Adopted from Advanced Cardiac Life Support (ACLS) Guidelines and 2003 American Stroke Association Scientific Statement

Abbreviations: SBP, systolic blood pressure; DBP, diastolic blood pressure; IVP, intravenous push; MAP, mean arterial pressure

strokes, strokes with hemorrhagic transformation and in the elderly. Edema and herniation are the most common causes of early death in patients with hemispheric stroke. Patient position, hyperventilation and hyperosmolar therapy may be used, as in patients with increased ICP secondary to closed head injury. Recent reports of hemicraniectomy to treat life-threatening ICP have suggested that these patients have a lower mortality rate, if surgery is performed before clinical deterioration. Selected patients with either hemorrhagic transformation or intracerebral hemorrhage after thrombolytic therapy may benefit from surgical evacuation of the hematoma, but this has not been proven prospectively in randomized, double-blind trials. If neurosurgical care is not available in house, a transfer policy is required to expedite patient transfer when neurosurgical expertise is needed.

Couple of surgical interventions are applicable to patients with cerebellar strokes:

1. Patients with acute hydrocephalus secondary to an ischemic stroke most commonly affecting the cerebellum can be treated with placement of a ventricular drain.
2. Decompressive surgical evacuation of a space occupying cerebellar infarction is a potentially lifesaving measure, and clinical recovery may be very good.

Consultations

In the first hours of acute stroke, an experienced professional sufficiently familiar with stroke or a stroke team should be available within 15 minutes of the patient's arrival in the emergency department. Physical medicine and rehabilitation (PM&R), occupational therapy, physical therapy, cognitive therapy and speech therapy experts are consulted within the first day of hospitalization. Consultation of cardiology and vascular surgery or neurosurgery may be warranted based on the results of TTE/TEE, carotid duplex scanning, neuroimaging, and clinical course. During hospitalization, additional useful consultations include home health care coordinator, rehabilitation coordinator, social worker, psychiatrist (commonly for depression), and dietitian.

Diet

Patients with acute stroke are at great risk of aspiration pneumonia. All patients should be given nothing by mouth (NPO) until a swallowing assessment is performed. This frequently involves careful switching of oral medication to parenteral preparation during this period. Oral Aspirin can be switched to per rectal suppository. Because of temporary dysphagia, a temporary feeding tube may be required. If the patient remains at a significant aspiration risk for the foreseeable future, a percutaneous endoscopic gastrostomy (PEG) feeding tube may be required. A dietitian can help identify a diet that not only addresses the aspiration risk but also ensures adequate caloric intake to help prevent poststroke malnutrition. The dietitian also must consider special dietary needs of patients with hypertension, diabetes mellitus, and hyperlipidemia. Based on a clinical trial on stroke patients who can swallow, supplemental nutrition is not necessary in this group.

Physical Activity

Physical activity is tailored to the severity of stroke. Aspiration precautions, with the head of the bed elevated to 30–45°, need to be observed. Physical therapy will test and suggest level of activity. This should be performed within the first 24 hours of hospitalization. Increase activity if tolerated as per the suggestions of the rehabilitation coordinator, with the goal of mobilizing the patient as early as possible. At discharge, encourage patients to increase activity as tolerated.

Further Inpatient Care

Inpatient care is tailored to the severity of the acute stroke and comorbid illnesses. Some recent studies suggest that admission to a dedicated stroke unit with specially trained staff may reduce both short and long-term morbidity and mortality rates. The goals of early supportive care after admission (adapted from the American Stroke Associations Guidelines) include the following:

1. The use of comprehensive specialized stroke care (stroke units) incorporating rehabilitation.
2. The use of standardized stroke care order sets to improve general management.
3. Early mobilization of less severely affected patients and measures to prevent subacute complications of stroke.
4. Assessment of swallowing before starting eating or drinking is recommended.
5. Patients with suspected pneumonia or urinary tract infections should be treated with antibiotics.
6. Subcutaneous administration of anticoagulants for treatment of immobilized patients to prevent deep vein thrombosis.
7. Treatment of concomitant medical diseases.
8. Early institution of interventions to prevent recurrent stroke.

Outpatient Care/Rehabilitation

Poststroke outpatient care largely focuses on rehabilitation and prevention of recurrent stroke. Rehabilitation planning begins within the first day of the acute stroke. The American Stroke Association guidelines for rehabilitation focus on 6 major areas, as follows:

1. Preventing, recognizing, and managing comorbid conditions and medical complications
2. Training for maximum independence

3. Facilitating maximum psychosocial coping and adaptation by patient and family
4. Preventing secondary disability by promoting community reintegration, including resumption of home, family, recreational, and vocational activities
5. Enhancing quality of life in view of residual disability
6. Preventing recurrent stroke and other vascular conditions.

In/Outpatient Measures in Secondary Prevention

The acute hospitalization is focused not only on treating the acute stroke but also on identifying risk factors for recurrent stroke and beginning to modify these risk factors if possible. Antiplatelet therapy (anticoagulation in strokes caused by atrial fibrillation), treatment of hypertension, hyperlipidemia, diabetes, cessation of smoking and lifestyle modifications (diet and exercise) have all been proven to be effective means of preventing secondary stroke over long-term. The combined result of all these measures can result in a 80% relative risk reduction of secondary stroke.

Patients discharged from the hospital after ischemic stroke should be considered for antiplatelet medications unless contraindicated. Current choices include the following: 1) Aspirin, taken daily in low-to-medium doses (50–325 mg), is an effective and inexpensive first-choice agent for reducing recurrent stroke risk. 2) Newer antiplatelet agents, such as clopidogrel (Plavix) and 3) aspirin/dipyridamole combinations (Aggrenox) are also effective in reducing recurrent stroke rate but may cause adverse effects that must be monitored. Initiating long-term anticoagulation (e.g. warfarin) reduces the risk of recurrent stroke in patients at risk for cardioembolic stroke. In patients with atrial fibrillation, the recommended target INR is in the range of 2–3. In patients with mechanical prosthetic valves, target INR is in the range of 2–3.5, depending on the type of valve. Patients with rheumatic valvular heart disease, cardiomyopathy, arrhythmias, or heart failure should be considered for long-term anticoagulation. Patients without one of these indications for anticoagulation do not appear to benefit from warfarin therapy, judging by results of the Warfarin Aspirin Recurrent Stroke Study (WARSS). Additional outpatient medications should be tailored to the patient's comorbid conditions and to risk factors identified during hospitalization. Use of HMG-coreductase inhibitors has been proven to be beneficial in reducing the rates of stroke in patients with coronary artery disease and elevated or high-normal levels of low-density lipoprotein (LDL) cholesterol. Medications to address hypertension, hyperlipidemia, and diabetes mellitus should be reviewed with the patient prior to discharge.

Transfer to a Stroke Capable Hospital

Emergency medical services (EMS) triage and transfer of patients with stroke is an important issue in stroke care. The recommendation for the establishment of stroke centers has helped define for consideration the elements of both primary and secondary stroke centers. EMS agencies are likely to be asked to triage patients with potential stroke to centers that have demonstrated capabilities to evaluate and treat these patients in a timely fashion. Hospitals without neuroimaging capabilities should stabilize and immediately transfer patients with potential stroke to centers with CT scan availability. Hospitals without intensive care units or access to timely neurosurgical expertise should transfer patients who are candidates for thrombolytics or who have received thrombolytics to institutions that can provide those services. Patients with large hemispheric strokes who may be at significant risk for edema and increased ICP and who may require neurosurgical expertise should be transferred before clinical deterioration occurs.

Complications

Complications following a stroke can be divided into those occurring acutely, typically within 72 hours, and those occurring later. Acute complications include cerebral edema, increased ICP and possible herniation, hemorrhagic transformation, aspiration pneumonia, and seizures. Post-thrombolytic complications center around bleeding. The greatest concern is intracerebral hemorrhage, typically occurring within the first 12 hours after treatment. Other potential sites of bleeding include GI tract, genitourinary tract (associated with Foley catheters), and skin, typically at sites of intravenous lines. Subacute complications include pneumonia, deep venous thrombosis and pulmonary emboli, urinary tract infections, decubitus ulcers, contractures, spasticity, joint problems such as the shoulder-hand syndrome, and malnutrition. A significant number of stroke survivors also experience depression. Identification and treatment of depression is extremely important in maximizing quality of life, not only for stroke survivors, but also for their families and care providers.

Patient and Health Personnel Education

Stroke is a major public health problem in both the developing and developed nations. Education is paramount in the fight to prevent and treat stroke. Education must include all elements of the stroke treatment and prevention. While medical education is often difficult and requires constant reinforcement, it has potential for minimizing the stroke burden. Public education is perhaps the hardest of all. Presently, several organizations are reaching out to the communities to promote stroke awareness and to develop coordinated stroke care within the region. Public education must involve all age groups. Incorporating stroke into basic life support (BLS) and cardiopulmonary resuscitation (CPR) curricula is just one way to reach the health personnel. Avenues to reach an audience with a higher stroke risk include using religious and cultural organizations, employers, and retirement communities to promote stroke risk and symptom awareness. Prehospital care providers are essential to timely stroke care. Course curriculum for prehospital care providers is beginning to include more information on stroke than ever before. Through certification and advance cardiac life support (ACLS) instruction, as well as continuing medical education classes, prehospital care providers can remain current on stroke and promote stroke awareness in their own communities. Physician and nursing staff involved in the care of patients who have had a stroke, both in the emergency department and in the hospital, should participate in scheduled stroke education. This will help them maintain the skills required to treat stroke patients effectively and to remain current on medical advances for all stroke types.

Palliative Care

Unfortunately, some patients with stroke have a fatal brain injury. Others have profound neurological impairments such as a persistent vegetative state or evidence of unstable vital signs. Other patients with stroke have serious preexisting medical or neurological illnesses, such as dementia, that have caused severe impairments, and the new cerebrovascular event may add more disability. Despite the interventions that are described in this outline, the prognosis of such patients often is very poor. Many people would not want to survive if a devastating stroke would lead to a persistent vegetative state or other condition of devastating incapacity.

Bibliography

1. Adams HP Jr, del Zoppo G, Alberts MJ, et al. Guidelines for the early management of adults with ischemic stroke. A guideline from the American Heart Association/ American Stroke Association Stroke Council, Clinical Cardiology Council, Cardiovascular Radiology and Intervention Council, and the Atherosclerotic Peripheral Vascular Disease and Quality of Care Outcomes in Research Interdisciplinary Working Groups. Stroke. 2007;38:1655-711[Medline].
2. Agarwal P, Eshkar N, Verro P, Sen S. Differential response to intravenous versus intra-arterial thrombolysis in acute ischemic stroke on the basis of hyperdense middle cerebral artery sign. Cerebrovascular Diseases. 2004;17:182-90.
3. Albers GW, Bates VE, Clark WM, et al. Intravenous tissue-type plasminogen activator for treatment of acute stroke: The Standard Treatment with Alteplase to Reverse Stroked (STARS) study. JAMA. 2000;283(9):1145-50 [Medline].
4. Alberts MJ, Hademenos G, Latchaw RE, et al. Recommendations for the establishment of primary stroke centers. Brain Attack Coalition. JAMA. 2000; 283(23):3102-09 [Medline].
5. American Heart Association: Textbook of Advanced Cardiac Life Support. American Heart Association; 1997.
6. Brott TG, Clark WM, Fagan SC. Stroke: The first hours Guidelines for Acute Treatment. National Stroke Association; 2000.
7. CAST investigators: Randomised placebo-controlled trial of early aspirin use in 20,000 patients with acute ischaemic stroke. CAST (Chinese Acute Stroke Trial) Collaborative Group. Lancet. 1997;349(9066):1641-9 [Medline].
8. Chen ZM, Sanderock P, Pan HC, et al. Indications for early aspirin use in acute ischemic stroke: a combined analysis of 40000 randomized patients from the Chinese acute stroke trial and the international stroke trial. On behalf of the CAST and IST collaborative groups. Stroke. 2000;31(6):1240-9 [Medline].

9. Hacke W, Kaste M, Bluhmki E, et al. Thrombolysis with alteplase 3 to 4.5 hours after acute ischemic stroke. N Engl J Med. 2008;359(13):1317-29 [Medline].
10. Katzan IL, Furlan AJ, Lloyd LE, et al. Use of tissue-type plasminogen activator for acute ischemic stroke: The Cleveland area experience. JAMA. 2000;283(9):1151-8 [Medline].
11. Kothari RU, Jauch EC, Broderick J, et al. Acute stroke: delays to presentation and emergency department evaluation. Ann Emerg Med. 1999;33:3-8 [Medline].
12. Kothari RU, Pancioli A, Liu T, et al. Cincinnati Prehospital Stroke Scale: Reproducibility and validity. Ann Emerg Med. 1999;33:373-8 [Medline].
13. Lattimore SU, Chalela J, Davis L, et al. Impact of establishing a primary stroke center at a community hospital on the use of thrombolytic therapy: The NINDS Suburban Hospital Stroke Center Experience. Stroke. 2003;34(6):e55-7 [Medline].
14. Lewandowski CA, Frankel M, Tomsick TA, et al. Combined intravenous and intra-arterial r-TPA versus intra-arterial therapy of acute ischemic stroke: Emergency Management of Stroke (EMS) Bridging Trial. Stroke. 1999;30(12):2598-605 [Medline].
15. Lyden P, Brott T, Tilley B, et al. Improved reliability of the NIH Stroke Scale using video training. NINDS TPA Stroke Study Group. Stroke. 1994;25(11):2220-6 [Medline].
16. Marler JR, Jones PW, Emr M. Proceedings of a National Symposium on Rapid Identification and Treatment of Acute Stroke. Bethesda, Maryland. The National Institute of Neurologic Disorders and Stroke (NINDS), National Institutes of Health. 1997; Publication No. (NIH): 97-4239.
17. Schneider AT, Kissela B, Woo D, et al. Ischemic stroke subtypes: A population-based study of incidence rates among blacks and whites. Stroke. 2004;35(7):1552-6 [Medline].
18. Sen S, Huang DY, Akhavan O, Wilson S, Verro P, Solander S. IV vs. IA TPA in Acute Ischemic Stroke with CT Angiographic Evidence of Major Vessel Occlusion: A Feasibility Study. Neurocrit Care. 2009;11(1):76-81 [Medline].
19. The National Institute of Neurological Disorders and Stroke rt-PA Stroke Study G: Tissue plasminogen activator for acute ischemic stroke. N Engl J Med. 1995;333(24):1581-7 [Medline].
20. Zweifler RM. Management of acute stroke. South Med J. 2003;96(4):380-5 [Medline].

5

Concepts in Stroke Rehabilitation

Mouli Madhab Ghatak

Stroke is a vascular insult, which results in cytoarchitectural damage in the highly qualified and sensitive cell population of the human brain. The critical and multidimensional psychophysical dysfunction caused by a stroke is till now partially conquered by the researchers, despite the revolutionary growth of this complex science. While the basic scientific invention has grown aggressive neuroprotective interventions in its acute phase, the integration of clinical neurorehabilitation has reached its excellence in dealing at least partially with the residues left by its uncontrolled aggression during its inception. The 'great brain' rehabilitates its royal generosity through generous cytogeneration operating its adaptive plasticity throughout the whole damaged neuropremises and multiphasic, multidisciplinary reinforced practice of stroke rehabilitation evolves to assist and encourage this neuroplasticity. In fact the foundation of stroke rehabilitation is no more challenged by the theory of 'spontaneous recovery' as 'learning-based-brain plasticity' is strongly appreciated in expanded scientific research on stroke survivors of our time.

Neural Plasticity: The Light in Rehabilitation

Brain has shown its unique plastic behavior through which any cellular loss is recovered or managed by structural and functional reorganization. It's a typical representation of cellular function, either by structural regenesis or reactivation of already present nonfunctional neuronal zones. This may be by *collateral sprouting* when a neighboring axon represents the damaged axon by generation of new adaptation. The branching of collateralized axon (called–Pruning) actually reactivates the lost area and the activity of these parallel synaptic routes yields positive response towards functional achievement. When the contributing axon is remote from the injured axon, the foreign target may result in some sensitive, adaptive or even maladaptive outcome, called 'ingrowth'. The sympathetic ingrowth is a typically known example in CVA/or brain injured patient. The 'regenesis' of mature brain cells is also seen in some areas like the subventricular zone of lateral ventricular wall area for Olfactory bulb (interneurons), subgranular zone of dentate gyrus, etc. But it is a fact that the CNS—neurons in most case do not regenerate and it is its intrinsic behavior.

The Learning: Plasticity Duet

Recent encouraging informations have been obtained from some studies on CNS plasticity directly induced by learning. During normal brain growth, the learning largely directs the functional performances of an individual and is evident that a 'Gold Medalist' shooter of 'Olympics', has developed his skill through learning and repetitive practice.

Documentation of neural response representation of specific inputs measured in auditory, somatosensory and motor cortices in animals before and after learning, is interesting and it is paired with behavioral studies of humans, which provides strong suggestions and inferences of capability of CNS to self-organize both during development in childhood as well as after injury in matured state.

The typical cortical plasticity process related to learning encounters the following factors:

1. Specialization—there must be specific sensory inputs/stimuli which helps 'specialization' in the functional representation, and finer distinctions with specific sensory training gradually develops the skilled performance by selective cortical representations.
2. Repetition—learning needs repetition. The sensory inputs are to repeatedly excite the reorganization process and a closely attended specific training progressively develops selective representation.
3. 'Learning to learn'—the perceptual, cognitive, motor and executive skills are largely processed by 'self-shaping' through specialized stored and manipulated-experience-related inputs, which helps reorganization in developmental as well as mature states.
4. Progressive re-mapping—there is gradual amplification of cell growth and increased coordination of distributed neuronal populations with networking which develops subject-specific performance level.
5. Plasticity is a competitive process, it needs processing time for proper integration, it depends both on extrinsic and intrinsic inputs, it is a complex and continuing process by reactivation, differentiation and synchronization.

Based on this interesting updated concept several rehab regimens are rapidly being popular and retested.

'Nonuse'—Willful Nonuse of unaffected limb encourages the early attempts to use the affected limb as the adaptation of various tasks cannot develop by the unaffected limb.

Basic Factors in Stroke Rehabilitation

The sudden onset catastrophy—'STROKE' not only physically weakens the patient, but the psychocognitive dysfunction, the metabolic and cardiovascular impairments complicate the whole scenario. Rehabilitation of such patient should be provided under great care with proper scientific outlook to combat all these incapability factors. Moreover, when the patient has already limited his lively function because of geriatric decay, the total program should be directed towards individualized, standardized, unique, safest, energy efficient, pleasurable, high quality and long-term care.

Goal of Stroke Rehabilitation Programs

1. Recognition, prevention, and minimization of
   a. Pre-existing medical complications,
   b. Ongoing general health problems,
   c. Secondary medical complications.
2. Training for maximal/physical functional independence.
3. Facilitation of maximal psychosocial/and professional adaptation.
4. Promotion of community/reintegration, resumption of prior life roles, including returning to home, family, recreational and vocational activities.
5. Improving and ensuring the quality of life.

Stroke Recovery Predictors (SRP)

1. The smaller the lesion, the smaller the deficit (except in brainstem)
2. Recovery is unfavorable in patients with diabetes mellitus, bowel and bladder incontinence lasting more than four weeks, flaccid paralysis lasting more than 2 months and gross perceptual deficit or poor motivation.
3. Initial deficits after stroke in young and very old tend to be less than those seen in middle aged, but the younger patients suffer from more deficits afterward than the patients of other age group.
4. Slowly developing stroke exhibits less functional loss than suddenly developed lesions.
5. Purely cerebellar lesions show higher recovery rates than lesions of other sites of brain.
6. Hemorrhagic strokes have better recovery than ischemic ones in most cases.
7. The earlier the initiation of integrated rehabilitation, the better the recovery. The most important period is 40 days after attack and the recovery is usually slow after 3 months of stroke.
8. Rehabilitation at home, in nursing homes or in general hospital is less effective than that performed in integrated rehabilitation centers where equipped, comprehensive, multidimensional and individualized rehab programs are followed.

When Rehabilitation?

1. As early as possible after the neurological stabilization, usually after 72 hours of stroke, rehabilitation should be started to prevent further complications and attain highest possible functional capabilities.
2. If the patient needs few days to few weeks to be treated in acute care hospital (for cardiological, medical, hemodynamic or/and neurological stability), rehabilitation should be started in acute care set ups and the moment the patient is stabilized, he/she should be transferred to any good rehabilitation center (or at home if suitable).
3. As because initiation of stroke rehabilitation after 3 months of onset yields poorer result, any such late entry should be handled cautiously with proper prognostic explanation to the party and patient to avoid unnecessary consumer's/insurer's claim and legal risks. However, late initiation/rehabilitation should be targeted more towards functional programs.
4. Various studies prove that a number of patients show recovery even after 6 months and may continue improving even after 2 years of stroke.
5. Though organic changes or central regeneration is far from reality after 2 years or long after stroke, rehabilitation has still something to do to correct or modify some peripheral impairments or complications. Starting educating the patient to live with disability has no time bar.

Where and Whom to Rehabilitate?

1. During the acute phase, stroke rehabilitation should be started in the acute care hospital with concomitant medical treatment.
   a. Patients severely ill out of large lesions or worse medical conditions such as electrolyte or sugar imbalance, renal, cardiovascular or pulmonary upsets, take longer period to stay in acute care hospital should have initiation and maintenance of proper rehabilitation programs along with medical treatment in the primary care hospital.
   b. Patients with less medical complications may be shifted to rehabilitation centers having modern treatment facilities as early as possible and all further rehabilitation and medical treatment may be continued there.
   c. Persons without significant residual disabilities (TIA) may return home with proper home rehabilitation guidelines.
   d. Patients who cannot opt for indoor rehabilitation in any exclusive rehabilitation center, due to poor affordability or any other psycho-sociological causes, may arrange for home rehabilitation with required manpower provision (PMR specialist, physiotherapist, occupational therapist, psychotherapist, speech therapist, etc). Though such arrangements may not ensure expected results because of poor coordination and unequipped rehabilitation services.

The selection of patient is rather less important than the selection of modes or items of the programs, as almost all patients having any sort of residual impairment after stroke should undergo rehabilitation. Even minor impairments which do not play any important role in general incapability is to be treated through rehabilitation medicine as early as possible. Stroke survivors are categorized on the basis of different disabilities and the rehabilitation programs are planned accordingly.

Phases of Poststroke Rehabilitation

Acute Inpatient Rehabilitation

This phase of rehabilitation refers to the effort of reactivation of the physiological functions of an acutely ill patient, who has just survived or is yet to be survived. So the rehabilitation program consists of maintenance of neuromuscular, circulatory, cognitive (perceptual and behavioral) and communicative conditioning services along with intensive nursing care and repetitive evaluation and continuous monitoring systems. The medical treatment ensures the preventive and curative aspect of consequences of stroke and its associated problems, like HTN, DM, electrolyte and hemodynamic imbalances, stress bleeds, renal, cardiac and respiratory hazards and neurogenic malfunctioning, of various body parts with an intensive supervision in a well equipped emergency-care set up. The nursing and rehabilitative care supports the adaptive life during the process of survival and struggle for functional regain.

This three way defense against the morbid reactions of a stroke patient is really a challenging battle. The combined medical, nursing and rehabilitative care must be coordinated and comprehensive and must include the following measures:

1. Medical and rehabilitative evaluation.
2. Continuous monitoring in respect to metabolic and organic functions, medications and disabling factors.
3. Proper limb and body positioning.
4. Bladder and bowel care rehabilitation.
5. Psychological support.
6. Communication evaluation and balanced speech therapeutic support.
7. Bedside therapeutic exercises including:
   a. Range of motion exercise.
   b. Breathing and respiratory exercises including postural drainage.
   c. Progressive functional measures like turning in bed, sitting on bed and chair to standing even initiation of walking.
   d. Conditioning exercises balancing the metabolic harmony with proper rest and exercise rhythms.
8. Nutritional support.
9. Educating the patient and family to cope up with the sudden catastrophy and incapability and the future measures.

10. Repetitive assessment of continuing rehabilitation and preparing the patient for next phase of rehabilitation.

The Intermediate Phase

When the storm is over the patient comes out from the emergency room with a clear picture of residual disabilities, the individualistic, patient centric scheme of rehabilitation is planned with detailed assessment of each and every medical, neuromuscular, cardiopulmonary and metabolic factor. All members of a stroke rehabilitation team assess the patient on their own. Identifying the specific deficits, a realistic goal is set by the team. Now a well planned rehabilitation program is considered and discussed among the members under the able guidance of a psychiatrist or related specialists.

The basic foundation of a rational rehabilitation management program is always a "stepped program" and aims toward maximum functional independence, irrespective of the intensity of the morbidity and disability and other complicating factors. A stroke survivor may belong to a wide range of disability starting from a minimal motor hemiparesis or a mild focal neurodeficit to a severely ill, comatose condition compounded with serious neurodeficits and hemodynamic or cardiopulmonary instability. This phase is a crucial period for deciding the appropriate choice of the mode of rehabilitation and so all the stroke survivors in this stage are divided into three subgroups with an ideal choice of rehabilitation placement namely indoor rehabilitation, day care rehabilitation and home rehabilitation.

The Stepped Program

The specific clinical picture with disabilities presented by the patient builds a practical basis of rehabilitation measures in this phase. The medical complication like diabetes, hypertension, cardiopulmonary, renal and metabolic disorders are effectively prepared in the one hand and a goal oriented multidisciplinary neurorecovery program is started on the other. With the advancement of stroke recovery rehabilitation programs, the previous concept of putting the patient under vigorous exercise programs are now revised. The modern approach deals with simultaneous application of definitive and stepped physical therapies, occupational therapies, cognitive and behavioral therapies, speech pathology modification, orthotic intervention, neuromedicinal intervention, proper nutritional guidelines and a skilled nursing care. All these management programs are coordinated and interlinked in order to reach the goal **(Fig. 5.1)**.

The physical therapy is framed with proper positioning of the limbs (antispastic), maintaining full range of movement of joints, regulated development of tone along with different neurodevelopmental techniques facilitating achievement of isolated and coordinated movement patterns of affected muscles. And thereby minimizing the future complications through preventive measures like development of tone in shoulder muscles, body weight supported antispastic training and stretching, etc. Different researchers

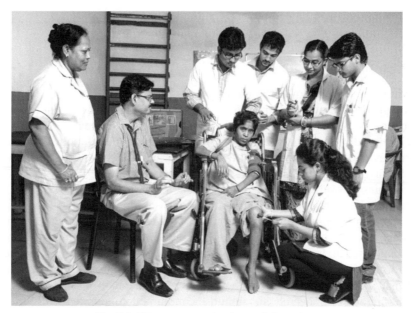

Fig. 5.1: The group examination and discussion
(For color version, see Plate 3)

have recommended various approaches—Brunnstrom highlighted the better effects and utilization of synergy (mass movement pattern of the muscles) to facilitate better recovery in the early stage. But Bobath is in favor of suppressing (preventing and breaking) the synergy in order to develop isolated movement of muscles. The recent researches are more concentrated towards effective motor relearning through various measures. Task specific motor skill development is suggested by Carr and Shepherd (some modern approaches are described in the next chapter).

The usual nature of flexion and adduction spasticity and flexor synergy in upper limb and extensor synergy in the lower limb become very important factors, which restrict, delay or even help the rehabilitation at times. It is controversial till date whether exercises and positioning can cure or prevent these peculiar neuromuscular changes. Stretching, splinting, mobilization, sensory stimulation and different exercises have limited effects over such centrally guided nature of limb musculature. But different physical therapies are recommended for prevention of various musculoskeletal complications from the early phase of rehabilitation program with a futuristic goal.

The recent slogan of physical rehabilitation is "only train and never exercise the muscles" so the physical therapies nowadays for stroke survivors mostly demand modification of the abnormal neuromuscular patterns along with advanced motor training and retraining through learning and relearning by various activities and tasks, activating CNS for cortical reorganization.

This specific goal oriented motor learning procedure is achieved by very scientific, sincere and target-oriented occupational therapy, functional re-orientation training, best performed in a functional rehabilitation gym. A stepped functional therapy starting from training for supine to sidelying, supine to sitting, improving sitting balance, sitting to standing, standing balance training (independent and stand-in-frame supported), gait training, maintaining proper gait sequence (heel strike, knee flexion, toe off and prevention of circumduction of hip) and eventually an intense ADL training are guided by an occupational therapist **(Fig. 5.2)**. A well-equipped hand therapy unit under an occupational therapist, takes care of the various abnormal and complicating factors of the hand, like abnormal neuromuscular patterns are scientifically assessed (the grasp, reach, prehension, sensory impairment, etc.) and sincere efforts are given in order to initiate minute changes gradually. Various kits and equipment including functional bandaging and splinting are introduced for proper hand training. Repeated practice of such training initiates the activation of learning module and triggers the plastic behavior of brain. However, patients having gross cognitive deficit cannot be trained with such instruments and activities. Training related to occupational therapies also supports cognitive therapies with some specific programs like peg activities, matching the colors, etc. Different finer work training substitutes a part of cognitive rehabilitation program. However, the best form of sensory motor learning programs always demands execution of cognitive and occupational therapy jointly.

Stroke survivors having gross cognitive impairments must be put in cognitive therapy unit. Effective neuromotor training is not possible unless

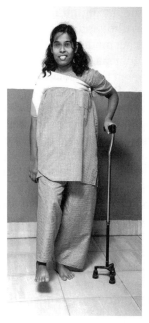

Fig. 5.2: Functional (gait) training in a stroke patient having
Bobath cuff in shoulder to prevent shoulder subluxation
(For color version, see Plate 3)

the cognitive deficits are encountered properly and in such cases, a stroke rehabilitation program usually faces a dark future (see the chapter on cognitive rehabilitation program). Other factors like psychological depression and instability is a barrier for positive motivation towards rehabilitation and if not handled cautiously may result in a poor outcome (see the chapter Psychiatric rehabilitation).

The various patterns of dysphasia are frequently associated with the cortical lesions, the pathogenesis are described in the chapter "Clinical presentation of stroke syndrome" and the diagnosis and management are described in the chapter "speech and language dysfunction".

Stroke patients may suffer from mild-to-moderate dysphagia, which also retards the rehabilitation outcome with a psychological set back and recurrent episodes of aspiration pneumonia seeks special medical treatment, nursing care and nutritionist's interventions (see the chapter swallowing disorders). Various other complicating problems arising from stroke and chronic immobilization and deconditioning situation are narrated in the next chapter.

The integrated team rehabilitation concept is vividly described with the activities and science related to all subspecialities or team members in the chapter "Models of Rehabilitation of Spinal Cord Injury and Stroke Patients".

Modern Approaches of Neurodevelopmental Rehabilitation in Stroke

The modern psychiatric approaches for stroke rehabilitation program is directed towards achieving maximum functional independence through newer strategies of control of spasticity and other complications and introducing different learning modules.

Different methods to counteract spasticity are stated in chapters "Medical/pharmacological management for spasticity" and "Therapeutic rehabilitation for spasticity management".

Neuromuscular blocks performed by botulinum toxin type A is proved to be effective in diffusing the flexor tone in upper extremity. It improves the disability restricting hygiene and dressing and decreases pain. The 'release' factor of hand evaluation may be improved by decreasing the flexor tone, which helps achieving better hand function. Such injection also decreases plantar flexor tone and hip adductor spasm, which improves the gait pattern. Brashear et al shows improvement in Ashworth scale scores without change in functional measures in some patients. Nerve blocks can also be performed by using Phenol in concentration of 26% in an aqua solution. Excessive elbow flexion in a stroke patient may be improved by musculocutaneous nerve block. Median nerve block may relax flexed wrist and fingers. While tibial nerve block reduces equinovarus posture.

The intrathecal pump and other procedures are described in other chapters.

Few studies offered *body weight supported (BWS) tread mill training* with better/faster process of recovery of walking. Such a gait training is performed

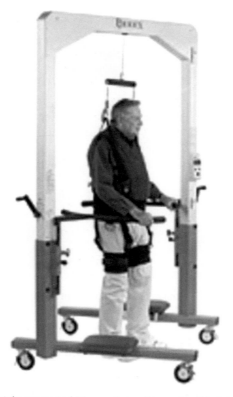

Fig. 5.3: Body weight supported (Harness) standing and gait training (on Treadmill) allows vertical shift of center of gravity and functional pelvic rotation. *Courtesy:* Hospimedica International *(For color version, see Plate 4)*

on a trademill with an overhead harness to support the body weight of the patient partially. Such a supported locomotion is usually sustained and transferred to walking over ground with full weight bearing. It allows upright posture, minimizes risk of fall and facilitates a reciprocal stepping pattern with improvement of motor and balance control. It is task specific with potential for multiple repetitions.

Hemiparetic ambulations are also being tried with different approaches like bodyweight supported treadmill walking, modified bicycle ergometer with proper monitoring of cardiovascular response **(Fig. 5.3)**.

Constraint-induced Movement Therapy

It is a method of forced and repetitive use of paretic hand engaging for a long time daily. The subject is asked not to use the normal hand and 'massed practice' with quick, attentive and closely observed practice sessions of different tasks has been reported to yield fairly positive results in respect to functional outcome in absence of conventional physiotherapy **(Fig. 5.4)**.

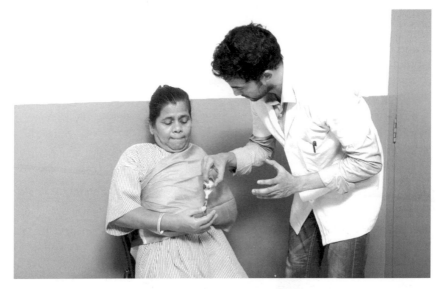

Fig. 5.4: Constraint-induced movement therapy (CIMT)
(For color version, see Plate 4)

Method of Training of Constraint-induced Movement Therapy

In constraint-induced movement therapy (CIMT), a mitt or sling is used on healthy hand for forced nonuse, and a series of tasks like grasping and releasing objects and pegs, turning pegs of books, moving light objects from one place to other, pinching fingers, feeding, writing, etc. This is to be forcefully recommended at least 6 hours a day and conventional physiotherapy is omitted for this patient. Patient is allowed to begin this training only after obtaining at least 20° voluntary extension of wrist, 10° voluntary extension of two fingers at MCP or IP joints of the paralytic hand.

The patient is asked to wear a mitt on the healthy hand throughout the working hours and 2 weeks of such 6 hours/day session (5 days/week) has shown positive functional result. Significant improvement in strength, ROM, task specific use of fingers is evident even in an old CVA patient.

The positive change is noted in functional MRI, which has proved the basis of application of CIMT.

Functional electrical stimulation (FES): Selected patients are also placed with FES along with conventional physical therapy, which have shown improvement of functional motor activities to some extent. FES may be described as a kind of electrical orthosis which may improve ankle dorsiflexion, wrist dorsiflexion by its sustained antispastic, stretching effect.

Studies with multichannel functional electrical stimulation (MEES) to get rehabilitation for nonambulatory hemiplegic patient have been shown to improve gait pattern and ground reaction forces.

Neuromuscular electrical stimulation has been used to augment range of motion and facilitation treatment and strengthening and scapular stabilization of and eventually correcting the shoulder subluxation for a laxed and hypotonic shoulder in a stroke patient.

Positional feedback and electrical stimulation were combined in new treatment modality for adult hemiparetic patient lacking normal voluntary wrist extension, four weeks positional feedback stimulation training (PFST) has been shown to improve isometric wrist and a repetitive isotonic exercise with facilitation wrist extension. Without continuous one-to-one therapist supervision is easily applied by such procedures.

EMG biofeedback has also been proved as an effective instrument for neuromuscular re-education. Some recreational therapy (discussed in another chapter), acupuncture and sensory stimulation are also used in some studies.

Virtual reality training: It is an advanced form of human computer interface that allows the user to interact with and become immersed in a computer generated environment. Such computer generated virtual environment can assess and rehabilitate cognitive and functional abilities by providing interactive scenarios that stimulate "real world task". Many activities of daily living such as driving may be hazardous to persons after stroke. A virtual reality system stimulates potentially hazardous situations without risk.

Stroke patients with balance disorder when given specific vestibular rehabilitation program has been shown to improve dizziness, the sensory organization deficit and the balance can be improved upto a great extent with an effective vestibular rehabilitation programs.

Exercise and Physical Activity Recommendation for Stroke Survivors

The recent study shows that about 14% of stroke survivors achieve full recovery in physical function, 25–50% needs some assistance during activity of daily living and the rest of the survivors have severe long-term paralytic disabilities. Ambulatory patients may perform at 50% of peak O_2 consumption and 70% of the peak power output, which can be achieved by age, and gender matched individual without history. This difference in tolerance is probably due to prolonged bed rest (deconditioning), reduced left ventricular function, associated neurodisability like flaccidity/plasticity of extremities impaired trunk balance and increased aerobic requirements during walking. Thus, the energy lost in walking is increased which is sometimes twice that of able-bodied persons. It in turn leads to more secondary complications like reduced circulation, muscular atrophy and poor cardiorespiratory function.

The activity and exercise prescription for a stroke patient should be designed to optimize functional motor performance through gradual partial body weight supported walking. Specialized training to develop skill, self-care and leisure time activities. The recent focus for rehabilitation of stroke patients aims to reduce prolonged inactive state and increase aerobic fitness. With

the limitations of neuromuscular and cardiorespiratory unfitness, a regular physical activity regime is promoted as follows:
   a. Submaximal exercise training monitored by blood pressure, pulse and TMT.
   b. Treadmill graded aerobic exercise training.
   c. Task oriented exercise protocols with complemented activities of daily living training.
   d. Cycle argometer training.
   e. Spirometric exercises.
   f. Graded gait training, coordination and balance training movements.
   Exercise recommendation should be judicious and requires an evaluation of primary and secondary risk factors and a pre-exercise evaluation of the various barriers like CAD, poor tolerance, risk of fall, mental confusion and cognitive impairments, age-related skeletal metabolic ophthalmological problems, etc. are mandatory.

Long-Term Rehabilitation

After the completion of the intermediate phase, the patient and the family members start thinking about what is preserved and what is lacking. A less number of unfortunate patients affected by a large, lesion who remain in comatose or semicomatose condition (evaluated by Glasgow coma scale) with very slow recovery, may be kept at home or a transitional living center (TLC) with good nursing care, frequent visit of a physician especially in cases of emergency and some low intensity maintenance, physical therapy are to be continued with a hopeful expectancy for return of higher motor function in future. These patients definitely remain totally dependant and live a vegetative life; rehabilitation has got very little access in conquering such situations.

On the other hand, patients with smaller lesions having minimal residual problems and achieving good functional independence within a few weeks, restarts a normal and healthy life at home and workplace too. They usually need very little assistance in the long-term rehabilitation phase when the patient is placed in the community.

The domain of disability consisting of a subgroup of patients between these two extremes of disability profile are usually the main concern for a good long-term rehabilitation program. As this subgroup consists of the highest number of patients having moderate degree of disability and poor to moderate return of self-ambulation with or without cognitive, speech or any other complications, the prime concern for long-term rehabilitation in these cases lies on adaptability of the patient at home, community or job with the existing residual disability. A wide variety of patient-population with varieties of medical and rehabilitative factors may turn up in this phase and a patient-centric program according to the needs of the individual should be planned. In this stage usually medical backup is reduced and the mobility factor becomes the greatest issue to avoid dependency in most of the cases.

The mobility related rehabilitation program includes functional training for mobility at bed, transfer techniques, wheel chair training (for selective patients), gait training and outdoor mobility training and these should be practiced stepwise from the early phase of rehabilitation. A goal directed mobility training which is initiated from the early days of the stroke, in anticipation of regain of maximum independence in mobility, is continued on a long-term basis. Gait training maintaining the proper sequences in swing and the stance phases is usually difficult due to poor voluntary movement of ankle dorsiflexors and increased tone of plantar flexors compounded with extensor synergy pattern in the lower extremity. AFO and functional crepe bandaging may reduce the effects of spastic plantar flexors and inverters. Patients with a poor regain of quadriceps movement resulting in buckling of the knee may take the advantage of gaiters which helps keep knee in extended position during gait training. The typical heel strike, flexion of the knee and toe off are usually absent in most of the cases, sometimes the increased adductor tone in absence of voluntary movement of flexor muscles helps in ambulation of the patient.

However, patient is trained scientifically step-by-step to overcome complex movements and newer barriers are to be faced by the patient as a challenge and proper training is necessary for this purpose.

The self-care activities including dressing, bathing, toileting, eating, etc. are trained by the occupational therapist when the patient seems to have good tone and voluntary movement and the assistance of the family members is important for accelerating this training. The patients who regain a good coordinated muscle movement patterns are trained for the finer activities like writing, cutting small objects, buttoning, unbuttoning, etc.

Patients not regaining such coordinated muscular movements eventually develop the habit of using the unaffected limbs for maintaining the activities. Persons with right hand dominance when affected by left hemisphere stroke usually suffer from aphasia and right hemiparesis and in this condition returning to work becomes more difficult because of poor activity in the dominant hand associated with speech disorder.

Different community support groups, friends and family members, the doctor and caregivers should inspire the patient with a positive outlook. A proper matching of improvement with the psychological expectation of the patient counteracts depression. A job site evaluation and vocational counseling are also important which are described in another chapter of this book.

Various adaptive devices are also used to overcome the impairment and to perform various household and personal care works in patients who are supposed to have an irreversible loss of function of a particular area.

Secondary Stroke Prevention

Stroke survivors usually have a greater risk of recurrent attacks. A good guideline and educational sessions must be provided to the patients to avoid the second attack.

The risk factors like hypertension, obesity, psychological stress, diabetes mellitus, inactivity, high lipids are modifiable risk factors, which are to be controlled with proper treatment and intervention.

Ischemic stroke sufferers must be put on aspirin and newer antiplatelet medications like clopidogrel, ticlopidine, etc. ACE inhibitors have been shown to have direct effects in lowering the incidence of a second attack.

Proper nutritional recommendations, daily session of exercises and a tension free lifestyle with regular intake of medications can keep a patient on the safe side.

Driving after Stroke

Stroke survivors who regain a good motor control and cognition are evaluated for driving. Driving evaluation tests basic cognitive skills like—memory, spatial organization, attention, concentration and reaction times. Driving skills are tested in simulators or behind the wheel with licensed instructors. Modification of particular part based on patient's impairment may also be done in selected cases. Adaptive devices like spinner knobs, accelerator, and extenders may be incorporated to compensate the motor deficits.

Vocational counseling and job related training as a long-term rehabilitation is described in another chapter of this book.

Bibliography

1. Bonita R, Beaglehole R. Recovery of motor function after stroke. Stroke. 1988;19:1497-500.
2. Bracewell RM Stroke: neuroplasticity and recent approaches to rehabilitions. J Neuro Neurosurg Psychiatry. 2003;74(11):1465.
3. Bracewell RM. Stroke: neuroplasticity and recent approaches to rehabilitation. J Neurol Neurosing Psychiatry. 220;74(11):1465.
4. Brosseau, et al. Post-Stroke Inpatient Rehabilitation: I. Predicting Length of Stay. AMJ Phys med Rehabil. 1996;75(6):422-30.
5. Brosseau, et al. Post-Stroke Inpatient Rehabilitation: II. Predicting Discharge Disposition. American Journal of Physical Medicine and Rehabilitation. 1996;75(6):431-6.
6. Bushnell, et al. Secondary Stroke Prevention Strategies for the Oldest Patients: Possibilities and Challenges, Drugs and Aging. 2009;26(3):209-30.
7. C Meek, et al. A systematic review of exercise trials post stroke. Clinical Rehabilitation. 2003;17:6-13.
8. C. Werner, et al. Treadmill Training with Partial Body Weight Support and an Electromechanical Gait Trainer for Restoration of Gait in Subacute Stroke Patients: A Randomized Crossover Study. Stroke. 2003;33:2895-901.
9. Caro JJ, et al. Management Patterns and Costs of Acute Ischemic Stroke: An International Study. Stroke. 2000;31:582-90.
10. Chen, et al. Facilitation of Sensory and Motor Recovery by Thermal Intervention for the Hemiplegic Upper Limb in Acute Stroke Patients: A Single-Blind Randomized Clinical Trial. Stroke. 2005;36(12):2665-9.
11. Clive ES. Recovery after stroke. Journal of Neurology, Neurosurgery, and Psychiatry. 1983;46:5-8.

12. Cramer, et al. Neuroplasticity and brain repair after stroke. Current Opinion in Neurology. 2008;21(1):76-82.
13. De Weerdt, et al. Group physiotherapy improves time use by patients with stroke in rehabilitation. Australian Journal of Physiotherapy. 2001;47(1):53-61.
14. Deborah S. Factors Influencing Stroke Survivors' Quality of Life During Subacute Recovery. Stroke. 2005;36:1480-4.
15. Derick, et al. Long-term survival after stroke. Age Ageing. 1984;13:76-82.
16. Dickstein, et al. Stroke Rehabilitation: Three Exercise Therapy Approaches. Physical Therapy. 1986;66:1233-8.
17. Dombovy, et al. Rehabilitation for Stroke: A Review. Stroke. 1986;17(3):363-9.
18. Godde, et al. Behavioral significance of input-dependent plasticity of human somatosensory cortex. Neuroreport. 2003;14(4):543-6.
19. Gordon, et al. Physical Activity and Exercise Recommendations for Stroke Survivors: An American Heart Association Scientific Statement from the Council on Clinical Cardiology. Stroke. 2004;35:1230-40.
20. Hackam, et al. Combining Multiple Approaches for the Secondary Prevention of Vascular Events After Stroke: A Quantitative Modeling Study. Stroke. 2007;38(6):1881-5.
21. Hakkennes, et al. Constraint-induced movement therapy following stroke: A systematic review of randomised controlled trials. Australian Journal of Physiotherapy. 2005;51(4):221-31.
22. Handschu, et al. Acute Stroke Management in the Local General Hospital. Stroke. 2001;32:866-70.
23. Hankey, et al. Rate, degree, and predictors of recovery from disability following ischemic stroke. Neurology. 2007;68(19):1583-7.
24. Henrik S, et al. What Determines Good Recovery in Patients with the Most Severe Strokes? The Copenhagen Stroke Study. Stroke. 1999;30:2008-12.
25. Hlustik, et al. Cortical Plasticity During Three-Week Motor Skill Learning. Journal of Clinical Neurophysiology. 2004;21(3):180-91.
26. Hummel, et al. Drivers of brain plasticity. Current Opinion in Neurology. 2005;18(6):667-74.
27. Ichiro Miyai, et al. Functional Outcome of Multidisciplinary Rehabilitation in Chronic Stroke. Neurorehabilitation and Neural Repair. 1998;12:95-9.
28. Indredavik, et al. Stroke Unit Treatment Improves Long-term Quality of Life: A Randomized Controlled Trial. Stroke. 1998;29:895-9.
29. J Legh-Smith, et al. Driving after a stroke. Journal of the Royal Society of Medicine. 1986;79:200-3.
30. John RF Gladman. Improving long-term rehabilitation. British Medical Bulletin. 2000;56:495-500.
31. Jørgensen, et al. Treatment and Rehabilitation on a Stroke Unit Improves 5-Year Survival: A Community-Based Study. Stroke. 1999;30:930-3.
32. Kalra, Eade. Role of Stroke Rehabilitation Units in Managing Severe Disability After Stroke. Stroke. 1995;26:2031-4.
33. Karni, et al. Functional MRI evidence for adult motor cortex plasticity during motor skill learning. Nature. 1995;377(6545):155-8.
34. Keir SD, Miller J, Yug, et al. Efficient gene transfer into primary and immortalized human fetal glial cells using adenoassociated virus vectors: establishment of a glial cell line with a functional CD4 receptor. J neuroviral. 1997;3(5):322-30.
35. Kollen, et al. The Effectiveness of the Bobath Concept in Stroke Rehabilitation: What is the Evidence? Stroke. 2009;40(4):e89-e97.
36. Kopp, et al. Plasticity in the motor system related to therapy-induced improvement of movement after stroke. Neuroreport. 1999;(4):807-10.

37. Kumar, et al. Perceptual Dysfunction in Hemiplegia and Automobile Driving Gerontologist. 1991;31:807-10.

38. Kwakkel, et al. Long term effects of intensity of upper and lower limb training after stroke: a randomised trial. Journal of Neurology Neurosurgery and Psychiatry. 2002;72:473-9.

39. Langhammer, et al. Stroke patients and long-term training: is it worthwhile? A randomized comparison of two different training strategies after rehabilitation. Clinical Rehabilitation. 2007;21:495-510.

40. Lindberg, et al. Use-Dependent Up- and Down-Regulation of Sensorimotor Brain Circuits in Stroke Patients. Neurorehabilitation and Neural Repair. 2007;21(43):315-26.

41. Loewen, Anderson. Predictors of stroke outcome using objective measurement scales. Stroke. 1990;21:78-81.

42. Lourencao, et al. Effect of biofeedback accompanying occupational therapy and functional electrical stimulation in hemiplegic patients. International Journal of Rehabilitation Research. 2008;31(1):33-41.

43. Luders, et al. Drug Therapy for the Secondary Prevention of Stroke in Hypertensive Patients: Current Issues and Options. Drugs. 2007;67(7):955-63.

44. M Dam, et al. The effects of long-term rehabilitation therapy on poststroke hemiplegic patients. Stroke. 1993;24:1186-91.

45. Mangold, et al. Motor Training of Upper Extremity with Functional Electrical Stimulation in Early Stroke Rehabilitation. Neurorehabilitation and Neural Repair. 2009;23:184-90.

46. Mark Hallett. Plasticity of the human motor cortex and recovery from stroke. Brain Research Reviews. 2001;36(2-3):169-74.

47. Mc Govern, et al. Management of stroke. Postgraduate Medical Journal. 2003;79(928):87-92.

48. McCarron, et al. Driving after a transient ischaemic attack or minor stroke. Emergency Medicine Journal. 2008;25:358-9.

49. MD Patel, et al. Relationships between long-term stroke disability, handicap and health-related quality of life. Age Ageing. 2006;35:273-9.

50. Mirelman, et al. Effects of Training with a Robot-Virtual Reality System Compared with a Robot alone on the Gait of Individuals after Stroke. Stroke. 2009;40(1): 169-74.

51. Noll, Stephen. Physical Medicine and Rehabilitation: State of Art Reviews. Long-Term Consequences of Stroke. Clinical Journal of Pain. 1993;9(2):147-8.

52. Ole Morten Rønning. Outcome of Subacute Stroke Rehabilitation. A Randomized Controlled Trial. Stroke. 1998;29:779-84.

53. Pamela D. Randomized Clinical Trial of Therapeutic Exercise in Subacute Stroke. Stroke. 2003;34:2173-80.

54. Pamela W. Management of Adult Stroke Rehabilitation Care A Clinical Practice Guideline. Stroke. 2005;36:e100.

55. Paolucci, et al. Functional Outcome of Ischemic and Hemorrhagic Stroke Patients After Inpatient Rehabilitation: A Matched Comparison. Stroke. 2003;34(12):2861-5.

56. Raymond KY Tong, et al. Gait Training of Patients after Stroke Using an Electromechanical Gait Trainer Combined with Simultaneous Functional Electrical Stimulation. Physical Therapy. 2006;86:1282-94.

57. Robert AK. Acute and subacute rehabilitation for stroke: A comparison. Archives of Physical Medicine and Rehabilitation. 1995;76(6):495-500.

58. Rønning, Guldvog. Outcome of Subacute Stroke Rehabilitation: A Randomized Controlled Trial. Stroke. 1998;29:779-84.

59. Rudd, et al. Randomised controlled trial to evaluate early discharge scheme for patients with stroke. British Medical Journal. 1997;315(7115):1039-44.

60. Satoru S, et al. Impact of factors indicating a poor prognosis on stroke rehabilitation effectiveness. Clinical Rehabilitation. 1993;7:99-104.

61. Sawaki, et al. Effects of Somatosensory Stimulation on Use-Dependent Plasticity in Chronic Stroke. Stroke. 2006;37(1):246-7.

62. Shinton R, Sagar G. Lifelong exercise and stroke. British Medical Journal. 1993;307:231-4.

63. Spillane. Stroke-Induced Trismus in a Pediatric Patient: Long-Term Resolution with Botulinum Toxin A. American Journal of Physical Medicine & Rehabilitation. 2003;82(6):485-8.

64. Stern, et al. Factors Influencing Stroke Rehabilitation. Stroke. 1971;2(3):213-8.

65. Studenski, et al. Daily Functioning and Quality of Life in a Randomized Controlled Trial of Therapeutic Exercise for Subacute Stroke Survivors. Stroke. 2005;36(8):1764-70.

66. Sulch, et al. Randomized Controlled Trial of Integrated (Managed) Care Pathway for Stroke Rehabilitation. Stroke. 2000;31(8):1929-34.

67. Tarkka, et al. Paretic Hand Rehabilitation with Constraint-Induced Movement Therapy after Stroke. American Journal of Physical Medicine & Rehabilitation. 2005;84(7):501-5.

68. Thanvi B, et al. Early neurological deterioration in acute ischaemic stroke: predictors, mechanisms and management. Postgraduate Medical Journal. 2008;84:412-7.

69. Toyoda K. Pharmacotherapy for the secondary prevention of stroke. Drugs. 2009;69(6):633-47.

70. Van Peppen, et al. Outcome measures in physiotherapy management of patients with stroke: a survey into self-reported use, and barriers to and facilitators for use. Physiotherapy Research International. 2008;13(4):255-70.

71. Wang, et al. Effect of Intramuscular Botulinum Toxin Injection on Upper Limb Spasticity in Stroke Patients. American Journal of Physical Medicine & Rehabilitation. 2002;81(4):272-8.

72. Wolf, et al. Repetitive Task Practice: A Critical Review of Constraint-Induced Movement Therapy in Stroke. Neurologist. 2002;8(6):325-38.

73. Wylie CM. The value of early rehabilitation in stroke. Nursing Research. 1970;19(6):556.

74. Yan, et al. Functional Electrical Stimulation Improves Motor Recovery of the Lower Extremity and Walking Ability of Subjects with First Acute Stroke: A Randomized Placebo-Controlled Trial. Stroke. 2005;36(1):80-5.

6

Management of Complications and Deconditioning Hazards of Stroke and Spinal Cord Injury Patients

Partha Pratim Pan, Mouli Madhab Ghatak

We discussed earlier that, stroke and spinal injury produce various generalized and focal neurodeficits and complications; however, many other systemic hazards arise out of the long-standing bed-ridden, morbid status in both these two conditions. These conditions because of neuroarchitectural damage initiate neuroresponsive-multisystem complications (like urological, dynamics in respiration, bony and arthrological, cardiovascular and vasomotor, etc.) and these complications are aggravated by a gross deconditioning due to bed rest which plays a great role in aggravating the complications.

Like most of the other medical problems, it is detrimental to prescribe bed rest in stroke patients. In spinal cord injury (SCI)—relative immobilization of the injured parts of the spine, with or without surgical fixation has been indicated for first few weeks. Apart from this prescription—bed rest and immobilization are quiet inevitable with associated motor weakness. Prolonged stay in hospital without proper rehabilitation also prevent the person from regaining motor function.

So, stroke and SCI are the two conditions where deconditioning is often unavoidable. But the detrimental effects of immobility can be prevented to a great extent; and in established cases of stroke and SCI complications triggered by deconditioning, pharmacological or rehabilitative measures should be applied to break the vicious cycle of complications → deconditioning → more complications **(Table 6.1)**.

Table 6.1: Various complications and deconditioning hazards of stroke and SCI	
Musculoskeletal system	Contracture
	Muscle weakness and atrophy
	Osteoporosis and disordered calcium metabolism
	Heterotrophic ossification
	Shoulder pain and reflex sympathetic dystrophy

Contd...

Contd...

Pulmonary complications	Decreased pulmonary compliances Aspiration pneumonia Atelectesis
Cardiovascular complications	Cardiac changes at rest Cardiac changes with exercise Postural hypotension Venous thromboembolism
Integumentery systems	Pressure ulcers Subcutaneous bursitis Dependent edema
Neurological complications	Pain syndromes Spasticity Compression neuropathies
Genitourinary complications	Stone formation Urinary tract infection Decreased libido
Gastrointestinal complications	Gastric atony Constipation Gastroesophageal reflux
Alteration of higher brain functions	Depression Lack of motivation Emotional liability

Musculoskeletal Changes

Contracture

Limitation of range of active and passive motion of a joint due to biomechanical or biochemical changes in muscles and connective tissue within or around the joint are called contracture. It is one of the most common complications of SCI and stroke patients. Muscle fibers and connective tissues which are maintained in a shortened position for a week or more, adapt to the shortened length by contraction of collagen fibers and reduction in muscle fiber sarcomeres. Immobilization causes decrease in activity of enzymes involved in collagen synthesis like prolyl-4-hydroxylase and galactosyl-hydroxylate-glucosyl-transferase.

One important factor that contributes largely for developing contracture in stroke and SCI is muscle imbalance due to paralysis and spasticity. Across a joint, when a muscle is paralyzed and its antagonist is stronger—the antagonist overpowers and it eventually becomes shortened. Similarly, in presence of spasticity resting length of the spactic muscle is reduced, which induces contracture formation.

Prevention

Contracture occurs most commonly in the lower limbs with involvement of muscles that cross two joints, because stretching of only one joint or the other may not adequately stretch the entire muscle. A person with lesion at C5 is particularly at risk of developing elbow flexion and supination contractures. Improper bed positioning aggravates tendoachilis, hamstring, hip flexor and shoulder contractures.

Very few contractures help in activities of daily living (ADL), one example is elbow flexion contracture may help in self-feeding. In general, contracture is detrimental foe against achieving good functional outcome. Contracture interferes with mobility, ADL and skin care. Multiple-joint contractures interfere significantly with bed positioning, standing upright, mobility and maintaining perennial hygiene. A hip flexion contracture accelerates knee and ankle joint contracture; stride length is shortened, walking become difficult, energy consumption is greatly increased.

Contractures are preventable. Selection of firm mattress, proper posture in bed and wheelchair, use of resting and dynamic splints, active and passive ROM exercises and early ambulation are the key points to prevent contracture. There are some specific preventive measures suitable for some specific contractures. These measures have been outlined below:

Contractures	Specific prevention
Tendoachilis	Use of foot board
Hip flexon	Occasional prone lying
Hip external rotation	Use of trochanter roll or derotation bar
Hand contracture	Use of palmer roll

Treatment

A careful clinical examination to see active and passive range of motion (ROM) is essential. X-ray may be needed to rule out bony ankylosis in cases of long standing contractures, as ankylosis is a contraindication for vigorous stretch. In presence of spasticity, nerve block may be needed to measure actual ROM and antispastic medications like Baclofen should be given concomitantly while treating contractures.

Active and passive ROM exercises combined with sustained terminal stretch at least twice a day, each session lasting 20–40 minutes is essential. Before applying stretch, deep heating with paraffin bath or ultrasound therapy may be helpful. Ultrasound therapy has the property to increase the extensibility of collagen.

For more severe contractures, sustained stretch lasting 2 hours or more can be given by static or dynamic splints. Plantar flexion, knee flexion and elbow contractures are preferably treated with serial casting, cast removed and reapplied every 2–5 days. Continuous passive mobilization (CPM) device is another option to provide sustained stretch.

In refractory cases, surgical treatment that includes capsular release, tenotomy or tendon-lengthening procedures may be necessary. In presence of muscular imbalance tendon transfer may be indicated.

Last but not least, important treatment of contracture is functional training. The use of the affected limbs for ambulation and other activities combined with strength and endurance program should be encouraged to reduce muscle imbalance across the joint and reduce contractures.

Muscle Weakness and Atrophy

Disuse causes a progressive decrease in muscle strength paralleled by a decrease in the cross-sectional area of the muscle fibers. Decline in maximal attainable tension and loss of muscle weight occurs rapidly. The muscle wasting is thought to be the result of decreased protein synthesis rather than increased protein breakdown. Antigravity muscles such as gastrocnemius soleus and back muscles appear to loose strength disproportionately, and large muscles seem to loose strength twice as quickly as smaller ones. Type I, slow twitch muscle fibers are more subject to immobilization atrophy than type II, fast twitch fibers. Immobilization in a shortened position promotes a more rapid deterioration. Patients with stroke or SCI are particularly more prone to develop all these phenomena due to associated neuronal injury.

Prevention

As muscle atrophy has been shown to begin after as little as one day of immobilization and once muscle strength is lost it is time consuming to regain the lost strength with rehabilitation measures, it is better to prevent, and to take preventive measures as early as possible. Proper positioning of joints is necessary in bedridden patients as immobilization in shortened positions causes more rapid deterioration. Routine stretching of the muscles prevents atrophy to some extent. Repeated isometrics with as little as 10% of maximal strength for 10 seconds may be useful to prevent atrophy.

Treatment

Once atrophy has set in progressive resistive exercise is valuable. Neuromuscular electrical stimulation increases strength and girth of the muscle—but should be used with caution as it may increase spasticity. Proprioceptive neuromuscular facilitation techniques, cycle ergometry, isokinetic strength training and functional training—all are helpful, individually as well as in combinations.

Osteoporosis and Disordered Calcium Metabolism

When a stress is applied to a bone, as in normal activities, particularly during weight bearing the strain is sensed, with subsequent increase in osteoblastic and decrease in osteoclastic activities. If no force is applied to skeleton—in immobilization—the reverse happens—osteoblastic activity predominates—urinary excretion of calcium and hydroxyproline and excretion of calcium in stool increases—bones become osteopenic. Disuse osteoporosis is more marked in subperiosteal region, involving the long bone epiphysis and metaphysis, and weight bearing bones are particularly vulnerable.

In neurogenic paralysis (Stroke/SCI), disuse osteoporosis is accelerated. In SCI, soon after injury, osteoblastic activity diminishes and rapid loss of bone mineral occurs, resulting in severe osteopenia in the paralyzed regions of the body. Total bone volume decreases rapidly over first few months after an injury, stabilizing at approximately 70% of baseline, a rate of decrease 100 times greater than that seen with aging. Pelvis, proximal femur and proximal tibia are affected the most. Bone loss reaches maximum after 16–18 months of injury—as much as 50% in upper tibia. Fractures can occur even with relatively nontraumatic events such as transfer activities. Fractures are reported in 4% of SCI patients. Majority of fractures are in distal femur or proximal tibia.

Adolescent boys after acute SCI may show a significant hypercalcemia due to bone resorption. Other risk factors for hypercalcemia include, complete injuries, tetraplegia, dehydration and prolonged immobilization. Symptoms of hypercalcemia include anorexia, abdominal pain, nausea, vomiting, constipation, confusion and in severe cases coma.

Prevention

Nonweight bearing exercise in bed is itself not much effective in preventing osteoporosis. A standing frame or a tilt table should be used for those who are unable to stand unsupported. As soon as the patient is stable, tilt table conditioning should begin at a 30° tilt for one minute, increased 10° every 3–5 days or earlier as tolerated until the patient is able to tolerate a 70° tilt for 30 minutes. The progression should be made in standing frame, parallel bars and finally to ambulation. General strengthening, stretching, endurance and coordination exercises and early resumption of activities of daily living, all are helpful to prevent immobilization osteoporosis.

Treatment

In established cases, bone density measurement techniques such as photon absorptiometry or CT scan are often needed to assess the severity of bone loss. Drugs such as calcitonin and bisphosponates are the most useful. Intranasal calcitonin given twice a day counteracts the bone resorption. Bisphosponates like alendronate, etidronate, pamidronate, clodronate, tiludronate—all inhibit bone resorption, in addition to inhibiting calcium phosphate crystal formation and dissolution. These drugs are now being given as preventive measures in SCI patients. Treatment of immobilization hypercalcemia is based on achieving adequate calcium excretion using intravenous fluids, loop diuretics and by pamidronate and calcitonin.

Heterotrophic Ossification

Abnormal formation of lamellar bone in para-articular soft tissue is heterotrophic ossification (HO). This condition, etiopathogenesis of which is still unsettled, has been linked with varieties of clinical conditions—SCI being one of them. About 16–53% patients with SCI develop heterotrophic ossification. A quarter of them have disabling ROM limitation, and some of them may develop ankylosis of the affected joint.

These complications are more common in immobilized patients. Therefore, apart from pharmacological intervention with etidronate, indomethacin or naproxen, ROM and stretching exercises may limit ROM loss. Seriously affected heterotrophic ossification (HO) cases, mostly having involvement of perihip areas is a challenge to rehabilitation outcome, as such cases restrict the flexion and adduction movements. Paraplegics or quadriplegics having good regain of upper limb power are good subjects for wheelchair training but hip flexion restriction limits sitting and wheelchair training and mobility with transfer training are affected much. For long-term rehabilitation issue, these cases may be chosen for surgical intervention with removal of extra bone growths followed by proper medications. As chance of recurrence is very high, girdle stone arthroplasty operation may be a choice after explaining its science and prognosis to the party in details. Such a surgery also helps take care of the hygienic limitations with bilateral HO in hips.

Complex Regional Pain Syndrome (Type I)

Complex regional pain syndrome type I (CRPS-I) was previously known as reflex sympathetic dystrophy (RSD). It is a clinical entity with neurovascular disturbances and abnormalities in the sensory motor nervous system of the upper limb, usually presenting with chronic painful hands and phasic changes of the soft tissue, skin and bones.

Prevalence

It is a complication frequently seen in stroke and cervical cord injury patients. About 12–21% of hemiplegic patients have been recorded to be the victims of CRPS type I. In any stroke or spinal injury rehabilitation ward, it is a common experience of the physiatrists and therapists to face this condition. It is prevalent in all age group of patients irrespective of gender; males, females and even children may have such problems. Statistics shows that people aged 40–60 years and the females are more prone to develop this complication.

Clinical Presentation

The symptoms begin with pain and swelling of distal part of the affected upper extremity, usually associated with pain and stiffness of shoulder joint (shoulder hand syndrome). The full course of the clinical picture can be divided into three stages:

1. *Stage I (Acute stage):* There is diffuse puffy swelling of fingers, dorsum of hand and wrist with moderate to severe pain, tenderness and redness with gradual development of restriction of joint movement. There is a change in the sweating pattern (hyperhydrosis), often very sensitive to touch. The areas is abnormally warm due to inflammatory alterations in

the regional blood flow. There may be faster than normal growth of nail and hair. The patient is usually anxious and shows personality changes often drawing attention towards such a condition. This stage usually persists for a few weeks to few months.

2. *Stage II (Dystrophic stage):* It lasts for a few months to one year. In this stage, swelling and pain is more persistent. The skin becomes cooler and fingernails become brittle, skin wrinkles disappear, the pain is more widespread with increased stiffness of fingers. Gradually osteoporotic changes in the bones with periarticular thickening become evident and the hair and nail growth is diminished.

3. *Stage III (Atrophic stage):* This stage persists for additional few months, the pain, swelling and warmth is usually reduced. Soft tissues show irreversible atrophic changes with severe loss of joint motion. The skin may appear smooth and glossy with ridged nails. The bones get osteoporotic changes, which may be extensive with an increased risk of fracture.

Diagnosis

Diagnosis is based on the clinical picture mostly, but the radiographic change is an important marker showing gradual increase of osteopenia and eventually severe osteoporosis. Triple phase bone scans may also be done to record increase uptake in the involved limb mostly in carpal and metacarpal joints. This may be related to the vasomotor disturbances.

Mechanism of CRPS (I)

Different hypothesis are suggested by different researchers in different places. The various theories behind the related pathogenesis of this condition are as follows:

1. This may be due to sympathetic dysfunction. Activation of SNS has been seen to cause lowering of body temperature resulting in increased pain in the affected area and such pain is relieved by sympathetic nerve block or sympathectomy (destruction of sympathetic innervation of the affected area).

2. Some types of neuropathic pain are seen with changes in pain signaling pathways including the neurons of spinal cord but research evidences prove that such pain in RSD is not purely a variety of neuropathic pain.

3. By the animal experimentation supported by human research presentations, the general hypothesis goes in favor of its relation with central nervous system. However, the RSD having a somatosensory response with sympathetic systems innervating blood vessels, sweat glands, etc. and the way these changes triggered by peripheral trauma makes the hypothesis unclear.

4. In chronic stage, the peripheral changes have been questioned with relation to the immunoinflammatory changes with involvement of endocrine and vascular systems.

Treatment

The treatment of such condition is focused on drugs, therapeutics and occasionally surgical interventions as follows:

Large majority of patients are treated with systemic corticosteroids in early phase. Prednisolone of 1 mg/kg body weight is administered with tapering doses. Patients having DM or other contraindications, prednisolone should be avoided. Antidepressants, NSAIDs, beta blockers, calcitonin, etc. are also in use for specific cases.

A sympathetic block is often a good choice with fair results. Typically, a stellate ganglia blockade with local anesthetics are used for temporary relief.

An early recognition of RSD is always preferred with selective treatment by various drugs and therapies, which may help avoid the irreversible changes of the affected limb.

Rehabilitative and Therapeutic Interventions

Various therapeutic measures have been suggested and studied in different centers with variable results. These are specifically targeted in relieving the pain and avoiding future complications as follows:

1. Proper positioning of the limb in optimal position with special attention in elevation of the limb for better drainage of edematous fluid and prevention of tissue contracture.
2. A crepe bandage application or using compressive pneumatic cuffs are also recommended for reducing the swelling in acute stage. Isotoner gloves are also used for the same purpose.
3. Aggressive and graded activities and movement are recommended for 'desensitization' of hypersensitive tissues. Vigorous massage (deep frictional) may release the soft tissues preventing dystrophic complications.
4. Trials with contrast bath, ice application in acute stage, using transcutaneous electrical nerve stimulation (TENS) and US therapy have also been reported with varied results.
5. Maintenance of joint range of motion (JROM) by passive movements and occupational therapeutic interventions including splinting or bandaging of the hand to improve flexion and extension of fingers are also in use. Occupational hand training in mild to moderate case in the stage II and stage III are also a common practice to improve ADL. Exercises improve JROM and vascular flow with less affection of decalcification of bones.

Surgery

Surgical release is not a common practice and has got limited results.

Hemiplegic Shoulder

Poststroke subluxation with pain in shoulder in the hemiplegic limb is a common phenomena. Although the exact cause of subluxation remains controversial, such a change may be attributed to the reduction of tone in shoulder girdle muscles especially the supraspinatous, altering glenohumeral joint alignment. The subluxation can be felt as a palpable gap (? dislocation) between the acromian and the humeral head in the affected side (easily recognizable when compared with the unaffected side). During the flaccid stage (usually the first 4 weeks) the subluxation is very prominent and may persist for a long period in absence of return of tone in supraspinatous muscle.

Subluxation is usually associated with pain, though direct correlation between these two is controversial. Almost 3/4th of stroke survivors experience shoulder pain within the first year after the stroke. Such pain is usually associated with limited range of motion and tenderness on joint, and willful avoidance of movement of the joint. There is significant stretching of capsule and the ligaments and handling the patient (say like transferring or changing the position) holding the patient's affected limb may dislocate the glenohumeral joint or may induce bursitis, or tendinitis or even tear of the soft tissue attachments, which may lead to a chronic painful shoulder syndrome. Patient with diabetes, large brain lesions having poor return of tone are more susceptible to such a condition.

Plane radiography, MRI of left shoulder may support the clinical findings of better assessments of the bony alignment and soft tissue damages.

Management

Conventional use of brace or support (like Bobath Calf, arm sling) may decrease the possibility of gravity assisted soft tissue stretching.

Range of motion exercises, local electrical nerve stimulation, use of NSAIDs, nerve blocks, intra-articular injections, etc. are recommended according to the condition. Malhandling the shoulder by family members, caregivers, therapists are to be avoided by proper training and education.

Central Pain Syndrome

Central pain syndrome is a complex pain feeling of different body parts after stroke or any damage to CNS especially thalamus, brainstem or spinal cord. It is also named as thalamic pain syndrome or Dejerine-Roussy syndrome or central poststroke syndrome.

Clinical Nature

It presents as a feeling of deep burning, tearing or aching, sometimes 'pins and needles' or distracting sensations like tingling, throbbing, itching, tightening, etc. patient may feel irritating pain by simply a light touch even by a beloved one. Such pain may also be triggered by various stimuli like movement, ROM exercises, exposure to sun, cold, breezes or touches of blankets, clothes, splints or by mental anger, depression, etc. CPS may develop months or even years after injury or damage to the CNS.

Management

Central pain syndrome (CPS) is not a fatal disorder anyway, but distressing to the patient as well as the caregivers, doctor and family members. Generally, NSAIDs or other pain medications provide little or no relief to CPS.

Various medications have been tried with varied results in CPS. The management focus goes mostly towards a good psychological support and favorable environment, along with tricyclic antidepressants, anti-convulsants, narcotics, etc. Narcotic analgesics like morphine are seen to be effective. Various sedatives are also used to manage acute conditions. Usually, it is self-limiting or it may persist for a long period in some cases.

Autonomic Dysreflexia

Autonomic dysreflexia (AD) is an acute condition with spinal cord lesion at or above T6 level (the level of sympathetic splanchnic outflow) due to massive sympathetic discharge triggered by some irritational stimulus. It is mostly experienced after 2 months of injury. About 48–83% of quadriplegic or high paraplegics face such sudden life-threatening situation.

The noxious stimulus is transmitted to the dorsal column of spinothalamic tract and generate a generalized sympathetic response. Due to the spinal lesion inhibitory impulses cannot descend through sympathetic chain to counteract the autonomic response and acute rise of blood pressure occurs due to splanchnic and peripheral vasoconstriction. The rise of blood pressure stimulates carotid sinus and aortic arch receptor, which eventually results vasodilatation and bradycardia. The sympathetic discharge also initiates sweating in the particular neurological segments.

Clinical Picture

- Sudden acute hypertension
- Pounding headache
- Sweating above the level of injury
- Flushing of face
- Nasal stuffiness
- Red blotching on chest
- Cool calmy skin
- Piloerection
- Reflex bradycardia
- Visual blurring
- Mental confusion.

In severe cases, there may be encephalopathy, seizures, loss of consciousness, myocardial failure, intracerebral hemorrhage, pulmonary edema, etc.

With the typical clinical picture and above-mentioned signs and symptoms, usually a bedside diagnosis is made. History of such previous episodes also favors diagnosis. However, ECG, frequent pulse, BP and temperature record and blood glucose level estimation are of immense importance for diagnosing as well as for monitoring the condition.

Noxious Stimuli, which can Cause AD

Any odd environment or uncomfortable condition stressing the patient's mind, body and disability may precipitate AD. The usual external or endogenous noxious stimuli causing AD are as follows:

1. Infection like urinary tract infection (UTI), respiratory infection, etc.
2. Gastrointestinal (GI) problems like distention due to neurogenic bowel and constipation due to impaction of fecal matter.
3. Pressure sore—pain and discomfort, aggravating mental tension.
4. Extreme hot or cold climate.
5. Irritation in any body part due to pressure of paralytic limbs, catheter, etc.
6. During any medical tests or procedures—drawing blood, cystoscopy, MRI, etc.
7. Any painful stimuli, cut, bite, burn of skin/nails.
8. Excessive physical strain like massive exercises, standing in stand-in-frame for a long time, etc.
9. Any psychological injury or anxious situation, etc.

How to Prevent AD?

Avoiding the strenuous factors, infections, discomfort producing situations are generally recommended to prevent such acute episode. An overall comfortable and free environment and regular psychotherapy may reduce the frequency of AD. General recommendations include:

1. Catheter to check regularly. Releasing the clamped catheter in regular intervals, removing any plugging or kinking in catheter is important.
2. Timed evacuation of bowel, prokinetic drugs and manual removal of impaction to avoid constipation are necessary.
3. Patient should wear loose and light clothings and should stay in airy and soothing environment.
4. Any sharp object, irritating agent in bed and room is to be avoided, routine skin assessment is helpful.
5. Relaxing the patient before any strainful procedure or exercise is mandatory.
6. Any possible source of infection like bed sore, urinary catheter, etc. should be detected earlier and treated effectively.

Treatment of AD

1. Allowing the patient to sit up—the orthostatic hypotension factor may counteract the raised BP.
2. Eliminating the cause and stimuli, which acts as the input. Painful areas may be anesthesized.
3. Treating the BP—should be done with extreme caution—because the reflex vasodilation and reduction of the episode by removing the noxious

stimuli may reduce the BP without any medication and administration of antihypertensives may cause serious hypotension. However, if BP rises much or chest pain or any cardiac episode is suspected, nitroglycerin patch with or without antihypertensives may be used.

4. Relaxing the patient psychologically and keeping a cool and calmy place.
5. Continuous monitoring of vitals and observation must be there.
6. In severe cases—hospitalizing the patient and treating for other medical complications like CVA, MI, seizures, etc.

Cardiovascular Hazards

Cardiovascular hazards may coexist with stroke in an elderly patient or may be triggered by prolonged bed rest.

Cardiac Changes at Rest

Bed rest causes tachycardia—increase by one-half beat per minute each day for first 3–4 weeks of immobilization, probably due to imbalance of autonomic nervous system function. However, tetraplegia is an exception, in up to 71% of patients with complete tetraplegia bradycardia is seen, the reason being unopposed action of vagus on heart, while SCI causes damage to sympathetic outflow. Apart from rate alteration, other cardiac changes of a resting heart are decrease in stroke volume, cardiac size and left ventricular end-diastolic volume.

Cardiac Changes with Exercise

Deconditioning causes increased heart rate response to submaximal exercise (up to 30–40 beats per minute greater than expected after 3 weeks of bed rest), decreased stroke volume in sub maximal and maximal exercises, decreased cardiac output, decreased maximal oxygen uptake ($VO_{2\,max}$)—which indicates reduced aerobic fitness.

Postural (Orthostatic) Hypotension

Prolonged bedridden condition alters normal autonomic response in upright position that leads to blood pooling in lower extremity and ineffective vasoconstriction during standing. As a result, blood pressure suddenly falls when the person moves from a reclining to an upright position. The symptoms are dizziness, light-headedness, fainting, and vertigo. Persons with SCI frequently have low baseline blood pressure. They commonly become symptomatic with postural changes and transfer activities.

Deep Vein Thrombosis and Pulmonary Embolism

A deep vein thrombosis (DVT) is an occlusion of deep vein of leg by a thrombus (clot) causing unilateral swelling of the involved extremity. It is a frequent complication in stroke and spinal injury patients.

Stroke and SCI patients having age over 40 years, past or family history of DVT, obesity, pregnancy, ladies in post natal period or on OCP, diabetes and hyperlipidemia or getting poor rehabilitation for SCI/stroke are more prone to develop DVT.

The patient usually presents with swelling of the calf, mid ankle and gradually in thigh along with pain in the calf, usually of sudden onset. It may manifest within a few hours of the occlusion of the vein or sometimes as gradual swelling of affected limb with pain and tenderness. Pain is worse on standing and walking. In chronic cases, there may be ulcers and damage of the tissues, distal to the thrombosed area. A Doppler ultrasound, venography provides confirmation of diagnosis.

Pulmonary Embolism

The thrombus may be dislodged from the veins of calf and may travel to the lungs through the bloodstreams and may occlude lung vessels. The patient complains of chest pain, shortness of breath, etc. which is an emergency condition and needs critical care intervention. It is potentially a fatal complication.

Prevention

Stroke and spinal injury patients usually have reduced blood flow in the paralytic limb because of poor functioning of the peripheral pump of the calf muscle and stasis mediates aggregation of platelets, which should be prevented effectively by the following measures:
1. Patient should be under antiplatelet or anticoagulant therapies. Prophylactic use of low molecular weight heparin (LMWH), warfarin may reduce the possibility of DVT.
2. Good rehabilitation programs including passive mobilization and exercises.
3. Frequent elevation of the limb.
4. Use of compression garments, stockinets those are specially made with increasing pressure effect towards the distal part of the limb.
5. Compression over the vulnerable area through a pneumatic pump.
6. If the patient is mobile, it is important to avoid sitting for a long time (say like during traveling by a train) with hanging legs.

Treatment

1. Low molecular weight heparin has reduced the complication of the DVT and pulmonary embolism upto a great extent in recent days. Enoxaparin 1 mg/kg body weight may be used twice a day.
2. Patient is usually shifted to oral anticoagulant after certain period of active management through LMWH. Warfarin of 0.1 mg/kg body weight may be started and altered according to the need of the patient as a maintenance therapy with regular monitoring of prothrombin time (PT), international

normalized ratio (INR), etc. However, any bleeding episode should be carefully noted before and during the treatment with heparin or warfarin.

3. Elastic compression stockings are to be used routinely.

4. Exercising the affected limb is to be avoided to prevent the possibility of dislodging the thrombus during the initial phase.

5. The chronic, uncared DVT patients having irreversible tissue damage and necrosis are usually at high risk and active medical treatment to reduce the complication along with surgery (amputation) is usually suggested as a life saving measure. However, chances of PE and other vascular thrombosis and embolism may be life-threatening in such a case.

Pulmonary Complications

Pulmonary complications of stroke and SCI patients may be due to pre-existing airway disorder or due to neural damage in SCI or due to immobility too. Pulmonary hazards in high SCI patients are described in another chapter. Let us discuss the immobility related chest and airway complications in cardiovascular accidents (CVA) and SCI patients.

Chest movement in supine position becomes restricted due to diminished diaphragmatic movement, decreased chest excursion, progressive reduction in ROM of costovertebral and costochondral joints. Pulmonary function parameters such as tidal volume, minute volume, vital capacity and maximum voluntary ventilation are all reduced. In supine position, mucocilliary clearing mechanism become ineffective, cough is impaired. Dependent areas become poorly ventilated and overperfused; there are regional changes in ventilation perfusion ratio, significant arteriovenus shunting with lowered arterial oxygenation. All these lead to atelectasis and hypostatic pneumonia.

In addition one-third to one-half of the stroke patient have dysphagia which may lead to aspiration pneumonia. Hemiparetic weakness of respiratory muscles also weakens cough.

Diseases of the respiratory system particularly pneumonia, is the primary cause of death in patients with SCI. In tetraplegics respiratory muscles are weak and may lead to ventilatory failure.

Preventive measures include early mobilization, frequent posture change in bed, chest physical therapy including breathing exercises, resistive inspiratory muscle training, incentive spirometry, assisted coughing, chest percussion and postural drainage.

Patients with stroke should be evaluated clinically to assess the strength and coordination of muscles involved in swallowing and to detect aspiration. Videofluoroscopy using a modified barium swallow is helpful. Aspiration may be prevented by increasing arousal, sitting upright, changing consistency of food and exercises of oral, lingual and laryngeal muscles. If swallowing is not safe, a nasogasrtic tube is indicated for feeding. Dysphagia, in general improves rapidly—most by the end of first month.

The pulmary rehabilitation is covered in another chapter in this book.

For patients who have developed pulmonary complications, appropriate antibiotics, bronchodilators, mucolytic therapy via nebulizer is required.

Adequate pulmonary hygiene is important. In case impending a ventilatory failures, ventilator is required.

Integumentary System

Pressure Ulcers Sore

Only a brief outline is presented here as anohter chapter on pressure sore is skin care is covered in this book (Chapter 9).

Localized areas of cellular necrosis occurring mostly over the bony prominences due to prolonged, unrelieved local external pressure are pressure ulcers. Immobility is the major risk factor. If pressure is applied over, a particular area of skin continuously for 6–12 hours irreversible change in the skin occurs, leading to necrosis and skin breakdown, ultimately ulcer formation. Other risk factors are advanced age, abnormal skin sensation, abnormal mental status and altered sensorium, muscle and skin atrophy, malnutrition, moist skin due to fecal or urinary incontinence, spasticity, heterotrophic ossification, etc.

As, in SCI and stroke patients, most of the above-mentioned risk factors are very common, they are highly vulnerable to develop pressure ulcers. Fuhrer et al in a community-based survey of SCI persons, noted that 33% had at least one pressure ulcer and 13.6% had a stage 3 or 4 ulcer.

Pressure ulcer formation increases morbidity and mortality, increases expenses of, and delays rehabilitation. Moreover, it can cause complications like bacteremia, septic arthritis, endocarditis, meningitis, cellulites, sinus tract or abscess formation, osteomyelitis, etc. So, it should be prevented and it is fairly preventable. For persons admitted to the model spinal cord care systems the incidences of severe pressure sores is only 2%. Prevention has following aspects:

i. *Skin inspection and care:* The patient's skin must be examined regularly to detect potential signs of impending ulcer formation, which include color variations, blisters, rashes, temperature variations, bruises, surface breaks and dry flaky skin. If found, all pressures from the area must be removed. Skin should be washed and dried twice daily, moisturizing creams should be applied over dry skins.

ii. *Care of posture by position:* Patients in bed should be turned and repositioned at least every 2 hours around the clock. If tolerated prone lying is preferable, as anterior part of the body has larger low-pressure areas and smaller high pressure areas. Sitting uninterrupted for more than 2 hours should not be allowed. During transfer, patients should not be dragged across the bed.

iii. *Skin protectors:* Use of padded dressings, sheep skin mats or pads, silicon gel pads, elbow pads, heel pads or pillow under the calf are helpful to prevent ulcer formation.

iv. *Pressure reducing support surface:* They are manufactured so that pressure over the skin is keept below the capillary closing pressure of 32 mm Hg. Different types are (A) Static type overlays like; (a) Polyurethane foam overlays; (b) Gel-filled overlays; (c) Water filled overlays; (d) Air filled overlays; or (B) Dynamic overlays using external power sources.

v. *Educating the patient and caregiver:* This is very important in preventing pressure ulcers.

For treating pressure ulcers important things are:
a. Restoration of nutrition by supplementing protein, vitamin C and zinc.
b. Treating anemia.
c. Relieve/spasticity or spasm.
d. Systemic antibiotics.
e. Pressure reducing devices.
f. Conservative wound care.
g. Surgical care of pressure ulcers including use of skin grafts (Chapter 9).

Subcutaneous blisters: Blister occurs where there is excessive pressure over bursas and is prevented by removing that pressure. Treatment is by NSAIDs, percutanious drainage, corticosteroid injection and surgical removal if necessary.

Dependent edema: It is a common complication of immobilization. It can be prevented with adequate mobilization, elevation, use of elastic stockings or gloves, pressure gradient compression or massage.

Neurological complications (detailed elaboration in other respective chapters is available)

Pain syndromes: Central poststroke pain, though relatively rare is often highly problematic. Nociceptive pain, radicular pain, segmental pain and deafferentation central pain are varieties of pain syndromes in SCI patients. Apart from drug management proper positioning, mobilization and early ambulation are parts of treatment of these conditions.

Spasticity: Stroke and SCI are UMN lesions, spasticity is almost associated with them, and immobilization aggravates spasticity seriously. Prevention and treatment are dealt in a separate chapter in this book.

Compression neuropathies: Common sites are peroneal nerve below the fibular head and ulnar nerve at the retrocondylar groove. Turning the patient every 2 hourly prevents compression neuropathy.

Genitourinary Complications (Vide Chapter 24)

Increased diuresis and mineral excretion leading to stone formation is common in immobilized patients. In supine position, voiding is difficult and post void residual volume is increased. Residual volume is increased in varieties of neurogenic bladder in stoke and SCI patients. Hypercalcuria in SCI promotes stone formation. Bladder stone and increased residual volume promotes bacterial growth leading to urinary tract infection. Long-term immobilization reduces spermatogenesis, androgenesis and libido.

Preventive measures include adequate fluid intake and use of upright posture for voiding. Intermittent clean catheterization is a very good system to prevent urinary infection and achieve bladder control.

Metabolic and Endocrine System Alteration

Immobilization results in a decrease in lean body mass and increase in body fat content, disorder of nitrogen balance and mineral and electrolyte losses (loss of nitrogen, calcium, phosphorus, sulfur, potassium). Hyponatremia is manifested by lethargy, confusion, disorientation, seizures. Endocrine changes are due to altered responsiveness of hormones and enzymes. Glucose intolerance occurs primarily due to reduced peripheral sensitivity to circulating insulin. Other immobility-induced changes are altered circadian rhythm, altered temperature and sweating response, altered regulation of hormones of parathyroid, thyroid, adrenal, pituitary glands. Glucose intolerance to some extent can be ameliorated with isotonic and isometric exercises.

Alteration of Higher Brain Functions

Stroke itself along with sensory deprivation during prolonged bed rest affects emotions and cognitive functions. Depression, anxiety, withdrawal, apathy and sleep disturbances are common emotional problems associated with immobilization. Patients may become restless, irritable, noncooperative and agitated. Psychomotor skills like ability to concentrate, motivation, judgment, problem solving, learning ability and memory are also affected. All these problems seriously hamper rehabilitation. There may be decreased visual acuity and a raised auditory threshold.

In addition, lesion in the brain in cerebrovascular accidents creates behavioral and psychological problems. Larger cortical lesions produce more psychological problems than smaller subcortical lesions. Problems vary from emotional lability, decreased insight, unilateral neglect, a sense of helplessness, etc. to dementia. Depression is very common and recorded in up to 50% of stroke patients.

Traumatic SCI is one of the most devastating calamities in life, almost every sphere of a person's life is affected and adjustment to SCI is a challenge to all persons. About 6% of death after SCI is related to suicide.

In preventing and treating these cognitive and psychosocial complications, it is important to apply appropriate physical and psychosocial stimulations early in the course of illness. Counseling in group therapy sessions, attention to socialization, encouragement of family interaction, recreational therapy and rehabilitation to achieve activities of daily living are the preventive measures.

Bibliography

1. Appell H. Muscular atrophy, following immobilization. Sports Med. 1990;10: 42-58.
2. Ashmore CR, Summers PJ. Stretch induced growth of chicken muscles: myofibrillar proliferation. Am J Physiol. 1981;241:C93-97.
3. Baker JH, Matrumoto DE. Adaptation of skeletal muscle to immobilization in a shortened position. Muscle Nerve. 1988;2:231-44.

4. Birk head NC, Bizard JJ, Daly JW, et al. Cardiodynamic and metabolic effects of prolonged bed rest with daily recumdias or sitting exercise and with sitting inactivity. Ohio Aerospace Medical Research Laboratories, Wright-Patterson Air Force Base, AMRL-TDR-64 - 61, August 1964.

5. Birkhead WC, Bizzard JJ, Daly JW, et al. Cardiodynamic and metabolic effects of prolonged bed rest. Ohio Aerospace Medical Research Laboratories, Wright-Patterson Air Force Base AMRL-TDR - 63 - 37, May 1963.

6. Blauer D. The natural history and functional consequences of dysphagia after hemispheric stroke. J Neurol Neurosurg Psychiatry. 1989;52:236-41.

7. Booth FW. Physiologic and biochemical effects of immobilization on muscle. Clin Orthop. 1987;219:15-20.

8. Buezynski A, Kedziora J, Wachowiez B, Zolynski K. Effect of bed rest on the adenine neucleotides concentration in human blood platelets. J Physiol Pharmacol. 1991;42:389-95.

9. Clagett GP, Anderson FA, Heit J, et al. Prevention of venous thromboembolism. Chest. 1995;108 (Suppl 4):312 S-34 S.

10. Craig DB, Wahha WM, Don HF. Airway closure and lung volume in surgical positions. Can Anaesth Soc J. 1971;18:92-99.

11. De Vivo M, Black K, Stover S. Causer of death during the first 12 years after spinal cord injury. Arch Phys Med Rehabil. 1993;74:248-54.

12. De Vivo MJ, Stover SL. Long-term survival and causes of death. In: Stover SL, De Lisa JA, Whiteneck GC (Eds). Spinal Cord Injury, Gaithesburg. MD: Aspen. 1995;289-316.

13. Dooley CP, Scholossmacher B, Valenzuela JE. Modulation of esophageal peristalsis by alterations of body position: effect of bolus viscosity. Dig Dis Sc. 1989;34:1664-67.

14. Fuhrer MF, Garber SL, Rintala DH, et al. Pressure ulcers in community resident persons with spinal cord injury: Prevalance and risk factors. Arch Phys Med Rehabil. 1993;74:1172-77.

15. Gcerts WH, Code KI, Jay RM, et al. A prospective study of venous thromboembolism after major trauma. N Eng J Med. 1994;331:1601-06.

16. Goldspink DF. The influence of immobilization and stretch on protein turnover of rat skeletal muscle. J Physiol (Lond). 1977;264:267-82.

17. Green D, Lee M, Lim A, et al. Prevention of thromboembolism after spinal cord injury using low molecular weight heparin. Amm Infern Med. 1990;113:571-74.

18. Greenleaf JE, Van Beaumont W, Convertino VA, Starr JC. Handgrip and general muscular strength and endurance during prolonged bed rest with isometric and isotonic leg exercise training. Aviat Space Environ Med. 1983;54:696-780.

19. Greenleaf JE. Physiological response to prolonged bed rest and fluid immersion in humans. J Appl Physiol. 1984;57:619-33.

20. Harper J, Amiel D, Harper E. Collagenase from periarticular ligaments and tendon: enzyme levels during the development of joint contracture. Matrix. 1989;9:200-05.

21. Lehmann KB, Lane JG, Piepmeier JM, et al. Cardiovascular abnormalities accompanying acute spinal cord injury humans: Incidence, time course and severity. J Am Coll Cardiol. 1987;10:46-52.

22. Maynard FM. Immobilization hypercalcemia following spinal cord injury. Arch Phys Med Rehabil. 1986;67:41-4.

23. Merli G, Herbison G, Ditunno J, et al. Deep vein thrombosis in acute spinal cord - injured patients. Arch Phys Med Rehabil. 1988;69:661-64.

24. Minarie P, Meunier P, Edoward C, et al. Quantitative histological data on disuse osteoporosis: comparison with biological data. Calcif Tissue Res. 1974;17:57-73.

25. Raab W, De Paula E, Silva P, et al. Cardiac adrenergic preponderance due to lack of physical exercise and its pathogenic implications. Am J Cardiol. 1960;5:300-20.

26. Robinson RG, Starr LB, Kuhos K. A two year longitudinal study of post stroke mood disorders: findings during the initial evaluation. Stroke. 1983;14:736-41.

27. Rognarsson KT. Sell GH: Lower extremity fractures after spinal cord injury a retrospective study. Arch Phy Med Rehabil. 1981;62:418-23.

28. Rubin CT, Lanyon LE. Regulation of bone formation by applied dynamic loads. J Bone Joint Surg. 1984;66A:397-402.

29. Ryhack RS, Lewis OF, Lessard CS. Psychobiologic effects of prolonged bed rest (weightlessness) in young, healthy volunteers (study II). Aerospace Med. 1971;42:529-35.

30. Salfer RB, Bell RS, Keeley FW. The protective effect of continuous passive motion on living articular cartilage in acute septic arthritis: an experimental investigation in the rabit. Clin Orthop. 1981;159:223-47.

31. Taylor HL, Henschel A, Brozakek J, Keys A. Effects of bedrest on cardiovascular function and work performance. J Appl Physiol. 1949;2:223-39.

32. Tepperman PS, Greyson ND, Hilbert L, Jimines J, Williams JL. Reflex sympathetic dystrophy in hemiplegia. Arch Phys Med Rehabil. 1984;65:442-47.

33. Tisi GM. Preoperative evaluation of pulmonary function. Am Rev Respir Dis. 1979;119:293-310.

34. Tribe C. Cause of death in the early and late stages of paraplegia. Paraplegia. 1963;1:19-47.

35. Van Onwenaller C, La Place PM. Chartrainee A: Painful shoulder in hemiplegia. Arch Phys Med Rehabil. 1985;67:23-26.

36. Vebelhart D, Damiaux-Domenea G, Roth M, Chantraine A. Bone metabolism in spinal cord injured individuals and in others who have prolonged immobilization. A review. Paraplegia. 1995;33:669-73.

37. Venier LH, Ditunno JF Jr. Heterotropic ossification in the paraplegic patient. Arch Phys Med Rehabil. 1971;52:475-79.

38. Williams PE. Use of intermittent stretch in the prevention of serial sarcomere loss in immobilized muscle. Am Rheum Dis. 1990;49:316-17.

39. Wise MF, Milani JC. Dysphagia in spinal cord injury (abstract). Presented at the 13th annual meeting of Americal Spinal Injury Association, Boston, March 1987, abstract 30.

40. Yarkony GM, Heinermann AW. Pressure ulcers. In: Stover SL, De Lisa JA, Whiteneck GG (Eds). Spinal Cord injury: Clinical Outcomes from the Model Systems. Gaithesburg. MD, Arpen, 1995. pp. 104-11.

7

Therapeutic Exercise Program for Stroke Patients

S Srinivas Rau

Introduction

For good functional recovery following a stroke, a goal oriented therapeutic exercise program should begin early in the acute stage or immediately following the stroke. This helps in minimizing the deconditioning effects of prolonged bed rest and the compensatory movements of the patient, using his unaffected side and also helps in preventing secondary impairments. The program also serves to enhance the patient's mental status.

Physiotherapy Immediately after Stroke

A physiotherapist may be called to intervene immediately following stroke provided the patient in medically stable and there are no contraindications. Usually this is after 48–72 hours.

Goals of Exercises during the Early Stage

1. Promote awareness and use of the hemiplegic side.
2. Prevent development of abnormal tone.
3. Maintain range of motion and prevent deformities.
4. Improve body symmetry and balance.
5. Monitor changes likely to develop with recovery.

Positioning the Patient

Proper positioning of the patient is vital and essential for good recovery of the patient. This should be given priority and be the foremost consideration of the staff attending to a stroke patient.

A regime of turning or changing positions every 2–3 hours is advisable.

Choice of Positioning

Considering that majority of the hemiplegics develop spasticity or hypertonicity, suitable positions that do not promote hypertonicity should be chosen.

Magnus (1926) suggested that reflex activity due to the influence of the tonic neck reflexes plays a significant role in development of spasticity and this is greatest in the supine lying position with neck extended (Bobath 1974)

The labyrinthine reflex decreases extensor tone throughout the body in a prone position and in side lying position when the neck is neither hyperextended nor rotated. The influence of tonic neck and labyrinthine reflexes is greatly reduced.

Therefore, the most suitable position for a hemiplegic is to place him in side lying or the affected side. This position has certain advantages as listed below:

 i. Spasticity in the affected side is reduced by elongation of the whole side in side lying.
 ii. Awareness of the affected side increases as the patient bears weight on his paralyzed side.
iii. The normal side is left free to perform tasks.

The patient is placed in the affected side lying position with the head placed comfortably without much extension.

The trunk is rotated slightly backwards and pillows placed behind for support. The hemiplegic arm is brought forward to a right angle to the body by protracting the scapula, which is maintained by the patient's body weight. The forearm is supinated and wrist left in passive dorsiflexion at the edge of the bed. Protraction of the scapula decreases the flexor spasticity in the entire arm **(Fig. 7.1)**.

Note: Nothing should be placed in the hand to avoid the grasp reflex.

The hemiplegic lower limb is maintained in a step position with slight flexion at hip and knee. A pillow may be placed between the legs to avoid pressure on bony areas.

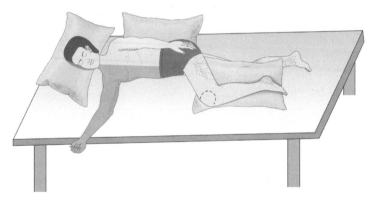

Fig. 7.1: Positioning choice 1: The affected right upper limb out stretched and normal left side is free for performances

The other upper limb is placed behind the patient or on his side.

The second position of choice is the side lying on the unaffected side.

The head is well supported, and the trunk is at right angles to the bed to avoid falling into a semiprone position.

The hemiplegic arm supported on a pillow in front in elevation of more than 100° to maintain protraction of the scapula, the normal arm may be placed anywhere as long as it is comfortable **(Fig. 7.2)**.

The hemiplegic lower limb is brought forward with pelvis protracted, supported on a pillow with hip and knee slightly flexed foot supported avoiding supination.

*Lastly the supine lying position (**Fig. 7.3**):* This position should be avoided for reasons given above and in case of hemiplegics, this is a position that involves the risk of pressure sores on the sacrum, heels and malleoli.

But, if for medical reasons other positions cannot be allowed, supine lying may be used but with precautions, i.e. head well supported on pillows and without flexing the thoracic spine.

A pillow is placed under the hemiplegic scapula to maintain protraction and elevation, elbow extended wrist in dorsiflexion with fingers extended.

A pillow under the hemiplegic buttock and thigh to protract the pelvis, legs extended. Feet placed in plantigrade position with support of pillows.

The above positioning serves to maintain the hemiplegic side in an antisynergistic posture which helps in the later stages of rehabilitation.

Maintenance of ROM, Prevent Deformities and Monitor Changes

In the early stages following stroke, there may be flaccidity with loss of function. It is important to maintain the normal length of muscles and keep the joint capsule free from adherence. Passive movement should be initiated early.

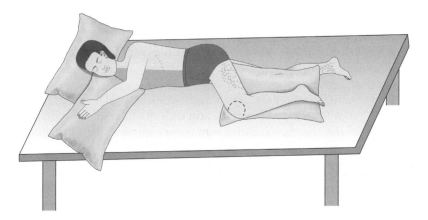

Fig. 7.2: Positioning choice 2: Head well supported, the hemiplegic hand over a pillow at 100° and hip and knee semiflexed

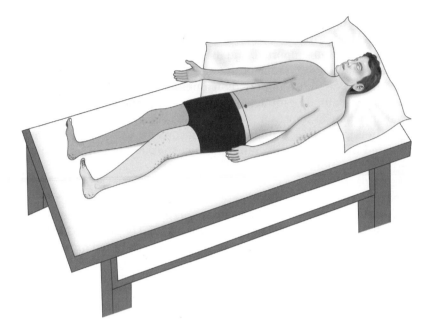

Fig. 7.3: Positioning choice 3: The supine lying and positioning of pillows

In the upper limb appropriate range of motion (ROM) exercises emphasizing on the shoulder external rotators and scapular elevation and protraction should be initiated to avoid the synergistic posture and also to prevent rotator cuff injury or impingement resulting into a painful shoulder. Tightness of wrist and finger flexors should be avoided. The use of splints may be beneficial.

Gradually as spasticity develops prolonged static postures of the arm, i.e. postures of internal rotation, adduction, pronation and wrist flexion should be avoided. Full range ROM exercises of muscles, prone to develop synergy is recommended **(Figs 7.4 and 7.5)**.

Weight bearing on the affected limb in sitting with the arm in extension and shoulder girdle elevated stimulates extension throughout the arm and weight transference on the affected side.

Weight bearing through the affected arm sideways and forwards in sitting or standing stimulates extension of the arm with shoulder in elevation. This is important for reaching out and also stimulates control around the shoulder.

Reflex Inhibiting Movement Patterns

These are movements, which have been found to have an effect on hypertonous, particularly spasticity following cerebral lesions (Bobath 1970):
- These movements alter tone by altering the abnormal postures and movements seen as a result of loss of central control over brain stem reflex activity.

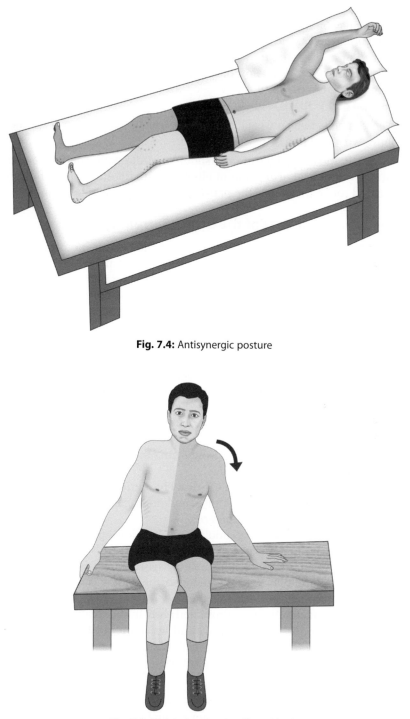

Fig. 7.4: Antisynergic posture

Fig. 7.5: Weight bearing in affected limb

Basic RIMP: Reflex inhibiting movement patterns (RIMP) for upper extremity.
- These may be modified as per individual needs.

For spastic flexor synergy of upper limb

Elevation and protraction of shoulder girdle abduction and external rotation of shoulder, extension of elbow, wrist and fingers, supination of forearm, abduction of thumb.

The use of this RIMP is illustrated below:

Problem: Inability to bear weight through the arm because of flexor spasticity at elbow, wrist and fingers.

Use of RIMP: In sitting, elevation of shoulder girdle with external rotation, abduction of the arm, extension of elbow, wrist and abduction of thumb. Extend and rotate the trunk. The patient attempts to reach the ceiling.

Selective Movements of the Upper Extremity

A selective movement is a movement out of the synergistic pattern. It is important for all hemiplegics to be able to voluntarily move their limbs out of the synergistic pattern.

The synergy of the upper extremity usually is scapular retraction, shoulder adduction, medial rotation, thus causing a disruption in the normal mechanics of the shoulder joint complex and a break of the normal scapulohumeral rhythm. This is generally the common cause for shoulder pain in hemiplegics.

To overcome the excess tone in the scapulohumeral muscles, it is essential that the hemiplegic shoulder is brought out of the synergy. A simple method to do so is to sit the patient on a plinth with the hemiplegic leg resting on the floor or on a stool.

The therapist kneels behind the patient with the patient's back resting on the therapist.

The therapist places his hand in front across the chest, with the thumb of the hand on the anterior axillary fold.

The other hand is used to hold the distal humerus.

With one hand the therapist elevates and protracts the scapula and with the other externally rotates the humerus.

The sequence of movement should be—elevation—protraction—lateral rotation all being done synchronously.

These movements are the opposite of the synergistic pattern.

Once tone around the muscles is reduced, the patient is taught to do this by himself by clasping his hands together.

This movement should be incorporated early in the treatment program.

Full ROM exercises for the elbow and wrist should be performed to maintain normal length of muscles. If necessary, wrist splints may be used to maintain the hand in a functional position.

The Lower Extremity

Normalizing postural tone is important to enable the hemiplegic to move selectively with minimum effort. The most difficult task of a therapist is to normalize tone because when the tone is too low, the patient cannot support himself or his body parts against gravity and when tone is too high with spasticity, the patient moves with effort in stereotyped patterns against resistance.

Therefore, from the beginning he should be assisted so that spasticity is reduced to minimum and abnormal movements do not become a habit.

Given below are a few activities for the lower extremity.

Inhibiting Extensor Spasticity in the Lower Limb (Fig. 7.6)

Have the patient lying with hips and knees flexed and hands encircling the knees. Rock the patient gently into flexion. This movement decreases extensor tone in the leg and at the same time maintains the scapula protracted to inhibit flexor tone of the upper limb. The activity may be repeated several times.

Control of Leg through Range

Hold the patient's leg with foot in dorsiflexion and eversion and leg flexed. Guide the leg into extension asking the patient to attempt to maintain the position of flexion of leg without abduction/external rotation at the hip. Gradually move the leg into extension, not allowing the patient to adduct/ internally rotate at the hip.

Placing the Hemiplegic Leg in Different Positions

The therapist places the patient's affected lower limb in different positions and the patient is asked to maintain that position. Initially, only flexion and extension may be trained and as the patient gains control, the positions can be made more complicated and demanding by adding abduction and rotation to flexion and extension.

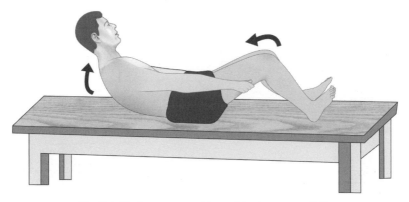

Fig. 7.6: Flexion movement to avoid extensor spasticity

Inhibition of Knee Extension with Hip in Extension

The hemiplegic lower limb is brought to the edge of the plinth to lie by the side.

The therapist fully dorsiflexes the toes to inhibit the plantar flexors and simultaneously facilitates knee flexion into its full ROM.

The patient is then encouraged to bring back the leg onto the plinth by extending the knee.

This activity is repeated several times. This ability to flex the knee while the hip is extended is essential for the start of the swing phase in walking.

Selective Hip Extension or Bridging (Fig. 7.7)

From the same starting position the patient is encouraged to lift his buttocks off the plinth maintaining the pelvis level.

The therapist facilitates movement by placing one hand on the patient's thigh on the affected side pushing down. Facilitation is provided by tapping the gluteal region to stimulate activity. Once this is accomplished with ease the patient is asked to lift his sound leg off the plinth so that all the weight is on the affected leg.

Trunk Mobilization in Hemiplegia

It is common for therapists to ignore the trunk and pelvis in the exercise program of hemiplegics. Considering the fact that one-half of the body is affected in hemiplegia, the trunk and pelvis are equally affected and need special attention.

Trunk mobilization is rotation of one set of key points against the other.

Key points of control is a term derived from the Bobath's concept of management.

A key point can best be described as a primary point within the body whereby postural tone can be controlled according to the demands of gravity or base of support and attainment of motor goals.

There are four key points: one central key point (CKP) and three proximal key points (PKP) which control tone centrally and proximally.

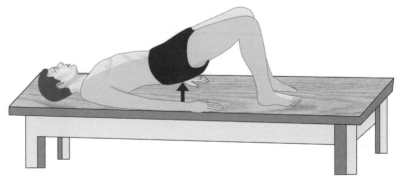

Fig. 7.7: Bridging and selective hip extension

The central key point (CKP): It is not anatomical but seen at a point of maximum facet joint rotation of spine (T7-T8) and has the following characters:

- It is anchored between the proximal key points.
- It moves in arcs of movement, i.e. up and forwards, down and backwards as seen in sitting. Up, forward and laterally and back medially to the midline as seen in weight transference.
- It is a point of maximum interplay.
- It facilitates balance interplay and pelvic tilt.

The proximal key points (PKP): The shoulder girdle and the pelvis constitute the proximal key points.

The shoulder girdle has the following characters:
- A large ROM, which is multidirectional.
- A large range of functional skills.
- Controls extremities involved in high level of skilled activity.
- These are two in number, which enable unilaterality and bilaterality of the upper extremities.

The pelvic girdle has the following characters:
- Small ROM.
- Involved more in weight transference and locomotion.

The synchronized movements of all the key points give us normal movement.

Why Mobilize the Trunk?

- To enable the patient to take up the base of support.
- To reduce tone or normalize tone from proximal to distal.
- To reintroduce movement between the CKP and PKP to achieve
    - Realignment of key points into symmetry.
    - Movement to symmetry through asymmetry.
- To facilitate the righting reactions and regaining balance activities.

How to Mobilize the Trunk?

Method: Patient sitting on edge of bed with feet on or off the floor (depends upon spastic or flaccid).

If spastic, feet off the floor as they tend to push against the support, thus evoking associated reactions.

If flaccid, the feet may rest on the floor to provide support and stability to the lower half of the body.

To gain rotation, we need extension.

Develop a pattern of flexion—extension—rotation. This can be achieved by first flexing the thoracic and lumbar spine, then guiding it into extension by facilitating over the control key point and then elongation by moving side-side, i.e. weight transference to each side. Take the patient down into flexion then rotate the trunk over to one side ensuring that there is elongation of the side flexors. Encourage the patient to 'let go' and gain extrastretch by holding the pelvis down.

The Pelvis in Hemiplegia

The pelvis has two roles:
1. To act as a stable area around which selective movement in the trunk, upper limb and lower limb can occur. It should be able to produce varying degrees of co-contraction depending upon the activity.
2. It acts as a moving structure over a moving leg producing mobility in terms of pelvic tilt and weight transference.

The pelvis also serves as a proximal key point and has the following characters:
- It provides more stability than mobility.
- It is concerned with balance and weight transference.
- It allows movement in the anteroposterior and lateral tilts.

The pelvis with a freely mobile lower limb can move multidirectionally, i.e. sinusoidally which, in turn, permits weight transference up and forwards over the weight bearing hip.

An extended pelvis allows us to come up against gravity, e.g. in slump sitting one needs to be able to extend the pelvis to sit straight. The problem that occurs directly at the pelvis is one of the flexions.

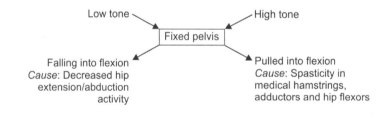

Gait and Gait Training

Most of the hemiplegics attending the physiotherapy departments are usually ambulatory either with the help of a walking aid or unsupported demonstrating a typical circumductory gait with a midline deviation.

Midline: In order to balance one needs to have a midline and be able to move away from it and return to it without falling thus initiating the righting and equilibrium reactions.

The midline of the body is taken as the correct alignment of the key points with an imaginary line passing through them. The line passes through the central key point which is midway between the key points of the shoulder girdles and through the midline of the pelvis.

Therefore, any deviation from this midline should initiate a balance reaction.

Possible Factors Leading to Deviation from Midline

- Flaccidity on one or both sides.
- Inability to recruit sufficient extensor activity.
- Lack of equilibrium and righting reactions.
- Overuse and compensation of the unaffected side.
- Sensory and perceptual problems.

The circumductory gait in hemiplegics is generally caused by the extensor synergy of the affected lower limb where the pelvis is retracted, hip and knee held in extension and the pull of the triceps surae muscle causing the ankle and foot to be maintained in plantar flexion and inversion.

Therefore, in order to facilitate gait in hemiplegics it is necessary to enable the patient to move selectively at these joints.

It is always better to initiate weight transference in standing and gaining the midline by re-establishing the equilibrium and righting reactions before allowing the patient to take a step.

To make walking functional, the components of normal gait should be understood and walking should be introduced early in the rehabilitation program. The use of wheel chairs or walking aids should be avoided. An important prerequisite for walking is the ability of the hemiplegic to stand up and sit down safely.

Management or Facilitation of Gait

Use your hands to prevent difficulties and provide suitable cues as and when required. The various phases of gait should be practised in standing. Emphasize on balance, stance and weight transfer.

Release spasticity at hip, knee and ankle to enable lifting the leg and taking a step.

Once these are achieved, then walking can be initiated.

Some Useful Methods to Facilitate Walking

- Therapist can place hands on either side of pelvis to facilitate hip extension and weight transference.
- Allow the patient to take the first step with the sound leg, then transfer weight to the hemiplegic foot, the therapist assists hip extension and weight transference with the hands on the affected side.
  Then the weight on the affected leg is brought forward over the sound limb, so that the affected limb is free to initiate the swing phase.
  Therapist may press down on the pelvis to prevent hitching of the pelvis.
- Making the patient walk with his arms held behind, extended and laterally rotated.
  Once control of hip and knee is gained, facilitate by holding both arms of the patient behind with wrist and fingers extended. This allows the patient

to extend the hip and trunk by counteracting the pull of flexor spasticity in trunk and other shoulders. This also checks associated reactions.
- Resting the hemiplegic arm on the therapist's shoulder.
The therapist places one hand on the scapula keeping it protracted.

Avoid pursuing with this method for long.

Avoid: Using walking sticks, tripods early in the rehabilitation process.
Do not prescribe orthosis too soon.
Do not initiate walking without achieving the prerequisites of gait.

Bibliography

1. Brigitta langhammer, Bobath or motor relearning program? A comparison of two different approaches of physiotherapy in stroke rehabilitation: a randomized controlled study. Clinical Rehabilitation. 2000;14:361-9.
2. Brunnstrom S. Movement therapy in hemiplegia, 1970.
3. Carre and Kenney, Positioning of the stroke patient: a review of the literature. International Journal of Nursing Studies. 1992;29(4):355-69.
4. Dickstein, et al. Stroke rehabilitation, three exercise therapy approaches. Physical Therapy. 1986;66(8):1233-6.
5. Duncan, et al. A randomized controlled pilot study of a home-based exercise program for individual with mild to moderate stroke. Stroke. 1998;29:2055-60.
6. Ernest E. A review of stroke rehabilitation and physiotherapy. Stroke. 1990;21: 1081-85.
7. Jones, Effect of recommended positioning on stroke out come at six months: a randomized controlled trial. Clinical Rehabilitation. 2005;19(2):138-45.
8. Judy W Griffin. Hemiplegic shoulder pain. Physical Therapy. 1986;66(12):1884-93.
9. Louise, et al. Thirty minutes positioning reduces the development of shoulder external rotation contracture after stroke: a randomized controlled trial. Archive of Physical Medicine and Rehabilitation. 2005;86:230-4.
10. Sackley and Lincoln. Physiotherapy treatment for stroke patients: a survey of current practice. Physiotherapy Theory and Practice. 1996;12(2):87-96.
11. Schwarz, et al. Effect of body positioning on intracranial pressure and cerebral perfusion in patient with large hemispheric stroke. Stroke. 2002;33:497-501.
12. Sheila Lennon. Gait Re-education based on the Bobath concept in two patients with hemiplegia following stroke. Physical Therapy. 2001;81(3):924-35.
13. Susan Burreca. Treatment interventions for the paretic upper limb of stroke survivors: a critical review. Neurorehabilitation and Neural Repair. 2003;17(4):220-6.
14. Tanaka, et al. Trunk rotatory muscle performance in post-stroke hemiplegic patients-1. American Journal of Physical Medicine and Rehabilitation. 1997;76(5):366-9.
15. Thielman, et al. Rehabilitation of reaching after stroke: task-related training versus progressive resistive exercise. Archive of Physical Medicine and Rehabilitation. 2004;85:1613-8.
16. True Blood, et al. Pelvic exercise and gait in hemiplegia. Physical Therapy. 1989;69(1).
17. Wellwood and langhorn, effect of augmented exercise therapy time after stroke: a meta analysis. Stroke. 2004;35:2529-39.

8

Speech and Language Dysfunction in Stroke: Diagnosis and Management

K Venugopal, Indu Marium Jacob

Stroke is one of the leading causes of disability and communication impairment in adults. Of the estimated 400,000 strokes, which occur, in a year, approximately 80,000 of those patients have some form of aphasia. Aphasia is a communication impairment that commonly follows stroke. This refers to the disturbance of any or all of the skills of language, i.e. comprehension, speech, reading and writing.[2] Darley[3] noted that aphasia is generally described as an impairment of language resulting from focal brain damage to the language-dominant cerebral hemisphere. This serves to distinguish aphasia from the language and cognitive-communication problems associated with nonlanguage-dominant hemisphere damage, dementia, and traumatic brain injury. Kertesz[4] clinically described aphasia as a "neurologically central disturbance of language characterized by paraphasias, word finding difficulty, and variably impaired comprehension, associated with disturbance in reading and writing, at times with dysarthria, nonverbal constructional and problem-solving difficulty and impairment of gesture."

Aphasia attacks an intricate part of a person's daily life—the simple act of communication and sharing. Communication is a dynamic process, which involves the act of giving to or receiving information about the person's needs, desires, perception, knowledge or effective state. The modes of communication are writing, gestures and the most common and unique form in humans is through the oral mode or speaking.[24,25] When the ability to communicate (give or receive) is impaired or absent, its impact on the person and his/her family is profound.[30] Therefore, therapy is very much warranted and any help the patient can receive to recover function in the communication domain is treasured.

This chapter focuses on the disabilities brought on after a stroke to the dominant hemisphere causing aphasia. It discusses the general characteristics of aphasia, the types of aphasias, differential diagnosis, assessment and most importantly the treatment approaches.

observation of a patient's communication skills in everyday situations or during interaction with caretakers. These tools tend to less standardized than traditional tests but allow for more informal and naturalistic measures of communication. Functional assessment of communication is especially useful in documenting treatment outcome.

1. Functional Communication Profile (Sarno, 1969 in[2, 5])
2. Communicative Abilities in Daily Living (Holland, 1980 in[2, 5])
3. The Communicative Effectiveness Index (CETI) (Lomas et al., 1989 in[2,5])
4. Communication Profile: A Functional Survey (Payne, 1994 in[2, 5])
5. Functional Assessment of Communication Skills for Adults (ASHA FACS) (Frattali, Thompson, Holland, Wohl and Ferketi, 1995 in[2, 5]).

Independent Test of Specific Skills

Comprehensive test batteries of aphasia provide subtests for most skills that need to be assessed. However, clinicians may use many independent tests that evaluate specific skills of patients with aphasia. The following are a few examples:

Auditory Comprehension

1. Token Test (DeRenzi and Vignolo, 1962 in[2,5])
2. Auditory Comprehension Test for Sentences (ACTS) (Shewan, 1979 in[2,5])
3. The Functional Auditory Comprehension Task (FACT) (LaPointeand Horner, 1978 in[2,5])
4. The Discourse Comprehension Test (DCT) (Brookshire and Nichols, 1993 in[2,5]).

Reading

1. The Reading Comprehension Battery for Aphasia (RCBA) (LaPointe and Horner, 1979 in[2,5])
2. Gates-MacGainitie Reading Test (Gates, 1978 in[2,5])
3. Nelson Reading Skills Test (Hanna, Schuell, and Schreiner, 1977 in[2,5]).

New Assessment Procedure

Psycholinguistic Assessment of Language Processing in Aphasia (PALPA).

PALPA[37] is designed to be a resource for speech and language therapists and cognitive and clinical neuropsychologists who wish to assess language processing skills in people with aphasia. It consists of 60 assessments designed to help to diagnose language processing difficulties in individuals with acquired brain damage. As its name suggests, PALPA applies a psycholinguistic approach to the interpretation of process concerned with the recognition, comprehension, and production of spoken and written words and sentences. The approach is based on the assumption that the mind's language system is organized in separate modules of processing, and that these can be impaired selectively by brain damage. PALPA aims to provide information about the integrity of these module, to find those in which the aphasic person seems to be functioning below normal and those which appears to continuing to function normally or near-normally. PALPA is not designed to be given in its entirety to an individual rather the assessment should be tailored to those that are appropriate to the hypothesis under investigation. Therefore, by deriving hypotheses about the nature of the processing disorder, the PALPA aims to provide a firm grounding on which further assessment of a person's difficulties and on which to plan directed treatment programs. Those aphasic therapists who have already started using the PALPA have reported it to be very informative and useful in the evaluation and management of aphasia.[37]

Treatment of Aphasia

The treatment goal when treating patients with aphasia is to rebuild their skills in the various speech and language deficits that they have acquired due to stroke. Importantly the aims are to make the patient independent, maximize communicative strengths and enable them to function again in the community.[1,2,5,9,10]

Many specialized therapeutic techniques and alternative means are used to help people with aphasia. Efficacy of treatment was in the past and still under much debate. This is because of the variety and heterogeneity of the aphasic syndromes and the different treatment approaches.[1,2,5,17] However, in the recent years through more thorough randomized, controlled studies, as well as through literature reviews and meta-analyses, aphasia interventions have been proven to be warranted and effective.[1,6,7,9,10,17]

Variables that Affect Treatment Outcome

Part of the difficulty in determining treatment outcome is that many variables affect outcome and controlling all of them are difficult. Experienced clinicians report that several variables seem to limit or enhance the chances of significant recovery with treatment. Although not all variables have been subjected to experimental analysis some of the important variables that affect treatment outcome include:

1. *Age of patients*: Younger patients may improve more than older patients.[2,5]
2. *Premorbid language skills and literacy*: Patients with higher premorbid language and literacy skills may improve better than those with limited premorbid skills.[2,5]
3. *Education and occupation*: Patients with a higher level of education and those have faced greater occupational demand for language use may improve better than those without such education and occupational demand.[2,5]
4. *Nature of neuropathology (extent and location of lesions)*: Patients with smaller lesions and those with no repeated infarcts may improve better than those with larger lesions and repeated infarcts.[2,5,9]
5. *Past medical and behavioral disorders*: Patients with significant history of such disorders improve less that those without such disorders.[2,5,9]

6. *Medical, neurological and behavioral status*: Patients with relatively healthy status improve better that those with comprised status.[2,5,9]
7. *Severity of aphasia*: Patients with less severe aphasia improve more than those with more severe aphasia.[2,5,9]
8. *Timing of treatment initiation*: Patients who receive early treatment may improve more than those whose treatment is significantly delayed.[1,2,5,9]
9. *Length of treatment*: Generally and within certain limits, longer treatments produce greater improvements than brief treatments.[2,5]
10. *Intensity of treatment*: Generally and within certain limits, more intensive treatments produce better results than less intensive treatments.[2,5,11,12]
11. *Family involvement*: Patients whose family members participate in the treatment and learn to help the patients in natural communication contexts improve better than those who do not receive such help from their family members.[2,5,9,30]
12. Motivation level of the patient.[2,5,32]
13. *Improvement or deterioration in general health during the course of treatment*: Patients who sustain their health during treatment improve more than those whose health deteriorates in the same period.[2,5]
14. *Spontaneous recovery*: Certain amount of function is regained without therapy due to brain plasticity. Researchers have proposed three theories on how this is achieved, (1) the area surrounding the damaged area takes over the function of the damaged area, (2) functional reorganization of the neuronal networks involved in language, and (3) the corresponding area in the right hemisphere are activated when the areas in the left hemisphere are damaged. Spontaneous recovery is reported within the first six months after the event where spontaneous improvements of language functions are expected.[2,5,13-16]

Principles of Treatment of Aphasic Patients

The following principles are basic in treating any disorder in communication, including those associated with aphasia:

1. Careful observation and detailed assessment of the client.[2,5,9,10]
2. Selection of client-specific target behaviors that, when taught provide the greatest improvement in functional communication in natural settings.[9,10]
3. Sequencing target behaviors appropriately to ensure patient's success in treatment (easier initial targets and progressively more difficult ones).[5,9,10]
4. Maximize on patient'[5] communicative strengths.[2,5]
5. Providing the maximum amount of stimulation control in the beginning, including instructions, modeling, pictures, objects, role playing, and other events that help establish the target language skills.[2,9]
6. Reducing the clinically manipulated stimulus control in gradual steps so that the target language skills are produced in response to more natural stimulus events.[2,5,9]
7. Arranging naturally occurring consequences for the patient's attempts to strengthen those attempts.[1,2,5]

8. Providing immediate, response-contingent, positive feedback to the patient to increase the target language skill and to maintain them at a minimum of 80% accuracy.[1,2,5]
9. Providing immediate corrective feedback for incorrect responses to reduce their frequency.[1,2,5]
10. Training the clients in self-monitoring skills to sustain the treatment gains.[2,5]
11. Training family members to evoke prompt, support, reinforce and maintain appropriate communicative behaviors of the client in natural and functional contexts.[2,5]
12. A follow-up schedule that allows periodic monitoring of the client's communicative behavior with a view to offer booster therapy when needed.[2]
13. Providing therapy during spontaneous recovery to gain maximum improvement.[5,14,15]

Therapy Approaches

The critical clinical issue in current approaches to aphasia therapy is the necessity to individualize the therapeutic modality for the specific aphasic sign or symptom being targeted and the specific person being treated. Traditional methods of aphasia therapy have been improved by careful selection of timing and frequency of treatment delivery, more precise delineation of which aphasic deficit to focus on, more reasoned matching of therapy technique to the deficit, and modification of treatment modality as the syndrome evolves.[1,2,5,8-10]

Output-focused Therapy

Most speech/language pathologists still use the technique known as stimulation-response or direct retraining of deficit, as one aspect of their therapy program. First, the aphasic deficit is identified and, then, repetitive drill through several modalities (e.g. reading or repetition) is encouraged. An endless array of sophisticated modifications of this traditional approach has been developed.[1,2,5]

Behavior Modification Therapy

Operant conditioning, a form of behavior modification was one of the traditional approaches to treat aphasia. This approach involves shaping the language behavior by helping patients progress through a series of task presented in fixed order, from least to most difficult.[5,9,10]

Cognitive Therapy

Schuell[5,10] was the first to take a cognitive approach to aphasia therapy. Schuell and colleagues[5,10] proposed that an extended period of intensive stimulation would improve the quality of the aphasia language behavior. Because it was believed at the time that language was naturally learned through the auditory modality alone, Schuell emphasized the use of auditory stimuli. Duffy[5] suggests a multimodality approach to rehabilitation for aphasic patients. Chapey[5] recommends among other things, the use of divergent thinking in aphasia therapy (in divergent thinking task, a patient is required to produce several creative responses to every stimulus, e.g. the patient might be asked to think of several unusual ways to make use of an everyday object).

Combination of Behavioral and Cognitive Therapy

Programmed stimulation approach to aphasia therapy combines behavioral and cognitive methods.[5] That is the use of a hierarchy of therapy tasks based on the level of difficulty employed by behaviorist, but uses the kind of stimuli employed by therapist with a cognitive orientation.[1,5] Some common programmed stimulation for aphasics are Melodic Intonation Therapy (MIT) (Sparks and Holland, in Chapey[5]) and Visual Action Therapy (VAT) (Fitzpatrick and Baresi, 1982, in Chapey[5]). Melodic intonation therapy is a formal, hierarchically structured treatment program based on the assumption that the stress, intonation, and melodic patterns of language output are controlled primarily by the right hemisphere and, thus, are available for use in the individual with aphasia with left hemisphere damage. Melodic intonation therapy, in essence, consists of intoning normal language with exaggerated rhythm, stress, and melody. VAT is a nonvocal approach, which ultimately trains patients to produce symbolic gestures for visually absent stimuli.

Pragmatic Therapy

Pragmatic approaches use social interaction to improve the communication abilities of aphasic patients.[1,2,5,9,10] Many different pragmatic approaches exist. For example teaching language in a naturalistic setting by taking an aphasic out to a restaurant and helping him/her order a meal.

Martha Taylor Sarno[5], one of the pioneers of modern aphasia therapy, has also been one of the strongest supporters of the effort to manage the whole patient, to help the patient recover functional communication using all techniques possible in a comprehensive therapy program. She says that "the condition of aphasia should not be limited by a definition which separates the language pathology from the person."

One of the most active movements in current aphasia therapy is related to Sarno's cautions. Group treatment, focusing on regaining conversational skills, and on developing alternative strategies for communicating despite aphasia, is becoming increasingly popular. Interpersonal social contexts for developing effective supported communication are themselves the focus of treatment.

Promoting Aphasics' Communicative Effectiveness (PACE) developed by Davis and Wilcox, 1981 is a well-known pragmatic therapy for aphasia. PACE is based on the pragmatic rule of reciprocity, the therapist and the patient participate in a conversation as equals, each taking turns sending and receiving messages. The emphasis is on enhancing communicative ability, nonverbal as well as verbal, in pragmatically realistic settings. Use of compensatory strategies are encouraged, with less of a focus on relearning a lost or deficient linguistic skill, and more on improving communication by any means possible.

The PACE, MIT and VAT are also published treatment programs. Another popular published treatment program is the Helm Elicited Language Program for Syntax Stimulation (Helm-Estabrooks and Albert, 1991). It helps in teaching sentence structure and grammatical elements of speech production.

Psycholinguistic Approach

The psycholinguistic approach to aphasia therapy applies information-processing models of normal cognition in understanding of language disorders. An attempt is made to identify the locus of the language deficit within the cognitive/linguistic structure of normal language.[37] An analogy might be the search for a missing or defective enzyme within a complex metabolic system. The premise underlying this approach is that a specific aphasic sign or symptom may be the surface clinical manifestation of different underlying deficits within the cognitive structure of language.[37] Only by uncovering the precise underlying psycholinguistic deficit can therapy be properly targeted. To date, the clinical phenomena of anomia and agrammatism have been most responsive to this approach.[37]

Cognitive Neurorehabilitation

A newer approach to aphasia therapy is based on the idea that the ability to communicate is dependent not only on linguistic competence but also on related neurobehavioral functions, such as attention and memory.[18,19] The assumption is that brain damage that produces aphasia also produces disturbance in other, language-related cognitive functions, and that treatment of these other cognitive deficits can facilitate communication.[18,19]

For example, virtually all individuals with aphasia develop perseveration, which interferes with communicative capability. In 1987 Helm-Estabrooks and colleagues[20] introduced treatment for Aphasic Perseveration, and demonstrated that cognitive therapy focused on related neurobehavioral deficits can improve language function in individuals with aphasia.

McNeil and colleagues[21] have long argued that individuals with aphasia suffer a deficit in allocation of attentional resources and proposed an "integrated attention theory of aphasia," asserting a relation among attention, arousal, and language processing. This argument receives support from contemporary research in cognitive neuroscience, in which a left hemisphere attentional system linked to language has been described by Posner. Indirect evidence exists that attempts to treat attentional dysfunction in individuals with aphasia may ameliorate the language disorder; and experimental studies are just beginning to test this hypothesis.[19,21]

New Therapeutic Approaches for Teaching Aphasia

Computer-aided Therapy

The newer treatment approaches use computers to improve the language abilities of people with aphasia.[5,22,23] These are usually computer-like clinical devices, or treatment software for general purpose computers, sometimes with associates print materials. Studies have shown that computer-assisted therapy can help people with aphasia retrieve and produce verbs.[22,23] People who have auditory problems perceiving the difference between phonemes can benefit from computers, which can be used for speech-therapeutic auditory discrimination exercises.[22,23] Research has been reporting benefits for the use of such tools.[22,23] Benefits include more consistent stimuli, self-paced practice, automatic results reporting, greater clinician productivity, and improved performance following treatment.

Pharmacotherapy

Pharmacotherapy for aphasia is a new, still experimental, and somewhat controversial adjunct to other therapeutic approaches, and one which may, at last, capture the attention of neurologists and rehabilitation physicians on behalf of their patients with aphasia.[26-28] In contemporary cognitive neuroscience, disorders of memory are being fractionated, with different components of memory systems correlated with abnormal levels of specific neurotransmitters. Similar attempts are being made to understand the cognitive neurochemistry of language. Grossly, and as yet without fully adequate experimental support, language output abnormalities have been linked to dopaminergic system deficiencies and anomia and auditory comprehension disorders have been linked to cholinergic system deficiencies.[27] Single-case studies, in which the patients serve as their own controls, have demonstrated remarkable improvement in language function following pharmacotherapy for aphasia using this chemicocognitive model.[26] Few well-controlled studies have been carried out, however, and these, to date, have been less convincing than the single-case studies. Nevertheless, a detailed and critical review of the topic concludes "when used as an adjunct to behavioral therapy, pharmacotherapy appears to have benefit."[26]

Alternative Augmentative Communication in Aphasia

Alternative augmentative communication (AAC) refers to ways (other than speech) that are used to send a message from one person to another. The goal of AAC is the most effective communication possible and, in turn, the greatest potential for personal achievement.[24,25] People who use AAC do so to supplement their own speech. They may be able to use speech to an extent, but may also have to rely on AAC in certain situations. There are four main needs of people who use AAC. These goals include expression of needs and wants, such as the need to use the restroom; transfer of information, example being what he/she did that day; social closeness, such as telling a child you love them; and social etiquette, for example, saying thank you.[24,25] By understanding the intentions of the stroke patient in communicating, the proper AAC device can be used.

There are many types of AAC devices, ranging from simple to complex. The number of words that can be communicated with each technique also varies. The specific device used depends on the individual's needs, their present level of communication, and their abilities; therefore, no prescription can be given for one that will work best. The types of AAC can best be broken down into two categories: unaided and aided communication systems.[24,25] Unaided communication systems are defined as those nonspeech systems that do not require any additional augmentative device other than the communicator in the conveying of messages.[24,25] The main form of unaided communication is gestures. This includes sign language, fingerspelling, common gestures such as head nodding, and unique gestures created by the individual. The unaided form can be used at any time in any setting because of their simplicity.

Aided communication systems are those that rely on a device or display to help the speaker communicate.[24,25] Communication boards are one type of aided communication system, and are designed specifically for an individual. They must include lexigrams, which are symbols or pictures that are meaningful to the user. These can be helpful if the picture that the person wants to use is on the board; however, there is limited space, the person must be able to physically point to the picture, he or she must also cognitively know what they want to say, and the meaning of each symbol must clear. Another simple aided communication system is through using representational objects. With these, a small object has a more elaborate meaning. For example, a small matchbox car can represent that the patient wants to go for a car ride, or a small drinking glass may mean the person is thirsty.

Electronic devices are the newest way to communicate, and there are an extremely large variety of these from which to choose.[24,25] An evaluation of the abilities of the person must be done to determine which device will work best. Some devices are simple and may contain slots for three or four pictures from which the patient can choose, which is called direct select. Other devices scroll through the selections and the individual stops scrolling when the desired choice is reached, called indirect selection. Selection can be achieved through pressing a button or may be as sophisticated as only requiring an eye blink or a puff of air. With the most complicated devices, there is large keypads in which words can be typed. Each of these devices speaks for the patient through generated output. With these devices, it is important to choose a method that will fit the vocabulary needs of the patient.[24,25]

People having aphasia can benefit from alternate and augmentative communication, especially those experiencing Broca's aphasia and global aphasia.[5,24,25] These people do not have fluent speech, but may know what they want to say. By teaching simple gestural signs and sign language, these people can state needs quickly. The key is that the listener must know the signs being used. Using the communication boards, these people are able to transfer information and gain social closeness. The speech pathologist works with the aphasia patient to help them understand the meanings of the pictures and when to use them. Electronic devices can be programmed for the individual's specific communication needs. Using one of these devices, the person can communicate what they are thinking by direct selection or scanning. Complicated electronic devices may not be ideal for aphasia patients because their organization is inhibited due to the language problems. Computerized visual communication (or C-VIC)[23-25] was designed as an alternative communication system for patients with severe aphasia and is based on the notion that those with severe aphasia can learn an alternative symbol system (alternative to the symbol system used in natural language) and can use this alternative system to communicate. Pictures or icons, representing meaningful concepts or things, are developed and loaded into a computer. The patient with aphasia learns to manipulate these icons on the computer screen for purposes of communication. Patients with severe aphasia could master the mechanics of the system, learn icons for proper and common nouns, and use them in simple sentences, although they produced their sentences agrammatically. Nevertheless, teaching patients with severe aphasia to communicate by computer, even with agrammatic output, is a remarkable achievement.

With the availability of many therapeutic approaches speech-language therapist may choose to adhere to any on conceptual framework, while others are more eclectic and draw on this or that approach as adjudged to be of likely benefit to patients. However, most clinicians nowadays expose the patient to various therapeutic approaches and not restrict them to one. In this way clinicians can find the therapeutic approach that best suits the patient and provide the maximum improvement. All patients even with similar lesions or symptoms may not show the same gains for a particular therapy approach.

Something that is overlooked most of the time or not addressed is those factors that is of great concern and importance to people with aphasia.[29,32,34,35] These include dealing with communication breakdowns returning to work, maintaining financial stability in the absence of employment, making decisions regarding the family, dealing with troubled relationships, limited access to leisure opportunities and therefore countering boredom and isolation.[31,33-35] People with aphasia often find themselves isolated from family, friends, unable to or not involved in decision-making of personnel and family matters due to their communication deficits. Unable to return to work, people with aphasia are faced with hours of enforced leisure time. Therefore, boredom is a major issue. They often feel that their life is meaningless or wasted. To those who do not understand the nature of deficits of aphasia (friends and family members) people with aphasia become a subject of teasing, scolding, disappointment and embarrassment. All these factors greatly impact on Quality of Life for the person with aphasia. Studies have shown that here is a gap between the services provided and what really matters to the patient.[32,34,35]

Clinician are realizing these needs of people with aphasia and putting forth strategies to overcome these problems.[32,35] Strategies or approaches include providing the aphasic patients with adequate communicative skills, educating the family members and friends regarding aphasia and the specific features of the patient. The speech-language therapist along with the rehabilitative team provides appropriate skills to return to employment or provide alternate employment opportunities that best suit the aphasic persons residual skills, organizes leisure activities and adapts the environment of the aphasic person to facilitate independent functioning and return to the community.[32,35]

Speech-language therapist also holds group activities for people with aphasia. Within these groups a person with aphasia meets other people with aphasia. They realise that they are not the only one with such problems. In the groups these people with aphasia communicate with each other or learn to communicate with each other, make new friends, learn from others and their experiences, give others advice, express their problems and emotions and have fun. The clinician acts as a guidance and occasionally engages the group in small activities to bring the group closer and work on some of the deficit skills.

While these activities are commonly seen in the Western countries, they are yet to be well established here in India. These activities are of great importance as they benefit the patient and greatly impact on quality of life.

Similar to the experiences of the person with aphasia, family members often find communicating with aphasic person difficult.[29,30] They describe the continuous and exhausting pressure of trying to resolve misunderstanding and determine the meaning of what was being expressed. As they care for the aphasic person they take on new tasks and responsibilities, experience social restriction and may suffer exhaustion, loneliness and depression. Secondary to this, relationship between the family member and aphasic person may breakdown.[29,30] Therefore, it is important for the rehabilitation team to educate family members regarding aphasia, the deficits seen and the prognosis. The family members should be involved in the therapy, so that they understand what is being done and continue the therapy at home.[30] With the family members conducting therapy, it provides a means of communication and strengthens the bond between the family members and the aphasic person.[30] The clinician should provide the family members with strategies to communicate and understand what the aphasic person says.[29,30]

Conclusion

Aphasia, commonly caused by stroke, is an acquired language disorder that impairs the various language processes (comprehension, expression, reading and writing) in varying degrees. It therefore, creates problems in communication, in that it restricts or unables the person from doing daily activities (conversation, decisions, indicating needs and wants, telling jokes, watching TV and writing letters), returning to job, taking part in social activities and enjoying leisure activities. These restrictions or inabilities greatly impact on the Quality of Life of the person with aphasia. Once a person has acquired aphasia, full recovery is unlikely. Therefore, speech and language rehabilitation is very important and warranted to improve the areas of speech and language deficit, provide coping strategies, maximize the persons strengths and thus enable the person to function independently and return to the community.

References

1. Rosenbek JC, LaPointe LL, Wertz RT. Aphasia Treatment: Its Efficacy. A Clinical Approach. San Diego, College Hill Press, 1989.
2. Hegde MN. A Coursebook on Aphasia and Other Neurogenic Language Disorders. (2nd edn). San Diego CA: Singular Publishing Group, 1996.
3. Darley FL. Aphasia. Philadelphia, Pa: WB Saunders, 1982.
4. Kertesz A. Aphasia and Associated Disorders: Taxonomy, Localization and Recovery. New York: Grune and Stratton, 1979.
5. Chapey R. Language Intervention Strategies in Adult Aphasia, 3rd edn. Baltimore, Md: Williams and Wilkins, 1994.
6. Tompkins CA. Applying Research Principles to Language Intervention. In: R. Chapey (Ed). Language Intervention Strategies in Adult Aphasia, 3rd edn. William and Wilkins, 1994.
7. Robey RR. A meta-analysis of clinical outcomes in the treatment of aphasia. Journal of Speech Language, Hearing and Research. 1998;41:172-87.
8. Shewan CM and Kertesz A. Effects of speech and language treatment on recovery from aphasia. Brain Language. 1984;23:272-99.
9. Albert ML. Treatment of aphasia. Archives of Neurology. 1998;55:1417-9.
10. Steele RD, Aftonomos LB and Munk MW. Evaluation and treatment of aphasia among the elderly with stroke. Topics in Geriatric Rehabilitation. 2003;19(2):98-108.
11. Bhogal SK, Teasell R and Speechley M. Intensity of aphasia therapy, impact on recovery. Stroke. 2003;34:987-93.
12. Page SJ. Intensity versus task-specificity after stroke: how important is intensity? American Journal Physical Medicine Rehabilitation. 2003;82:730-2.
13. Goldenberg G and Spatt J. Influence of size and site of cerebral lesions on spontaneous recovery of aphasia and on success of language therapy. Brain and Language. 1994;47(4):684-98.
14. Lendrem W and Lincoln NB. Spontaneous recovery of language in patients with aphasia between 4 and 34 weeks after stroke. J Neurol Neurosurg Psychiatry. 1985;48(8):743-8.
15. Heiss WD, Kessler J, Thiel A, Ghaemi M and Karbe H. Differential capacity of left and right hemispheric areas for compensation of poststroke aphasia. Annals of Neurology. 1999;45(4):430-8.
16. Meinzer M, Elbert T, Wienbruch C, Barthel DD and Rockstroh B. Intensive Language Training Enhances Brain Plasticity in Aphasia. BMC Biology. 2004;2(20).
17. Holland A, Fromm D, DeRuyter F and Stein M. Treatment efficacy: aphasia. Journal of Speech Hearing and Research. 1996;39(Suppl):27-36.
18. Alladi S, Meena AK and Kaul S. Cognitive Rehabilitation in Stroke: therapy and Techniques. Neurology India. 2002;50(Suppl):102-08.
19. Helm-Estabrooks N. Cognition and aphasia. A Discussion and A Study. Journal of Communication Disorders. 2002;35(2):171-86.
20. Helm-Estabrooks N, Emery P and Albert ML. Treatment of aphasic perseveration (TAP) program: a new approach to aphasia therapy. Archives of Neurology. 1987;44:1253-5.

21. McNeil M, Odell K and Tseng CH. Toward the integration of resource allocation into a general theory of aphasia. Clinical Aphasiology. 1991;20:21-39.
22. Adrian JA, Gonzalez M and Buiza JJ. The use of computer-assisted therapy in anomia rehabilitation: a single-case report. Aphasiology. 2003;17(10):981-1002.
23. Weinrich M. Computer rehabilitation in aphasia. Clinical Neuroscience. 1997;4(2):103-7.
24. Glennen S and DeCoste D. Handbook of Augmentative and Alternative Communication. San Diego, CA: Singular Publishing Group, 1997.
25. Beukelman DR and Mirenda P. Augmentative and Alternative Communication: Management of Severe Communication Disorders in Children and Adults, 2nd edn. Baltimore: Paul H. Brookes Publishing Co., Inc., 1998.
26. Small S. Pharmacotherapy of aphasia: a critical review. Stroke 1994;25:1282-89.
27. Albert ML, Bachman D, Morgan A and Helm-Estabrooks N. Pharmacotherapy for aphasia. Neurology. 1988;38:877-9.
28. Walker-Batson D, Curtis S, Natarajan R, Ford J, Dronkers N, Salmeron E, Lai J and Unwin DH. A double-blind, placebo-controlled study of the use of amphetamine in the treatment of aphasia. Stroke. 2001;32:2093-97.
29. Lyon J, Cariski D, Keisler L, et al. Communication partner: enhancing participation in life and communication for adults with aphasia in natural settings. Aphasiology. 1997;11:693-708.
30. Burns MS, Dong KY, Oehring AK. Family involvement in the treatment of aphasia. Topics in Stroke Rehabilitation. 1995;2(1):68-77.
31. Le Dorze G and Brassard C. A description of the consequences of aphasia on aphasic persons and their relatives and friends, based on the WHO model of chronic diseases. Aphasiology. 1995;9:239-55.
32. Parr S, Byng S and Gilpin S. Talking About Aphasia. Buckingham, UK: Open University Press, 1997.
33. King P and Barrowclough C. Rating the motivation of elderly patients on a rehabilitation ward. Clinical Rehabilitation. 1989;3:289-91.
34. Hilari K and Byng S. Measuring quality of life in people with aphasia: the stroke specific quality of life scale. International Journal of Language and Communication Disorders. 2001;36(Suppl):86-91.
35. Sneeuw KCA, Aaronson NK, DeHaan RJ and Limburg M. Assessing quality of life after stroke: the value and limitations of proxy ratings. Stroke. 1997;28:1541-9.
36. Kertesz A. Western Aphasic Battery. New York, Grune and Stratton, 1982.
37. Kay J, Lesser R and Coltheart M. Psycholinguistic Assessment of Language Processing in Aphasia. Hove, Lawrence Erlbaum Associates, 1992.

9

Pressure Sore and Skin Care in Stroke and Spinal Cord Injuries

Rupnarayan Bhattacharya

Introduction

Skin care of a patient with hemiplegia, paraplegia or quadriplegia due to any reason is a very important aspect of the total management. If not managed properly almost all such patients end up with large pressure sore(s), which delay recovery or makes rehabilitation much difficult and raise the morbidity of the patient to a much higher level. Proper knowledge about pathophysiology of formation of pressure sore is important for its prevention and management. Every team member involved in rehabilitation of such patients must be aware of the sincere approaches to prevent sores. Especially, the nursing staffs, bed side attendant and the therapists should be careful in handling these patients.

Etiology of Pressure Sore

The cause of developing sore in a patient with spinal cord injury is multifactorial. These can be divided into two:
1. Primary factor
2. Associated factors

Primary Factor: Pressure (Intensity + Duration)

For viability, a cell depends on metabolism, which is entirely dependent on supply of oxygen and removal of carbon dioxide and waste products via microcirculation and tissue perfusion. The arteriolar pressure is around 32 mm Hg and at the venule end it is about 15 mm Hg. If due to any reason the tissue pressure rises, first there will be obstruction to venous outflow, which will lead to further rise in capillary pressure, leading to obstruction of arteriolar inflow, resulting in ischemia and subsequently tissue damage.

Tissue can withstand much higher pressure, if it is applied for a short interval followed by relief. But if it is applied for a prolonged time—tissues suffer from irreversible ischemia.

Not only intensity, but duration of pressure exerted on a particular area is important for developing pressure sore.

Normal pressures in different position

Supine	**Prone**
Occiput—40 mm Hg	Thorax—40 mm Hg
Sacrum—40-60 mm Hg	Patella—45 mm Hg
Ischial tuberosity—50 mm Hg	
Heel—40 mm Hg	

Sitting
Ischial tuberosities—70-400 mm Hg

Normally an individual frequently changes posture and position to avoid constant pressure on a particular area, but if there are sensory/motor paralysis (due to spinal injury/cerebrovascular accident, etc.) or in conditions in which patients lie immobile (as in shock/sepsis/coma/prolonged anesthesia), the chances of pressure necrosis of tissues are very high.

Associated Factors

1. Loss of mobility—head injury/unconsciousness
   Shock/sepsis (impaired microcirculation)
2. Diminished sensory function
3. Autonomic sympathetic dysfunction (loss of vascular tone, diminished/blood supply and venous return)
4. Metabolic disturbances, e.g. diabetes mellitus (neuropathy, infection)
5. Loss of bladder and bowel control
6. Severe anemia
7. Malnutrition, proteinuria
8. Infection
9. Psychological—depression (prolonged immobility, nutritional deficiency)
10. Mechanical insult—friction, wrinkles in bed, moist linen.

Pathology

Acute phase:	Erythema and then swelling, cyanosis, blister formation, loss of epidermis.
Incipient pressure sore:	Loss of epidermis, exposure of dermis, abscess formation, exposure of necrotic fat.
Chronic phase:	Deep destruction extending from skin and fat through fascia, muscle and synovial membrane, or even involving joint. Osteitis or osteomyelitis, dislocation or pathological fractures.

Long standing ulcer:	Inverted cone shape, i.e. superficially the ulcer is smaller in diameter, but much larger in depth. Most often the floor of the ulcer is formed by bone covered by a membrane. The edge of ulcer may show evidence of healing and repeated breakdown. Floor is covered by unhealthy/pale granulation tissues.
Infection:	Bacterial invasion leads to tissue breakdown and production of foul smelling purulent discharge. In long-standing cases, this leads to protein deficiency, anemia, fever, poor general health.
Bacteriology:	Usually staphylococci, streptococci, *Pseudomonas aeruginosa, Proteus, E. coli.*
Complicated ulcers:	In long-standing cases, there are multiple sinus formation, may communicate with urinary bladder or rectum. Secondary amyloidosis occurs in 30% cases by about one year. Ultimately leads to chronic renal failure.

Pressure Sore Grading

Grade I: Involving epidermis and dermis.
Heat, swelling, induration redness.
Erythema/absence of blanching.
Healing time: 10–14 days for re-epithelialization
Reversible lesion.

Grade II: Involves epidermis, dermis and subcutaneous fat.
Full thickness ulcer with increased inflammatory and fibrotic involvement. Surrounding area—inflamed.
Healing time: 3 weeks to 3 months.
Re-epithelialization—with collagen and fibrosis leading to scar tissue.
Reversible lesion.

Grade III (Fig. 9.1): Involving epidermis, dermis and adipose tissue and involving muscle.
Extensive undermining.
Edges: Rolled out.
Infection: Present.
Bone: Subperiosteal new bone formation and local osteoporosis.
Joints: Synovial effusion, restriction of movement.
Healing time: Variable, may need surgical repair.
Life-threatening.

Grade IV: Soft tissue necrosis down to bone and joint
Extensive undermining, bursa formation.

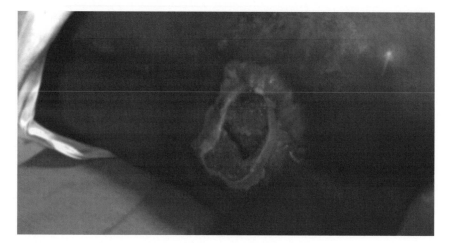

Fig. 9.1: Grade III pressure sore (sacral) in a paraplegic
(For color version, see Plate 5)

Osteomyelitis, septic arthritis, subluxation and dislocation in joints.
Systemic involvement: Anemia, hypoproteinuria, fluid loss.
X-ray: Evidence of bone involvement with osteomyelitis.
Healing: Always needs surgical treatment.
Life-threatening.
[From Eris JE Sarmiento A. The physiology and management of pressure sores. Orthop Rev. 1973;2(10):25-34.]

Distribution of Pressure Sore

In different studies it is seen that majority of the patients develop pressure sores while in hospital and sacral, trochanteric and ischial pressure sores are the most common. Following anatomical sites are important **(Fig. 9.2)**:
- Sacrum = 29%
- Trochanter = 19%
- Ischial tuberosity = 18%
- Heel
- Pretibial
- Malleolus
- Patella
- Foot
- Anterior superior iliac spine
- Elbow
- Other places

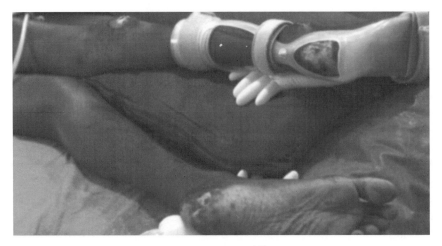

Fig. 9.2: Pressure sores at different sites
(For color version, see Plate 5)

Management of Pressure Sore

It can be divided as follows:
1. Systemic
2. Local
   a. Conservative
   b. Surgical

Systemic Measures

Nutrition: The measures undertaken may vary with chronicity of lesion and patient's nutritional status. In the presence of hypoproteinuria, the formation of ulcer is rapid and healing is slow. Patients need high protein, high calorie diet with adequate vitamin and mineral supplementation leading to positive nitrogen balance.

Anemia: Every effort should be made to maintain hemoglobin level around 11–12 g/dL by a combination of diet, drugs and blood transfusion.

Treatment of underlying disease: As for example, diabetes, chronic renal failure, infection, etc. must be treated accordingly.

Relief of spasm: The presence of spasm in the paraplegic patients has an adverse effect on them. When there are no ulcers, measures should be taken to prevent and correct spasm. In presence of sores, spasmodic movement of that part interferes with the healing of ulcers. Surgical treatment is going to fail invariably in presence of spasms. There are various methods to correct spasm:
   a. *Pharmacological agents:* Diazepam, baclofen, dantrolene sodium, dimethothiazine, mephemisin carbonate, etc.

b. *Surgical:* Intrathecal injection of alcohol, selective anterior rootlet rhizotomy, bilateral anterior rootlet rhizotomy, peripheral obturator neurectomy with adductor tenotomy.

[The different measures have been discussed in other chapters.]

Local Treatment

Conservative:

1. Early detection
2. Pressure relief
3. Hygiene
4. Dressing of sore
5. Care of linen beds

1. *Early detection:* This is very important step in management. Following are the early signs:
   a. Blanching
   b. Appearance of pressure mark
   c. Erythema
   d. Edema of skin and subcutaneous, blister formation
   e. Loss of epidermis and then varying thickness of tissue.

2. *Pressure relief:* This must be started as early as possible. This will be discussed in short.
   a. Change of posture every 1-2 hours.
      i. Avoid positioning over involved area.
      ii. Take proper precaution and splintage of spine during turning (splintage of spine).
      iii. Turning intervals are increased as patient tolerance improves.
   b. Use of proper mattress and pillows to protect bony prominences, i.e. sacrum, heels, ankles (when supine) and around knee, iliac spines, shoulder, chest (when prone).
   c. Shearing and friction—should be avoided.
   d. Bedsheets and linen should be kept free from wrinkles.
   e. Wheel chairs
      Ischial pressure must be relieved using the following techniques:
      i. *Raises:* Periodic raises from seat at an interval of 15 minutes.
      ii. *Weight shift techniques:* Pushups, leaning, sideways or reclining backwards.
      iii. Positioning in chair
         — Proper alignment of body with chair.
         — Keeping footrests properly positioned.
         — Adjusting wheelchair arm support.
   f. Mechanical means a variety of devices are available:
      i. Foam mattress
      ii. Air fluidized mattress
      iii. Circle—electric and striker frame
      iv. Riple mattress
      v. Different types of wheelchair cushions.

3. *Hygiene:* Daily cleaning with soap and water in a tub or shower to reduce the bacterial population on the body surface. The skin of perineum, axilla, buttocks, anal and genital regions need special care for these areas continuously remain wet with sweat, urine, feces or secretion from vagina. Cotton linen and garments are preferable to synthetic one. Tight external catheters should be avoided.

4. *Dressing:* Superficial ulcers or grade I sore can be kept exposed with application of antiseptic lotion. But deep pressure sores must be covered by well padded dressing so that the discharged fluid gets soaked in the dressing and linen remains dry. Frequency of the change of dressing will depend on amount of discharge from the ulcer. Large cavities should be packed lightly with gauze soaked in antiseptic solution till the patient is prepared for surgery. If the dressing is contaminated with stool or urine it should be changed immediately.

5. *Care of linen:*
   Linen — should be made of cotton and smooth.
          — should be kept dry and wrinkle free.
          — should be changed daily and immediately when it is soiled.

Surgical Treatment

Objective: The objective of surgical treatment of pressure sores are as follows:
1. Excision of wound, the fibrous tissue, bursa and infected scar tissue right up to healthy bleeding surface.
2. Resection of body prominences at the base of the ulcer.
3. Coverage of the defect with a composite tissue flap, which is capable to withstand the pressure.

Timing: Surgery should be done when:
1. General condition of the patient improves.
2. Ulcer is covered by healthy granulation tissue and evidence of peripheral healing.
3. Biological parameters are satisfactory, i.e. Hb level is 10 g/dL and above, no protein deficiency, diabetes is controlled, etc.

General Principles

Preoperative preparation—thorough assessment of the patient.
- Optimization of any deficiency.
- Pulmonary function test and optimization.
- Cardiac assessment and optimization.
- Correction of hemoglobin and protein deficiency.
- Antibiotics.
- Care of bowel and bladder.
- Planning of surgery—flap design (keeping in mind the lifestyle of the patient in future).

Anesthesia

Keeping in mind that there is sensory loss, most of the surgeons prefer—operation under sedation by an experienced anesthetist and strict monitoring over fluid and blood loss (replacement).

However, general anesthesia may be preferred when the patient has severe muscle spasm.

During positioning on the table, special care should be taken about the spine (especially cervical spine), ventilation, catheters, and pressure areas on the body (with the operating tables).

The skin is prepared with antiseptic lotion, and draped properly.

Surgery

a. *Wound excision and determination of actual extent of ulcer:* The ulcer should be excised with a healthy margin. The excised material is comprised of ulcer margin, bursa, fibrous wall and base, necrotic tissues and bony prominences at the base and any osteomyelitic bone. Any cone shaped ulcer—after excision should appear a saucer shaped wound with base and wall comprising of healthy granulation tissue.

b. *Flap planning:* Following things should be kept in mind:
   1. Size of the defect.
   2. Depth of the defect.
   3. Area surrounding the defect.
   4. Muscle/musculocutaneous flaps are better than fasciocutaneous flap because it provides better vascularity and withstand more pressure.

Area-wise Preference of Method of Wound Resurfacing

Sacral pressure sore:
- Primary closure
- Skin graft
- Gluteus maximus myocutaneous flap
- Gluteus maximus myocutaneous island flap
- Gluteus maximus V-Y myocutaneous flap
- Gluteal thigh flap.

Ischial pressure sore:
- Primary closure
- Gluteal thigh flap
- Inferior gluteus maximus myocutaneous flap
- Hamstring muscle or myocutaneous flap
- Biceps femoris myocutaneous flap
- Medially-based posterior thigh flap.

Trochanteric pressure sore:
- Tensor fascia lata myocutaneous flap
- Vastus lateralis myocutaneous flap
- Gluteal thigh flap

- Gluteus maximus (distally based flap)
- Anteriorly-based random thigh flap.

Multiple pressure sore: Amputation is considered at a suitable level.

Malignant change: Though rare, it may occur in an ulcer of long-standing duration (i.e. 10–15 years). Most often it is squamous cell carcinoma. Prognosis is poor.

Complications

1. Hematoma and seroma
2. Wound infection
3. Wound gaping
4. Flap necrosis
5. Recurrence.

Postoperative Management

1. Maintenance of Hb level and adequate hydration, nutrition.
2. Care of drain—which should be kept for a longer time, i.e. as long as serous fluid comes out.
3. Care of catheters.
4. Care of wound—flaps must be inspected periodically and dressed. Grafted areas should be managed very carefully as friction and mobilization of the patient may dislodge the graft resulting in graft loss.

   Patient should be positioned in bed in such a way so that pressure on the flap can be avoided.

Psychological Factors/Counseling of the Patient

There is no doubt that it plays a very important role in development and healing of pressure sore. Almost all patients after spinal injury, remain depressed and it is very difficult to mobilize the patient because they refuse to cooperate and to learn the self-care methods. Psychological counseling helps them to motivate and to arouse strong will to lead a meaningful life.

Patient education: After psychological counseling, proper steps for self care will be helpful for prevention and management of pressure ulcers. Daily skin care, inspection, transfer and shifting of weight, use of different orthosis and wheelchair—all of these should be taught by a team of therapists and nursing staffs by proper demonstration, audio-visual aids and motivating the patient.

Staff education: Care of these unfortunate patients is very much specialized one—and needs multidisciplinary approach. All the staffs like ward boys, nurses, doctors, therapists, ward cleaners—must be trained properly regarding their basic responsibilities.

Informed consent: Treating a patient of bed sore with spinal injury is more of bed sore than managing a simple ulcer. Treatment is formulated according to the family's financial ability and the degree of their active participation. The outcome of treatment is largely dependant on patients motivation and will.

Properly informed consent must cover the following topics:
1. Diagnosis or probable diagnosis.
2. Description of treatment and its purpose.
3. Inherent risks and complications.
4. Probable outcome.
5. Duration of treatment, future lifestyle of patient.
6. Alternative treatment, if available.
7. Consequences of refusing treatment.
8. Gross idea regarding cost of treatment.

Patient party must be explained that there is no warranty for cure, however, the warranty is for service.

BIBLIOGRAPHY

1. Bale S, Regnard C. Pressure sores in advanced disease: A flow diagram. Palliative Medicine. 1989;3:263-65.
2. Bouten, et al. The etiology of pressure ulcers: Skin deep or muscle bound? Archive of Physical Medicine and Rehabilitation. 2003;84(4):616-19.
3. Braden B, Bergstorm N. A conceptual schema for the study of the etiology of pressure sore, Rehabilitation Nursing. 1987;12(1):8-12.
4. Breslow, et al. The importance of dietary protein in healing pressure ulcers. Journal of American Geriatric Society. 1993;41(4):357-62.
5. Campbell RM. The surgical management of pressure sores. The Surgical Clinics of North America. 1959;39(2):509-30.
6. Daniel, et al. Etiologic factor in pressure sore: an experimental model. Archive of Physical Medicine and Rehabilitation. 1981;62(10):492-96.
7. Daniel, et al. Pressure sores and paraplegia: An experimental model. Annals of Plastic Surgery. 1985;15(1):1-88.
8. Knight AL. Medical management of pressure sores. The Journal of Family Practice. 1988;27(1):95-100.
9. Maklebust J. Pressure ulcers: Etiology and prevention. The Nursing Clinics of North America. 1987;22(2):359-77.
10. Mawson, et al. Risk factors for early occurring pressure ulcers following spinal cord injury. American Journal of Physical Medicine and Rehabilitation. 1988;67(3):93-133.
11. Reddy, et al. Treatment of pressure ulcers: A systemic review. The Journal of the American Medical Association. 2008;300(22):2647-62.
12. Reuler JB, Cooney TG. The pressure sore: Pathophysiology and principles of management. Annals of Internal Medicine. 1981;94(5):661-66.
13. Shea JD. Pressure sore: Classification and management. Clinical Orthopaedics and Related Research. 1975;112:89-100.
14. Theaker, et al. Risk factors for pressure sore in the critically ill. Anesthesia. 2000;55(3):221-24.
15. Yarkong GM. Pressure ulcers: A review. Archive of Physical Medicine and Rehabilitation. 1994;75(8):908-17.
16. Yarkony, et al. Classification of pressure ulcers. Archive of Dermatology. 1990;126(9):1218-19.

10

Swallowing Problems in Stroke and Brain Injury

K Venugopal, Indu Marium Jacob

Normal swallowing is a complex, dynamic neuromuscular activity that depends on a set of physiological activities resulting in liquid and solid material moving efficiently and safely from the mouth to the stomach.[1,2,13] It is also additionally concerned with protection of the airway, rejection of noxious ingested substances and the preparation of foods.[1-3] When swallowing is disrupted, the consequences can be devastating for the sufferer, with complications such as malnutrition, pulmonary aspiration and associated psychosocial stigma of being unable to eat. The implications of swallowing difficulty are, therefore of considerable importance to clinicians of all discipline.[2,8,9,13]

The causes of swallowing impairment (dysphagia) can be divided into neurological and mechanical/systemic causes.[1,2] Neurological causes include stroke, traumatic brain injury, progressive neurological disorders (Parkinson's disease, dementia) tumors in the central nervous system, meningitis, cerebral palsy, neurosurgery, and many more. Mechanical/systemic causes include infection, edema, obstruction (abscess, tumor or physical object), stricture (pharyngeal or esophageal) pharyngeal pouch, congenital, aging and drug induced.

This chapter focuses on swallowing impairment caused mainly by traumatic brain injury (TBI). Dysphagia is one of the most serious deficits in function that can result from brain injury, the consequences of which, at best, may hinder a patient's recovery to normal function, and at worst lead to death. Therefore, it is of utmost importance that the brain-injured persons are evaluated and necessary management is provided to ensure that they get adequate and safe oral nutrition and hydration either by oral or alternative non-oral methods of feeding.[8,9,13]

This chapter discusses the physiology of normal swallowing, the central control for swallowing, assessment of swallowing dysfunction and management of swallowing dysfunction in the brain-injured person.

Oral Preparatory Phase

This part of the swallowing is voluntary. It is a mechanical phase that can be by-passed by dropping liquid or food into the back of the throat.[1] In this stage, the food is chewed into smaller pieces and tasted. It is also mixed with saliva from three pairs of salivary glands, which are innervated by the glossopharyngeal nerve.[2,3] The food and saliva form a bolus of material.

The bolus is kept in the front of the mouth, against the hard palate by the tongue. The front of the tongue is elevated with its tip on the alveolar ridge. The back of the tongue is elevated and the soft palate is pulled anteriorly against it to keep the food in the oral cavity (the airway is open and nasal breathing continues during this phase). Labial seal is maintained to prevent food from leaking out of the mouth. Buccal muscles are tense. This prevents pocketing of food. Duration of the oral-preparatory stage is variable.

Oral Transport Stage

This stage of the swallowing is also voluntary. It starts with the jaws and lips closed, and the tongue tip on the alveolar ridge.[1] The pattern-elicited response is initiated at the end of this phase. Inspiration is reflexively inhibited at the beginning of this stage. The food is moved to the back of the mouth by the tongue by an anterior to posterior rolling motion. The anterior portion of the tongue is retracted and depressed while the posterior portion is retracted and elevated against the hard palate. When the bolus passes the anterior faucial pillars or touches the posterior wall of the pharynx, the oral stage ends and the pharyngeal stage begins as the tongue's driving force or the tongue's plunger action, forces the bolus into the pharynx. Logemann[2] describes the "pharyngeal tongue" which extends from the velum to the hyoid bone and valleculae. The "oral tongue" which extends from the tip to the back, adjacent to the velum, functions during the oral stage of the swallow while the "pharyngeal tongue" functions during the pharyngeal stage. The oral transport stage lasts one second.

Pharyngeal Stage

The pharyngeal phase of the swallow is involuntary. It is the most critical stage of the swallow; airway closure must occur to prevent the bolus from entering the respiratory system.[1,2] A number of things occur almost simultaneously.[2,3]

1. Sensory information from receptors in the back of the mouth and in the pharynx goes to the swallowing center in the medulla via IX cranial nerve. The palatopharyngeal folds pull together medially to form a slit in the upper pharynx. The bolus passes through this slit.
2. The velum is raised, primarily by the levator and tensor veli palatini muscles. This prevents the entry of food into the nasopharynx. The narrowing of the upper pharynx due to the contraction of superior pharyngeal constrictor muscle helps to close the velopharyngeal port.
3. The tongue is retracted, preventing the food from re-entering the mouth.

Laryngeal Substage

Three actions occur simultaneously to protect the airway.[2,3] (Obviously, inspiration is inhibited during the pharyngeal stage of the swallow.)

1. The larynx and the hyoid bone are pulled both upward and forward. This movement enlarges the pharynx. It also creates a vacuum in the hypopharynx, pulling the bolus downward. Finally, it contributes to the relaxation of the cricopharyngeous muscle.
2. The true and false vocal folds adduct. (Closure begins at the level of the true vocal folds and progresses up to the false vocal folds and then to the ari-epiglottic folds.)
3. The epiglottis drops down over the top of the larynx, protecting the airway and diverting the bolus into the pyriform sinuses. The bolus passes down on both sides of the epiglottis. If the bolus is liquid, the epiglottis acts as a ledge to slow its movement through the pharynx, giving the vocal folds time to adduct and the larynx time to elevate. (Nevertheless, the action of the epiglottis is the least important of these three movements.)

Three factors cause food to move down the pharynx during the rest of the pharyngeal stage:[2,3]

1. The tongue driving force using the "pharyngeal tongue".
2. The stripping action of the pharyngeal constrictors .
3. The presence of negative pressure in the laryngopharynx.

It is believed by some that the tongue driving force (TDF) is the most important of these factors. This generates pressure in the upper pharynx.

The pharyngeal stage ends when the cricopharyngeus muscle relaxes, allowing the bolus to enter the esophageus. It is believed that the following three factors affect the opening of the pharyngeal esophageal segment, although the process is not currently well understood:[2,3]

1. Innervation by the vagus nerve.
2. The timing of the stripping action in the pharynx may somehow trigger the relaxation of the pharyngoesophageal (PE) segment.
3. The elevation of the larynx may pull the muscle upward, causing it to open by stretching it and therefore causing it to relax.

Esophageal Stage

In this phase, which is of course involuntary, the bolus is moved down the esophageus via peristaltic wave motion with some help from gravity.[1-3]

At the beginning of the phase, the larynx lowers, returning to its normal position. The cricopharyngeus muscle contracts to prevent reflux and respiration resumes.

This stage normally lasts between three and twenty seconds, but in elderly persons peristalsis is slower.

Esophageal problems can cause the reflux of food back into the pharynx, leading to aspiration. It is important to differentiate these problems.

Central Control of Swallowing

Stimulation studies have shown that regions in the brainstem, specifically in the pons and the medulla that will evoke a swallowing reflex when stimulated.[4,5] The motor nuclei for many of the muscles involved in swallowing also are located in the brainstem.[1-5] However, direct stimulation of these nuclei produces a contraction of only a specific muscle group and does not generate a complete swallowing reflex.[5] Therefore, the motor nuclei themselves are distal to the interneurons that are responsible for initiating the swallow reflex.

Within the pons, regions dorsal and ventral to the trigeminal nucleus will evoke swallowing, when stimulated.[4] The dorsal region is a reticular formation that receives ascending sensory input from the pharynx and in turn transmits this information to the thalamus. The region ventral to the trigeminal nucleus is the part of the descending cortical-subcortical pathway. Both of these regions are responsible for conveying information about swallowing rather than its actual control.

Two areas lower in the brainstem are more closely associated with the control of swallowing.[4,5] One of these, the nucleus tractus solitarius (NTS), lies in the dorsal medulla. Many of the peripheral nerves that initiate swallowing when stimulated, such as the superior laryngeal nerve, synapse in the NTS and in the adjacent reticular formation.[4,5] The NTS also contains synapses from the cortical region that evoke swallowing. Synapses to the interneurons have very short latencies. When they fire, a burst of activity is sent to the motor nuclei with a specific timing sequence that evokes a coordinated swallow.[5]

Between the NTS and the dorsal motor nuclei of the vagus nerve is a separate region that receives input from pharyngeal receptors and is crucial for generating the esophageal phase of swallowing.[5] Unilateral lesions here or in the NTS do not prevent a swallow if the contralateral superior laryngeal nerve is stimulated, implying that there is bilateral duplication of this control.[4,5]

The second region in the medulla, lying more ventrally, that plays a role in swallowing is the nucleus ambiguous (NA). Stimulation of the NA will produce the esophageal, but not the pharyngeal phase of swallowing.[5] The NA receives sensory input from the superior laryngeal nerve, but the latencies of these signals are greater that the NTS (7 millisecond versus 2-4 milliseconds in the NTS).[5] Cortical input to this region is more extensive than in the NTS. These cortical inputs are believed to be primarily involved in the modulation of activity during swallowing.[4,5] The NA has multiple synaptic connections with ipsilateral and contralateral motor nuclei and brainstem regions that are involved in swallowing. The NA has been called the "switching" nuclei for swallowing, compared with the "master" neurons in the NTS.[5]

Role of the Cerebral Cortex

The cerebral cortex is known to play a major role in the initiation of the voluntary and pharyngeal phase of swallowing.[4,5] Muscle contraction during the involuntary phase of swallowing often has considered to be primarily influenced by lower brainstem activity.[5] Because these brainstem regions receive bilateral cortical input, bilateral injury was previously felt necessary to impair swallowing.[5] Recent work has shown, however, that the cortex may play a more significant role in facilitating swallowing and that unilateral lesions may be more damaging than previously believed. These findings are based both on stimulation and on observations of changes following stroke.[5]

Stimulation of a region immediately in front of the precentral cortex evokes swallowing that often is associated with mastication.[4,5] Surface electrodes stimulation of the lateral precentral and sylvian cortex during awake craniotomies for epilepsy surgery produces swallowing that is accompanied with orofacial movement, salivation, and vocalisation.[5] In experimental animals, the greatest disruption of swallowing was produced with lesions in the lowest part of the precentral gyrus and the posterior portion of the inferior frontal gyrus.[5] These cortical regions are felt to modify the duration and intensity of swallowing and to coordinate the interaction of facial, tongue, and masticatory muscles. The actions involves are related to tongue movement, elevation of the hyoid bone, adduction of the vocal folds, and contraction of the upper esophagus. The pathways of these cortical regions descend through the internal capsule and subthalamic region to the substantia nigra and the mesencephalic reticular formation. Stimulation of these regions also produces swallowing that is associated with mastication.[5] Reflex swallowing is facilitated by input from the hypothalamus and the midbrain ventral tegmental field, and exposing these regions to dopamine will increase this facilitation.[5]

Characteristics of Swallowing Disorders in the Brain Injury

Neurological impairment caused by brain injury may affect oral, pharyngeal and esophageal function of the swallowing mechanism. Each of these stages will be taken separately and the disorders that occur after brain injury in each will be enumerated.

Oral Stage

The abnormalities in swallowing seen after head injury in the oral stage include, inability or poor opening of mouth due to damage to the trigeminal nerve and primitive oral reflex such as bite reflex, which involves involuntary biting with difficulty in releasing.[10-12] Both of the above will interfere with the entry of food into the mouth and chewing of the food. Poor lip seal and spillage of food is commonly seen with facial nerve palsy.[13] Usually it is unilateral and sometimes associated with neglect where the patient is not aware of the leakage of food. The most frequent problem identified in the oral stage is reduced tongue movement and control which results in loss of bolus control or manipulation, pocketing of food in the mouth, poor anterior-posterior transition of the bolus and inability to generate force to push the bolus into the pharynx.[10-12]

Pharyngeal Stage

The main feature in the pharyngeal stage is the swallow reflex. Therefore, the problems that may occur are, nasal regurgitation or entry or food into the nasal cavity due to poor closure of the soft palate during the swallow reflex and delayed trigger of the swallow reflex due to reduced sensation or delay in relaying the message to the swallowing center.[12,13] Total absence of the swallow reflex is less frequently seen. Silent aspiration is common in severe brain injury where there is reduced or no pharyngolaryngeal sensation and weak or no cough reflex. The other common problem that increases the risk of aspiration is decreased laryngeal closure and decreased laryngeal elevation.[13] Unilateral or bilateral pharyngeal paralysis results in reduced peristaltic movement of the pharyngeal muscles and therefore inability to push the food to the next stage. Dysfunction of the cricopharyngeal segment, though not commonly seen, in combination with pharyngeal paralysis results in poor clearance and pooling of food in the pharynx, which increases the risk of aspiration.[2,12,13]

Esophageal Stage

The common neurological problem seen in this stage is the poor motility or peristaltic motion, therefore food not transported properly and person feels a sensation of the food getting stuck in the neck.[2]

The above entails many of the swallowing problems faced after head injury. However, there are other factors that interfere with the swallowing function and makes swallowing management challenging. These are, poor cognition, behavioral problems, severity of the injury, low consciousness level indicated by the Glasgow Coma Scale (GCS), and the presence of tracheostomy.

Impaired Cognition

Due to the high frequency of diffuse axonal injury, combined with localized frontal and temporal lobe damage, TBI tends to result in a characteristic range of cognitive impairments.[7] These include deficits in attention, and speed of information processing, learning and memory, executive function and the inability to think in abstract terms, reduced initiative, inflexible thought processes and impairment of the ability to control and monitor thought and behavior.[6,7] The precise nature and extent of these problems varies widely, depending on the function of the location and severity of injury, as well as premorbid factors. As many follow-up studies have demonstrated, they may affect the TBI individual's capacity to preform many of the activities that are necessary and relevant in daily life including swallowing.[6]

In relation to swallowing, cognitive problems interfere with the swallowing functioning because they have poor insight and comprehension and so might hold food in their mouth and swallow the food without chewing.[6,10,12] Poor attending skills make the patient very distractable and not to concentrate on the task of eating or focus on what the clinician has told them to do.[6] Frequently seen in TBI is short-term memory deficit. In this case putting forth strategies to swallow safely becomes very difficult, the patient may not be able to remember them and has to be reminded every time.[6,10,12] Many of these behaviors as a result of the cognitive impairment make the evaluation and management of swallowing very challenging.[6,8-10,12,13]

Behavioral Problems

The behavioral changes most frequently documented include the development of impulsivity, a low frustration tolerance, verbally threatening or physically aggressive behaviors, disinhibited inappropriate, irresponsible social behavior, self-centeredness leading to attention seeking and/or manipulative behavior, change in emotional expression and at the other end of the spectrum, reduced drive and motivation often accompanied by extreme slowness.[7] Such changes occur alone or in combination, and in widely varying degrees. In many instances they are also accompanied by a lack of insight on the part of the injured person, who may therefore fail to acknowledge or understand the differences others perceive.[7] This can result in a willingness or inability to modify the difficult behavior.

These behavioral problems greatly impact on swallowing because the patient may not be cooperative or refuse to take food, spit food out, shows adamant, impulsiveness (stuff food into mouth) or lack of interest, often after few mouthfuls refuse to take more and if compelled becomes aggressive. It is a great challenge for the clinician to overcome these behavior problems and ensure that the patient is swallowing safely.[10,12,13]

Severity of Injury

The greater the neurologic injury, the greater the risk for swallowing and aspirations. Though many studies have not investigated what type of lesion causes greater swallowing impairment, Rowe, based on clinical experience and anecdotal evidence proposed that patients with epidural hematomas have fewer swallowing problems than those with subdural hemorrhages due to the depth of injury.

Low Consciousness Level or Low GCS Scores

The brain-injured persons with low GCS scores display more swallowing impairment than those with a higher GCS score.[8-13] This is because with a higher GCS, the patient is more alert and has better motor control. Studies have revealed that a risk factor for abnormal swallowing and aspiration is a lower admitting GCS score.[8,9,13]

Presence of Tracheotomy

Studies have shown that a number of patients with tracheotomies had abnormal swallowing.[13] This is because the presence of a tracheotomy tube can contribute to aspiration. It prevents the use of air from the lungs to clear the larynx of matter and can restrict laryngeal elevation and diminish protection of the airway. Although a tracheotomy increases the risk of abnormal swallowing, its physical presence is not the sole or primary causative factor, because some patients with tracheotomy are able to swallow well.[13]

A brain-injured person may have varying difficulties in the different stages of the swallow function (oral, pharyngeal and esophageal). It is further complicated by poor alertness, impaired cognition, behavioral problems and presence of tracheostomy, etc. Therefore, dysphagia in persons with brain injury may pose a great threat to the patient's nutritional status and may slow or restrict patient's recovery progress. The speech pathologist in collaboration with other professionals in rehabilitation team such as the dietician, occupational therapist, physiotherapist, and the consulting doctor ensure that the patient is getting adequate and safe nutrition and hydration. This is done by thoroughly assessing the patient's swallowing function and then providing the appropriate management strategies.

Assessment of Swallowing

Assessment of the swallowing is very important in determining efficacy of the patient's swallow, what problems the patient exhibits and which all consistencies patient are able to tolerate or swallow well.[2,8,9] Swallowing assessment consists of clinical bedside evaluation and objective measures.[2,3] Both may be done separately or in combination. Clinical bedside assessment of swallowing (see Appendix) can provide the clinician with an indication of the nature and severity of dysphagia, establish a baseline oral-motor function, explore the impact of associated cognitive function and enable non-invasive evaluation of the various management options.[2] However, the drawback of clinical bedside swallowing assessment is that it cannot detect silent aspiration as this is commonly seen in head-injured patients.[2,8,9] Objective swallowing assessments can be used in detecting this. They include, barium swallow and its important derivative the videofluoroscopic swallowing study (VFSS), fiberoptic endoscopic evaluation of swallowing (FEES), manometry, manofluorography, bolus scintigraphy, ultrasonography, and videoendoscopic swallowing study. These allow the clinician to view the anatomy and physiology of the swallow and also pinpoint the area or areas of dysfunction within the swallowing process and therefore help in the process of selecting the appropriate management for the swallowing dysfunction.[2]

The most commonly used and more popular objective swallowing assessments are the fiberoptic endoscopic evaluation of swallowing (FEES) and the modified barium swallow MBS.[2,8,9] The FEES is a standard test using a small flexible fiberoptic endoscope (a small tube with a light on the end of it).[2] The endoscope is passed through the nose over the back of the velum to a position slightly above the voice box. In order to make the patient more comfortable, the inside of the nose is coated with a local anesthetic gel to reduce the sensation of the endoscope being passed. Once the patient is comfortable, he or she is given foods or liquids that are tinted with food dye so the examiner can follow their passage. The examiner then watches the material as it passes from the base of the tongue into the esophagus (swallowing passageway). Careful observation is made of foods and liquids that are retained in various areas. In addition, careful observation is made of any of the food substances that drip into the airway causing the patient to cough or choke. Important aspects such as the speed of the swallow, the amount of food or liquid that is not swallowed on the first swallow, and amounts of foods or liquids that drop near or into the airway can be observed under clear vision. At the same time, a recording of the entire examination is made so that the treatment team can view the results with the patient as often as necessary and offer a plan of treatment.

The MBS (or videofluoroscopy) is an X-ray study of swallowing.[1,2] That means it is done with a radiologist using a camera capable of taking video recording. This examination is well suited for patients with complaints of choking or regurgitating, or for patients who have had past episodes of pneumonia. Under X-ray observation, the patient ingests substances of varying consistencies coated with barium. The study usually starts with thin barium and, if the patient is able, proceeds to barium with thicker consistencies such as pudding or even a cookie. Frontal and lateral views of the swallow are obtained during the modified barium swallow with the patient in standing or sitting. The MBS is a purely dynamic study of swallowing and is recorded on videotape. Still film images are usually not made, although for specific disorders, still pictures may be obtained as well. The MBS identifies problems that occur in the mouth, at the base of the tongue, in the pharynx, or in the esophageus. In addition, this study also provides information about tongue motion and coordination and timing of the swallow. This study is useful not only to identify the problem, but it also offers information as to how to treat the problem.[2] The modified barium swallow has been used for almost 20 years to identify problems of swallowing.[1,2]

Assessment of swallowing function in patients with head injury may pose to be a great challenge because of the associated poor alertness, impaired comprehension skills, poor cognitive skills, and behavioral problems. During a clinical bedside examination patients may not be alert, may not cooperate and may not understand the tasks of the assessment. Therefore, the clinician may find it difficult to assess those skills such as oral motors skills, checking for cough reflex and dry swallow so that the clinician may have an idea of the swallowing mechanism before trialing with different consistencies of food. In these cases, the clinician may start straight with the swallowing trial with thick semisolids (such as honey or gungee/gruel). This is because to start the trial with fluids and solids may be unsafe as the clinician is unsure of the patient's oral motor control and swallow reflex. Once the clinician obtains an idea of the patient's swallowing skills he/she can then try with different consistencies and evaluate the efficacy of the swallowing function.

Formal objective assessments are useful in detecting silent aspiration and by viewing the swallow taking place, area of dysfunction can be determined.

However, in patients with TBI, these objective measures may be difficult to conduct because of the lower levels of consciousness, impaired cognition and behavioral problems.[8,9]

O'Neil-Pirozzi and colleagues[9] have suggested that objective swallowing assessment should be considered more regularly with these patients. This is because of the high incidence of aspiration and documented risk for silent aspiration in these cases and also limitations of a bedside swallowing assessment especially regarding its inability to identify silent aspiration. They conducted a study subjecting 12 tracheotomized patients with TBI with severely disordered levels of consciousness (Rancho Los Amigos II or vegetative state and Rancho Los Amigos III or minimally conscious state) to objective swallowing assessment. In their study all 12 patients were able to participate in the objective testing. Three of the 12 subjects aspirated and they did so silently. The rest of the nine subjects were able to swallow some of the different consistencies without aspirating. In addition based on the swallowing function viewed, the speech pathologists were able to give appropriate and better therapeutic strategies. The authors concluded by saying that tracheostomized individuals with severely disordered levels of consciousness following TBI who are in the acute rehabilitation stage are appropriate candidates for objective swallowing assessment. They suggest that they may be poor candidates when: swallow is not observed spontaneously and cannot be elicited using digital stimulation to the laryngeal area; a profound bite reflex is present and/or the patient cannot tolerate an upright position for a minimum of 15 minutes. Through their study they proved that objective swallowing assessment helps in detecting silent aspiration and not placing patients at unnecessary risk for aspiration. It also helps in the decision of the rehabilitation programs for these individuals. More similar studies with larger number of patients are needed to support the present study.

Many have recommended that objective swallowing assessment should be a routine testing procedure for dysphagic patients.[2,3,8,9] Though this may be feasible in the western countries it may not be feasible in developing and underdeveloped countries because of the high cost for the test especially when majority of the patients come from a very low socioeconomic status.

Management of Dysphagia

Once the speech pathologist has thoroughly assessed the swallowing function of the person with brain injury, it should be clear which of the management strategies would be appropriate.[1, 2] Further options available to choose are: 1. To initiate or continue oral feeding as the sole means of intake, 2. Initiate oral feeding with the nasogastric tube still in place, implement swallowing management and gradually increase reliance on oral intake, 3. Initiate indirect treatment with a view to introducing oral feeding when patient is more able, 4. Postpone intervention and reassess the patient after a further period of recovery, and 5. Discuss the provision of a permanent alternative or aid to oral feeding.

In patients with TBI when the clinician decides to initiate oral feeding with the nasogastric tube in place, implement swallowing management and gradually increase reliance on oral intake, the line of management will usually be compensatory swallowing strategies.[2,3,8,9,13] This is because the level of cognitive and behavioral impairments impacts on the complexity of the intervention. Therefore, when using techniques such as indirect swallowing therapy (oral motor exercises) and swallowing maneuvers, it may be difficult in patients with brain injury because they have to be cooperative, understand the technique, remember to use the technique each time they swallow and be motivated to initiate these techniques without prompting. Thus, compensatory swallowing techniques are commonly used in the management of swallowing in patients with brain injury because of its simplicity (yet effective) and minimal or no participation from the patient. The compensatory swallowing techniques include behavioral, postural and dietary modification.

Behavioral Modification

Behavioral modification includes changing or creating a quite, nondistracting environment.[2,8] Making the environment pleasurable for eating. Supervision during feeding is required in order to ensure that the patient is not impulsive with the food, making sure that the patient clears the mouth before the next mouthful and prompting for repeated swallows per mouthful for proper clearance.[1,2,8] Altering or modifying the texture, taste, volume or temperature of food can be tried to increase sensation and initiation of the swallow reflex.[2] Finally having visual or written cues to help patient during feeding times.[2,8]

Postural Modifications

The recommended posture for feeding is to be seated in a chair with feet placed firmly on the floor at a comfortable distance apart.[1,2] The spine should be erect and central and the head and neck lightly flexed. Whenever the patient cannot achieve this position, the best possible approximation should be arranged. Mobile arm supports for the chair arms can be helpful. Propping with pillows may be necessary as an expedient. If the patient cannot maintain head control, the feeder stands beside him on one side and passes her arm behind his chair so that her hand can support his chin on the other side. Other postural changes that facilitate safe swallow include[1-3]:

1. Chin-down posture involves touching the chin to the neck. It pushes the anterior pharyngeal wall posteriorly, the tongue base and epiglottis are pushed closer to the pharyngeal wall, airway entrance (space between epiglottic base and arytenoid cartilage) is narrowed and vallecular space is widened. It is helpful for those who have a delay in triggering the pharyngeal swallow, reduced tongue base retraction, and/or reduced airway entrance closure.

2. Chin-up posture involves tilting the head back. It allows food to drain from the oral cavity using gravity. It is helpful to patients with reduced tongue control.

3. Head rotation involves turning the head to the damaged side. It twists the pharynx and closes the damaged side of the pharynx, it pushes the damaged vocal fold toward midline improving adduction and food flows down the stronger side. It is helpful for patients with unilateral pharyngeal wall impairment or unilateral vocal fold weakness.

4. Chin down and head rotation: can combine these positions to protect the airway.

5. Head tilt in which the head is tilted to the stronger side. It uses gravity to drain food down stronger side and have better control. It is helpful for patients with both unilateral oral impairment and a unilateral pharyngeal impairment on the same side. If the patient is not able to maintain these positions, the caregiver can manually hold it. Postural modifications are simple and effective in repositioning the oropharyngeal structures and redirecting food boluses away from the airway.

Dietary Modification

Patients with swallowing difficulties of neurological origin usually find semi-solids easier to manage, while patients with a mechanical cause for dysphagia often do better with liquids.[2] Patients with reduced pharyngeal peristalsis or with a tight cricopharyngeal sphincter may do best by alternating a small amount of semi-solids with a sip of liquid to wash it down.[1,2] If the problem is at the oral stage, and no effective manipulation of food can take place, liquids, puree and semi-solids may easiest to project into the pharynx. Patients with delayed swallow reflex may do well with substance such as semi-solids, puree or of thick consistency so that it gives them enough time to initiate the swallow and without entering into the airway.[1,2] Dietary modifications require little or no participation from the patient.[1,2,8] The changes are extremely helpful when penetration and aspiration is documented with specific consistencies.

Alternatives to Rehabilitation of Oral Feeding

Alternatives are necessary when patients are unable to feed orally either because it is unsafe or because the patient cannot obtain adequate nutrition and hydration by the oral route.[1-3]

The alternative is temporary in cases where recovery is expected.[1] Patients who may be expected to make a recovery in time include the majority of those with non-progressive neurological etiology, and those postsurgical and traumatic patients who have shown no permanent mechanical obstacle to recovery during radiographic examination. However, not all patients who are expected to recover achieve oral feeding, and a temporary alternative is sometimes replaced with a more permanent method.[1,2]

The alternative methods include nasogastric tube and gastrostomy. The nasogastric tube is the most common temporary expedient for bypassing oral intake.[1-3] Generally these tubes are inserted through the nose and passed down the pharynx and esophagus into the stomach, while the patient is supine. The nasogastric tubes are of varying sizes. Feeds, which are prepared by the dietician, must be given continuously. The tube may be left in place for a period of weeks or even months but problems of irritation, discomfort and infection increase with time.[1] Nasogastric tube feeding is also known to cause high incidence of gastroesophageal reflux and aspirations.[1,2]

Gastrostomy feeding is an alternative, which may be considered for permanent use, for example, when dysphagia is severe and is a symptom of progressive neurological disease.[1,2] Gastrostomy feeding significantly reduces gastroesophageal reflux and risk of aspirations.[1] Open surgical gastrostomy is a surgical procedure designed to provide permanent opening for passage of food into the stomach. This is first described in 1837[1] and was the main stay of direct enteral feeding for many decades. It is usually performed under anesthesia. An opening is made in the abdomen and in the stomach and tube is inserted. This tube is of sufficient diameter to allow the passage of puree consistencies. The site of the stoma has to be dressed regularly to prevent infection. Endoscopy assisted percutaneous gastrostomy (PEG) first described in 1980 is becoming popular and has largely replaced surgical gastrostomy. This procedure is minimally invasive and is usually done under local anesthesia. Though there are two techniques for doing PEG, pull technique is commonly used by gastroenterologist. This technique is also used to place a wider bore catheter. Gastrojejunostomy or Jejunostomy is reserved for patients with very high aspiration risk. These techniques are more complicated and technically demanding.

Conclusion

After stroke TBI is one of the leading causes of dysphagia. The swallowing dysfunction commonly seen after TBI are, loss of bolus control, reduced tongue movement/control, delayed trigger of the swallow reflex, decreased laryngeal protection, decreased laryngeal elevation and unilateral pharyngeal paralysis. In addition to the obvious physiological deficits that affect the swallowing mechanism it is further complicated by poor level of consciousness, impaired cognition and behavioral problems that interfere with successful oral intake.

Assessment of swallowing deficits includes both clinical bedside swallowing assessment and objective swallowing assessment (FEES and MBS). There is more emphasis on conducting objective swallowing assessment in these patients in spite of the poor consciousness level, impaired cognition and behavioral problems to detect silent aspiration, which cannot be detected on the clinical bedside swallowing assessment. Silent aspiration can be commonly seen in patients with severe brain injury.

Due to the cognitive and behavioral problems the common line of management of swallowing impairment in patients with TBI includes behavioral, postural and dietary modifications. These management strategies are less complex and require minimal or no participation from the patients. With the increased awareness and benefit of early rehabilitation intervention, evaluation and treatment of swallowing disorders become vital in the acute management of patients with traumatic brain injury.

References

1. Langley J. Working with Swallowing Disorders. Oxon: Winslow Press Limited, 1987.
2. Logemann JA. Evaluation and Treatment of Swallowing Disorders. Austin, TX: Pro-Ed, 1998.
3. Goher ME. Dysphagia: Diagnosis and Management. Butterworths, 1987.
4. Hamdy S, Rothwell JC, Aziz Q, Thompson DG. Organization and reorganization of human swallowing motor cortex: implications for recovery after stroke. Clinical Science. 2000;98:151-7.
5. Plant RL. Anatomy and Physiology of Swallowing in Adults and Geriatrics. Otolaryngologic Clinics of North America. 1998;31(3):477-88.
6. Halper AS, Cherney LR, Cichowski K, Zhang M. Dysphagia after head trauma: the effects of cognitive-communicative impairments on functional outcomes. Journal of Head Trauma Rehabilitation. 1999;14(5):486-96.
7. Ponsford J. Traumatic Brain Injury: Rehabilitation for Everyday Adaptive Living. Hove, UK: Lawrence Erlbaum Associates.
8. Schurr MJ, Ebner KA, Maser AL, Sperling KB, Helegerson RB, Harms B. Formal swallowing evaluation and therapy after traumatic brain injury improves dysphagia outcomes. Journal of Trauma: Injury, Infection, and Critical Care. 1999;46(5):817-23.
9. O'Neil-Pirozzi TM, Momose KJ, Mello J, Lepak P, McCabe M, Connors JJ, Lisiecki DJ. Feasibility of swallowing interventions for tracheostomized individuals with severely disordered consciousness following traumatic brain injury. Brain Injury. 2003;17(5):389-99.
10. Morgan A, Ward E, Murdoch B, Kennedy B, Murison R. Incidence, characteristics, and predictive factors for dysphagia after pediatric traumatic brain injury. Journal of Head Trauma Rehabilitation. 2003;18(3):239-51.
11. Morgan A, Ward E, Murdoch B. Clinical progression and outcome of dysphagia following paediatric traumatic brain injury: a prospective study. Brain Injury. 2004;18(4):359-76.
12. Morgan A, Ward E, Murdoch B. Clinical characteristics of acute dysphagia in paediatric patients following traumatic brain injury. Journal of Head Trauma Rehabilitation. 2004;19(3):226-40.
13. Mackay LE, Morgan AS, Bernstein BR. Swallowing disorders in severe brain injury: risk factors affecting return to oral intake. Archive of Physical Medicine and Rehabilitation. 1999;80:365-71.

11

Psychiatric Rehabilitation in Stroke

Srilekha Biswas

Strokes or cerebrovascular accidents are characterized by rapidly developing science of focal disturbance of cerebral function. They occur when blood flow to a region of the brain is obstructed and may result in death or destruction of brain issue.

With increased awareness of the need of proper rehabilitation one can find more and more societies and websites which try to help stroke patients and their families. But unfortunately, there is still inadequate awareness of the fact that the disabilities resulting from stroke are both physical and mental. *Psychological handicaps may be of paramount importance in determining the outcome of rehabilitation program. So, it is important to include psychologists, psychiatrists and expert counselors in the rehabilitation team to get satisfactory result in the rehabilitation program.*

Psychological Consequences of Stroke and their Management

1. Stroke, like any other sudden traumatic event, may give rise to a series of responses which are considered essential for the process of living through the traumatic period and working through a reconstruction of personality structure. In this process the distressful events are displaced, delayed or disguised giving a mental picture of their absence.

   Initially, the patient goes through a stage of DENIAL, which may last up to two weeks during this stage most stroke patients hopes to return to normal. This prevents depression or anxiety and helps the body to adjust to the new situation.

   Next stage is *Grief Reaction Stage* when one sees depression and mourning often complicated by self-blame.

   This is followed by stage of *Anger* in the form of projections of blame, opposition, rebellion, noncompliance which makes the work of a rehabilitation team difficult.

Resolution of this stage culminates either in adaptive reconciliation and acceptance of disability or maladaptive regression which may lead to syndrome of post-traumatic stress disorder.

This is perhaps a generalization and in case of stroke, confusion and cognitive problems may mask or modify the stages. Yet it is helpful for the therapists to understand the cause of a patient's apparently unreasonable behavior. An expert counselor can help the patient to resolve these reactions which are traumatic to the patient and frustrating for the staff. Counselor first has to establish an emotional contact with the stroke patient and then gradually help him to resolve these reactions after establishing a therapeutic relationship based on genuineness, empathy, nonpossessive warmth and congruence. Cognitive behavior therapy may be helpful for patients showing post-traumatic stress disorder.

2. Fear, restlessness and aggressive behavior during the initial stage of confusion may be due to diminished perception at this stage leading to sensory misinterpretation of perceptual objects.

   By standing facing the patient, talking clearly in a moderately loud but gentle voice, it may be possible to pacify the patient and to establish contact (Fish).

3. Problems with personality and learning are caused by damage to various areas of brain, especially frontal lobe damage. These may be misinterpreted as stubbornness, lack of cooperation, rudeness or depression. This problems interfere with rehabilitation process in various ways as follows:
   - Poor attention, mood changes, low frustration tolerance interfere with learning.
   - Difficult tasks may lead to catastrophic reactions.
   - Problems with starting a job may be mistaken as laziness.
   - Problems with stopping together with poor judgment and impulsiveness can lead to accidents.
   - Lack of attention, inability to recognize errors, lack of ability to plan or to use foresight all interferes with patient's ability to return to his former job, with ability to drive and with ability to lead an independent life.
   - Extreme dependence, exploitation of disabilities to manipulate, lack of feeling for others may make relatives unsympathetic.

   These disabilities diminish somewhat with passage of time. It is important to look for these disabilities and to be aware of them when planning rehabilitation. Also counseling is needed for the patient and the family to cope with the disabilities.

4. *Cognitive problems:* Types of cognitive problems after stroke depends on site and side of the lesion. Problems may be:
   - Problems with comprehension.
   - Spatial relation syndromes such as problems with figure ground discrimination, problems with understanding position in space, etc.
   - Agnosias such as visual, auditory or tactile agnosia.

- Apraxias such as ideational apraxia, ideomotor apraxia, constructional apraxia and dressing apraxia.
- Problems with memory.

These problems may be less obvious than a paralyzed limb but together with problems of personality and learning may form "mental barriers" which may contribute patients becoming long stay invalids than the paralysis itself, by interfering with the process of rehabilitation.

Recognition and management of these problems may cause remarkable improvement in an apparently nonresponding patient. Lots of new thoughts are now emerging on methods of diagnosis and management of cognitive problems and this has become a specialized subject for occupational and physical therapists in a stroke rehabilitation team.

In short, the treatment consists of recognition of defects, proper treatment planning, making patient and relatives aware of the problem, using simple language when giving instructions, methodical repetitions, practical demonstrations, accepting slow progress, reassuring and informing patient about his/her progress. When required, specialized methods such as transfer of training approach, neurodevelopmental approach, or functional approach may be applied by trained therapist.

5. *Depression:* It is found in about 33% of poststroke patients. Peak incidence found in the period of six months to two years after the stroke.

Definite relationship found between stroke and depression in various studies where higher incidence of depression is found in poststroke patients when compared with controls suffering from traumatic brain injuries or orthopedic problems giving rise to similar problems with activities of daily living (ADL).

Left hemisphere lesions reportedly to result in significantly more depression than right hemisphere strokes. Proximity to frontal pole has proved to be an influential factor on development of poststroke depression. Other factors which may contribute to depression:
- Premorbid personality, e.g. those with self-sufficient nature may react more than those with strong dependency needs.
- Female sex.
- Greater age.
- More functional impairment.
- Absence of close relatives like spouse or children.
- Lack of social support.

Treatment
a. Nonpharmacological treatment consists of individual and group psychotherapy, cognitive behavior therapy, music therapy, social groups, etc.

Help of family and marriage counselor may be needed to repair the disorganized family and marital life.

Combination of psychotherapy and pharmacotherapy may have a better outcome.

   b. Pharmacological treatment mainly consists of use of antidepressant drugs.

Most studies reported use of heterocyclic compounds such as amitriptyline, nortriptyline and trazadone. Though found useful, their use is often limited by anticholinergic and cardiac side effects, sleepiness and orthostatic hypotension. Secondary amines (nortriptyline, desipramine) and trazodone are found to have less side effects than tertiary amines such as amitriptyline or imipramine. Low dose doxipin also reported to be useful with less side effects.

Selective serotonin reuptake inhibitors (SSRIs) like fluoxetine, paroxetine, sortilin, citalopram, escitalopram have improved safety profile but their use in elderly are sometimes limited by gastric upset and weight loss because elderly are more prone to extrapyramidal side effects of SSRIs.

Studies with both fluoxetine and citalopram showed improvement of symptoms. But for those stroke patients who are having other co-prescribed drugs like citalopram or sertralin may be safer because fluoxetine, fluvoxamine or paroxetine has an inhibiting effect on hepatic cytochrome P450 metabolic system and are more prone to drug interaction.

6. *Pathological emotionalism:* Increased tendency to cry or laugh without warning with inability to control them seen in about 21% of stroke patients. Episodes may be precipitated by visits by relatives, enquiry about health, TV, etc.

Relationship reported with strokes of anterior left hemispheres.

The problem is usually seen in the first four to six weeks following stroke and usually diminishes over the year. Counseling relatives to make them more understanding, avoiding situations which provokes attacks helps to reduce this problem. Tricyclic antidepressants reported to be helpful but their use is limited by side effects.

7. *Poststroke anxiety:* It is seen in about 32% of stroke patients and seen commonly with cortical stroke. Anxiety with fear of being alone or of going out with anticipation of fresh attacks with any episode of headache reported in patients with subarachnoid hemorrhage.

Counseling and psychotherapy is helpful. Benzodiazepine group of anxiolytics are helpful but may cause cognitive problems. Anxiolytics Buspiron have not proven to be useful.

8. *Psychosis:* Depression with psychotic symptoms, hypomanic episodes, bipolar disorder are all reported after cerebrovascular accidents. Levine and Finklestein (1982) reported relationship between lesions of right hemisphere especially of temperoparieto-occipital areas and psychosis. Peducular hallucinosis consisting of visual of auditory hallucinations with insight about their unreal nature occasionally seen after midbrain lesion.

Symptoms may resolve spontaneously or with treatment of the cause. Treatment with antipsychotics required, if symptoms are disturbing.

Typical antipsychotics such as haloperidol are useful but their use is limited on brain damaged person's susceptibility to extrapyramidal side effects. Typical antipsychotics such as olanzapine are helpful but cannot be given to stroke patients with diabetes. Mood stabilizers such as sodium valporate and carbamazepine are useful in selected cases.

9. *Social problems:* Social problems faced by stroke patients may be that of:
   - Social isolation
   - Economic strain due to cost of treatment, loss of job and skill
   - Poor family support in some cases
   - Loss of role in the family and in workplace
   - Disruption of marital and family life
   - Decrease in community involvement
   - Dependency.

For proper rehabilitation, this problem has to be recognized.

Attempts have to be made to keep the family functioning by spousal and family counseling. Depression in spouses of stroke patients is 2.5–3.5 times more than controls, that problem, if present have to be recognized and treated. Liberal community service is required at least for the first poststroke year to help the patient to live a useful life and to prevent the family from breaking down. The society and state have to understand the special needs of stroke victims.

Bibliography

1. Astrom, et al. Psychosocial function and life satisfaction after stroke. Stroke. 1992;23:527-31.
2. Carota, et al. A prospective study of predictors of poststroke depression. Neurology. 2005;64:428-33.
3. Chen, et al. Treatment effects of antidepressants in patients with poststroke depression: a meta-analysis. Annals of Pharmacotherapy. 2006;40:2115-22.
4. H Dam, et al. Depression among patients with stroke. Acta Psychiatrica Scandinavica. 2007;80(2):118-24.
5. Hackett, et al. Management of depression after stroke: a systemic review of pharmacological therapies. Stroke. 2005;36:1092-7.
6. Han and Haley. Family caregiving for patients with stroke: review and analysis. Stroke. 1999;30:1478-85.
7. Hanger, et al. Stroke patients view on stroke outcome: death versus disability. Clinical Rehabilitation. 2000;14:417-24.
8. House, et al. Mood disorders in the year after stoke. The British Journal of Psychiatry. 1991;158:83-92.
9. Huffman and Theodore. Acute psychiatric manifestations of stroke: a clinical case conference. Psychosomatics. 2003;45:65-75.
10. Jonathan Michael Bird. Psychiatric management in neurological disease. The British Journal of Psychiatry. 2001;179:278-9.
11. Linn and Ebrahim. Depression after stroke: a hospital treatment survey, Postgraduate Medical Journal. 1983;59:489-91.
12. Narushima, et al. Effect of antidepressant therapy on executive function after stroke. The British Journal of Psychiatry. 2007;190:260-5.

13. NB Lincon. Evaluation of cognitive behavioral treatment for depression after stroke: a pilot study. Clinical Rehabilitation. 1997;11(2):114-22.
14. Renee D, et al. Stroke, depression, and functional health outcome among adults in the community. Journal of Geriatric Psychiatry and Neurology. 2008;21(1): 41-6.
15. Robinson, Price. Poststroke depressive disorders: a followup study of 103 patients. Stroke. 1982;13:635-41.
16. Robinson, et al. Mood disorders in stroke patients: importance of location of lesion. Brain. 1984;107(1):81-93.
17. Teitelbaum, Ketfi. Psychiatric consultation with a nonoperative, depressed stroke patient. Psychosomatics. 1985;26:145-6.
18. Weisberg, et al. Psychiatric treatment in primary care patients with anxiety disorders: a comparison of care received from primary care providers and psychiatrists. American Journal of Psychiatry. 2007;164:276-82.

12

Nature, Impact and Retraining of Cognitive Deficits in Stroke

Shobini L Rao

The nature of cognitive deficits in stroke patients range from deficits of attention, information processing speed, executive dysfunction, presence of neglect and apraxia. Cognitive deficits are widely prevalent after stroke. Prevalence ranges between 40% and 50%. The deficits impact outcome at several levels. Cognitive functions assessed in the acute stage predict long-term global functional outcome, motor recovery, the rehabilitation process, caregiver's burden and return to work. Specific cognitive functions have an effect on specific outcomes. Cognitive retraining is the process of restoring functional normalcy to the brain damaged patients. The process of cognitive retraining targets the deficient functions and their constituent components through graded daily practice. Task specific improvements generalize to everyday behavior. The necessity for cognitive rehabilitation is being felt in stroke patients. Techniques for the treatment of neglect and apraxia are being used. Newer techniques, including motor imagery for improving motor functions and virtual reality for reducing neglect, are showing promise. Cognitive retraining procedures to retrain specific deficits, which impact specific outcome in stroke, need to be developed.

Nature of Cognitive Deficits in Stroke

Cognitive deficits are specific to the site of the brain infarction. Infarctions of the left middle cerebral artery territory (destruction of left perisylvian cortex) are associated with aphasias and damage to the left parietal convexity with motor apraxias. Infarctions of the right middle cerebral artery territory especially parietal lobes are associated with disorders of visuospatial perception, constructional apraxia, anosognosia, asomotagnosia, dressing apraxia and hemiinattention. Infarctions in the territory of the anterior cerebral artery with damage to the supplementary motor cortex cause speech disturbances and damage to the anterior corpus callosum causes apraxia of the left arm. Damage to bilateral anterior cerebral artery territory causes abulia with profound apathy, motor inertia and muteness. Infarction of the posterior cerebral artery territory may cause alexia if the posterior corpus callosum is damaged and memory disturbances if the bilateral inferomedial temporal lobes are damaged. Bilateral and numerous lacunar infarcts in the deeper white matter and diencephalons are associated with progressive dementia.[1]

Prevalence of Cognitive Deficits

Cognitive deficits are common after stroke. A multiethnic population of 1259 first-ever stroke patients in UK assessed 1-week poststroke had impaired cognition in 44%. Patients with anterior cerebral artery territory infarctions were most affected.[2] A prospective study of 4264 patients with acute ischemic stroke in Germany assessed 100 days poststroke by the Extended Barthel Index found presence of higher cognitive deficits in 55% of patients.[3] In stroke associated with small vessel disease, i.e. SSVD, 52% of 75 patients complained of cognitive symptoms 3 months poststroke.[4] Even patients with a single symptomatic lacunar infarct in the internal capsule or corona radiata have emotional disturbances and subtle cognitive impairments in demanding conditions.[5]

Assessment of Cognitive Deficits

Neuropsychological assessment is used to arrive at a profile of brain dysfunction in brain-damaged individuals. The procedure involves a detailed assessment of domains of attention, speed, language, executive functions, Visuospatial perception, learning and memory and focal signs. Deficits of attention, motivation can limit the comprehensiveness of assessment. The NIMHANS Neuropsychology battery–2004 is a comprehensive battery for adults with gender, age and education specific normative data for the Indian population.[6] Stroke patients may not be able to undergo a formal neuropsychological assessment soon after stroke due to clinical conditions and later due to residual impairments.

A variety of *scales* are used to rate the cognitive functioning in stroke patients. The scales are based on ratings by the treating staff, relatives or by the patients. Mini Mental Status Examination (MMSE), cognitive subscales of Functional Independence Measure (FIM), Lowenstein Occupational Therapy Cognitive Assessment (LOTCA) are used to assess cognitive status. Comparison of the scales found intertest correlations, which ranges between 0.47 and 0.67. The LOTCA was time consuming and exhausting. The FIM subscale required a better overall understanding of the patient's situation at the time of administration and was less convenient, while MMSE was simple to unseat the initial assessment.[7] The Functional Independence Measure (FIM) is often used to assess outcome in stroke. The FIM yields a total score (sum of all the scales); individual scale scores and physical and cognitive score (a two-dimensional interpretation). A multidimensional analysis on ischemic and hemorrhagic stroke patients yielded a three dimensional solution in both groups. The dimensions were self-care, cognitive function and toileting.[8]

Subjective experience of the patients is assessed through questionnaires. European Brain Injury Questionnaire administered on 214 stroke patients yielded 3 factors, i.e. depressive mood, cognitive difficulties and difficulties in social interactions.[9]

Informant's ratings of patient's difficulties are another measure. Partners of right hemisphere stroke patients reported more frequent and more severe changes than patients; while partners of left hemisphere patients tended to agree with the patient's ratings. The level of observability of the altered behavior, distress of the partner, distress of left sided stroke patients and hemispatial neglect of right sided stroke patients were factors leading to disagreement between the patient and the partner.[10] However, objective tests of cognitive functions correlated significantly with (0.42) informant-rated scale of estimated cognitive decline assessed using IQCODE.[11]

Newer procedures have been developed to assess specific functions. Assessment of *neglect* was conducted in 206 subacute right hemisphere stroke patients using anosognosia, visual extinction, and clinical assessment of gaze orientation and personal neglect, paper and pencil tests of spatial neglect in the peripersonal space. The automatic rightward orientation bias was the most sensitive clinical measure of neglect. Behavioral assessment was more sensitive than any single paper and pencil test.[12] Computer recording of 'process' measures of a cancelation task to measure neglect found that time between cancelations, components of cancelation time including pre movement, movement and drawing time and the starting point of cancelation significantly differentiated between neglect (N = 30) and non-neglect patients (N-57).[13] Comparison of tests of *apraxia* in 17 patients with left hemisphere lesions found different tests identified different patients as apraxic, indicating that tests could be sensitive to different subtypes of apraxia. The use of multiple tests is recommended for measurement of apraxia.[14] Another recent test, useful field of view (UFOV) measures the processing speed, divided attention and selective attention aspects of visual attention related to driving. Visual attention skills were poor in 52 stroke patients but improved after retraining.[15]

Functional imaging techniques using *Transcranial Doppler Ultrasonography* was used to monitor cerebral perfusion during object recognition in 29 ischemic stroke patients 4 weeks poststroke. Bilateral activation was associated with subsequent recovery at 2 months. Patients with no recovery showed activation on the side contralateral to brain lesion.[16] *Event–related brain potentials* (ERPs) were used to assess receptive language functions independent of behavior. N400 was elicited by names, which were incongruent to pictures in 10 left hemisphere stroke patients. The N400 derivative scores correlated with neuropsychological test scores.[17]

Assessment of *affect expression, perception and spontaneity* are new areas in the assessment procedure in stroke. Stoke patients (N = 27) were impaired in all the 3 areas compared with normal controls, but more so in affect perception.[18] Disturbances of integrality of brain functioning is evident in the assessment of *cognitive-motor interference* (CMI). Length covered during a one-minute walk or number of words generated in one minute is recorded singly and under dual ask conditions. There is a decrement in both parameters in dual task condition. Reduction of dual task gait decrement or of word generation was used as measures of functional recovery. Stride duration improved to a greater extent than cognitive performance.[19]

Impact of Cognitive Deficits on Stroke Outcome

Cognitive deficits in stroke are illustrative of the nature and severity of brain dysfunction. Theoretically, as stroke cause clean lesions, cognitive deficits throw light on the nature of brain behavior relationships. Clinically cognitive deficits have a significant association with stroke outcome such as spontaneous recovery, rehabilitation process, and caregiver's burden. Specific cognitive deficits have a bearing on specific functional capacities.

Effect of Cognitive Deficits on Spontaneous Recovery

Survival after stroke, length of hospital stay, dependent living and return to work are influenced by cognitive deficits. Cognitive impairment was an independent predictor of *survival* with a relative risk of 2.69 among 99 elderly stroke survivors. Patients with both cognitive and mobility impairments had a 2–3 fold greater risk of mortality than those with only a single abnormality.[20] Cognitive abilities such as judgment, comprehension and repetition had moderate positive correlation (r = 0.35) with *motor functional performance* in 37 first stroke patients with a mean age of 62 years. Balance and judgment abilities at admission or balance and lower extremity abilities at 2 weeks, or repetition abilities and lower extremity abilities at 4 weeks best predicted motor functional performance at discharge. The lower extremity and cognitive abilities at admission were the best predictors of patients' length of hospital stay.[21] Pre-existing cognitive decline and previous stroke predicted cognitive impairment poststroke in 75 patients with SSVD. Stroke severity and executive dysfunctions contributed to a poor *functional outcome*.[4] The Helsinki Stroke Aging Memory study cohort (N = 486) showed that worsening of cognition measured by MMSE between 3–15 months poststroke had an independent effect on *dependent living* at 15 months after ischemic stroke.[22] On the other hand, preserved cognition was associated with *return to work* (odds ratio = 2.64) in 120 stroke patients. Being able to walk (odds ratio = 3.98) and white-collar worker (odds ratio = 2.99) were the other factors associated with return to work.[23]

Effect on Rehabilitation Process

Cognitive deficits affect the course and outcome of rehabilitation, achievement of rehabilitation goals, and activity levels during the rehabilitation process. In a study on 177 stroke patients, cognitive problems of the patients was the major reason for nonachievement of *long-term rehabilitation goals*.[24]

Cognitive impairments accounted for 29% of variance in the *ratings of patients' activity levels* by staff members.[25] Dual task decrements arising when walking was combined with either word generation or paired associate learning, correlated significantly (r = 0.45) with disabilities in *activities of daily living.*[26] In a sample of 272 patients, even after rehabilitation cognitively impaired patients had worse outcome on *instrumental activities of daily living* at 6 months follow-up.[27] Decrements of speed of information processing assessed by a computerized test were associated with poorer *functional independence* in 37 acute stroke patients.[28] *Overall outcome* after rehabilitation measured by FIM was better in patients who had better cognitive status at admission to the rehabilitation center, in a group of 315 elderly first acute stroke patients.[29]

Effects of Cognitive Deficits on Caregivers' Burden

Stroke patients require long-term care even after discharge from the rehabilitation hospital. The caregivers may be spouses, children or other family members. The different aspects of their burden are disturbed sleep, disorganized household routines, restrictions on holidays and social life. Cognitive function was the only baseline patient characteristic which predicted subsequent psychosocial caregivers' burden among 68 patients living at home with a caregiver 6 months poststroke.[30] The same group of researchers in another study found that even when the caregivers was a spouse, the lower cognitive function of patients with stroke (N = 36) was associated with higher psychosocial burden.[31] The Relatives Stress Scale in both these studies assessed the caregivers burden.

Effects of Specific Cognitive Deficits on Specific Functional Capacities

Specific cognitive deficits are associated with reduction in specific functional capacities. Hence, cognitive deficits affect global and specific outcomes.

Attention: Stroke patients (N = 14) undergoing rehabilitation were found to have deficits of sustained auditory attention (N = 6), selective auditory attention (N = 8), visual selective attention (N = 12) and visual inattention (N = 7). Among these, initial auditory selective attention scores correlated with balance measures, wherein normal attention was associated with better balance.[32] Reductions of divided attention, i.e. the capacity for concurrent performance on two tasks and switching attention, i.e. alternate performance between two tasks were seen in elderly stroke patients. The reductions in attention were associated with poor physical and social outcome measures.[33]

Neglect: Unilateral neglect or hemi-inattention prevalent in right hemisphere stroke is an important cognitive modulator of outcome. A follow-up study on 52 right hemisphere stroke patients found that severity of neglect was correlated with total motor and cognitive FIM scores at admission, discharge and 3 months follow-up. Presence and severity of neglect also significantly impaired functional outcomes for reading and writing.[34] In a larger sample of 178 patients with first right hemisphere stroke, neglect was associated with severe baseline and neurological functional status at admission, less efficient and effective ADL and mobility, a higher percentage of patients with persistent incontinence at discharge. Despite physiotherapy and cognitive retraining to treat neglect, the outcome was poor for both ADL and mobility in patients with neglect compared to patients without neglect.[35] The association of poor mobility with neglect is again found in a retrospective analysis of 152 young severely disabled stroke patients, with a mean age of 54 years. Time taken to regain independent walking from stroke onset (range of 3-11 months) was longer in patients with cognitive impairments and neglect.[36]

Unawareness: Unawareness of deficits is associated with functional outcome. Unawareness was assessed through interview in 36 right hemisphere and 24 left hemisphere first-ever stroke patients. Standardized tests and procedures were used to document cognitive and neurological deficits. Unawareness of cognitive deficits was high, while that of motor and sensory deficits was low. In the right hemisphere group, higher total unawareness scores were associated with poorer functional outcome at discharge. Significantly, unawareness at admission was a significant predictor of discharge FIM motor scores.[37] Unawareness of illness together with hemiparesis and presence of a relative at home were the best predictors of time from right hemisphere stroke to discharge to home among 57 patients with first right hemisphere stroke. The best single predictor of the same was neglect.[38]

Apraxia: The severity of ideomotor apraxia assessed by a verbal gestureto command (pantomine) task was associated with dependency in physical functioning in 10 left hemisphere stroke patients. The dependency was greater for grooming, bathing and toileting.[39] Upper body dressing indexed by the capacity to put on a shirt was influenced by neglect and apraxia. Three out of 30 stroke patients who could not put on a polo shirt had neglect or apraxia and persistent arm paresis.[40] The presence of apraxia and cognitive deficits was greater in stroke patients who suffered falls compared with those who did not, in a total sample of 238 stroke patients undergoing rehabilitation.[41]

Executive Functions: Executive dysfunction assessed by detailed neuropsychological examination was present in 40% of a group of 256 ischemic stroke patients assessed 3-4 months poststroke. The executive dysfunction was associated with impairments in complex activities of daily living, greater cognitive impairments and stroke in the posterior circulation area.[42] The need for supervision on discharge was predicted in the acute rehabilitation stage in 44 stroke patients by deficits of reasoning and verbal learning assessed through neuropsychological tests.[43] Judgment abilities and balance at admission predicted motor functional performance at discharge in 37 first stroke patients. Judgment, comprehension and repetition had moderate positive relationships ($r = 0.35 - 0.62$) with functional performance.[21] Abstraction and concept learning measured by the Category test was associated with recovery in the hemiplegic upper limb. Initial scores on the upper extremity function test and the category test explained 81% of the variance of the discharge upper extremity function score. In another sample, of 16 stroke patients, survivors who made fewest errors on the category test showed the greatest amount of change in arm and hand function.[44]

Cognitive Retraining to Restore Functional Normalcy

Cognitive retraining is the treatment for restoring functional normalcy to brain damaged individuals, by reducing cognitive and behavioral impairments. Improvement of cognitive functions is associated with reduction of impairments and disability. Functioning of the patient improves and the patients are restored to functional normalcy. The goal of cognitive retraining is to restore the patient to as close as possible to levels of premorbid functioning. The process of cognitive retraining improves the components of psychological processes, which are impaired due to brain damage. Psychological processes are composed of components, which are integrated together to form the total process. An example would be the psychological process of attention, which is composed of the components of arousal, focusing, sustenance and division of attention. Each of these components would have to be trained using suitable tasks. Graded practice, is given daily on tasks, which target the component that has to be improved. The task difficulty increases over time to enable the patient to master the component, which is being trained. The progress of cognitive retraining is marked by increasing number of components for retraining, as well as training on an increasing number of processes. Psychological processes that are targeted for retraining are also graded. Psychological processes that have a pervasive effect on behavior such as attention are targeted earlier to higher-level processes like planning and organization.

In practice, a range of processes are targeted for retraining from the outset for the following reasons:

1. Patient's time at the hospital either as an inpatient or outpatient needs to be optimized.
2. Therapists' time and effort also has to be optimized.
3. The retraining program to be clinically viable has to be time and cost efficient.
4. It is hypothesized that cognitive retraining activates discrete brain regions and functional networks by giving graded practice on tasks, which require the functions that are mediated by those brain regions or functional networks, for effective performance.
5. Targeting multiple psychological processes has a synergistic effect, to improve behavior. The psychological processes are mediated by functional networks, which connect brain structures. The discrete brain regions mediate specific components of the total psychological process; hence a functional network is needed to mediate the composite process. In this scenario, a given brain region may participate in multiple psychological processes, provided the components mediated by the regions are shared by the psychological processes. Therefore, improving the functioning of a brain region through a particular task has a synergistic effect on the

performance of tasks, which require the component, mediated by that brain region.

6. The patient is encouraged to resume family roles and employment to the degree possible as he/she starts feeling better. The resumption of family and occupational roles reinforces and extends the improvement accrued during the retraining.

7. If necessary psychoeducation is given to the family and patient about the effects of brain damage on behavior. Counseling is given to family members regarding gradual nature of improvement, need for recognizing even small levels of improvement, and being supportive of the patient when the roles are resumed.

8. Inpatients with severe brain damage, behavior therapy may be combined with cognitive retraining and family counseling.

Need for Cognitive Retraining in the Treatment of Stroke Patients

The previous sections have made it abundantly clear that cognitive deficits are prevalent in stroke patients and impact on the global outcome as well as specific outcomes. Functional outcome in the spheres of motor functions, social functioning, return to work, discharge from hospital or the process of rehabilitation is influenced by cognitive deficits. Further, research has demonstrated that the presence of specific deficits have a bearing on specific functional outcomes. In view of this widespread impact, cognitive retraining should form an essential component of the rehabilitation process following stroke. Restoration of motor functions has been emphasized in stroke rehabilitation. Recent trends in rehabilitation have started the retraining of cognitive deficits in stroke patients. Even in the developed countries wherein specialized rehabilitation hospitals are available for patient care, cognitive retraining is still not the norm but physiotherapy therapy is. In the developing countries with fewer resources being available for long-term care of brain-damaged individuals, the initiation of cognitive retraining in the treatment of stroke patients is not widespread. The aim of this chapter is that it should be so.

Methods of Cognitive Retraining

Tasks are available for the retraining of attention, learning and memory, language, visuospatial functions and executive functions. The tasks have been devised in the context of rehabilitation of head injured patients. Application of the programs developed for treating cognitive deficits in traumatic brain injury to the treatment of stroke patients has to be viewed with caution, as the brain injured patient would have multiple deficits, while the stroke leads to discrete brain lesions. The documented benefits from treatment for cognitive dysfunction are sparse.[45]

The scenario of cognitive remediation in stroke is not rich in studies but the core deficits of aphasia, neglect, and apraxia have been addressed. Tasks for the improvement of language functions are not discussed, as they would form the corpus of aphasia therapy. Treatment of *neglect* has been attempted with the attention remediation module. It is a computerized procedure aimed to retrain components of attention, such as orientation, scanning and focusing of attention.[46] This module, wherein the patients are trained to scan increasingly distant regions of the neglected half for a target, has also treated neglect. Neglect is also improved by giving cancelation tasks, line bisection tasks and drawing tasks. The mainstay of therapy for neglect is improving visual scanning and improving the patient's capacity to attend to the neglected field. The procedures have limited efficacy. Newer approaches that are being tried include eye-patching techniques, use of video feedback during therapy, and training in visual imagery.[47] Use of hemiblinding goggles is a new technique for the treatment of neglect. Patients with right hemisphere stroke and with neglect wore specially designed hemiblinding goggles, which abolished all visual inputs form the right hemispace for one week. Compared to a control group with similar neglect but who did not wear the goggles, patients in the treatment group had amelioration of the visuospatial neglect, which was maintained for a further one-week period even after the suspension of treatment.[48] Another attempt is the use of virtual reality to reduce neglect. The virtual reality uses computers and multimedia peripherals to simulate an environment that users perceive as comparable to real world objects and events. Stroke patients (N = 16) were subjected to a virtual city street environment to improve the patient's capacity to cross streets. The program was feasible for the patients in terms of its cognitive and motor demands and showed promise in helping the patients to cross streets.[49] Limb activation is yet another new entrant to the treatment of neglect. Right hemisphere stroke patients (N = 9) one and half years poststroke were subjected to left limb movements while performing a visual scanning task involving the naming of letters and numbers. Active limb movement requiring a button push by the left hand was given to three patients. Passive left limb movement with functional electric stimulation was given to 8 patients. Positive results of improving the scanning while undergoing left limb activation was observed in 2/3 active movement patients; and 6/8 passive movement patients.[50] Visuomotor feedback training to reduce neglect was given by asking patients to lift rods. It was hypothesized that the task would involve appreciation of the left-right extension of the objects. A 3-day experimenter administered practice was followed by a 2-week self-administered practice. Assessment after 3 days and even at the one month follow-up showed that neglect reduced in patients at 12-month poststroke after the treatment.[51]

The increasing recognition of the influence of cognitive functions on functional recovery, has led to the development of programs using cognitive process to improve motor functions. Motor imagery is a cognitive process, which has been used to improve motor functions. Three patients with hemiparesis after stroke were trained to trace a horizontal line mentally. Compared with the deviation errors in the baseline tracing of the actual horizontal line, after mental practice subjects had reduced deviations in tracing the actual horizontal line. Further, the accuracy generalized modestly to the tracing of a curved line as well.[52] Motor imagery has been used as a cognitive strategy for functional recovery form hemiparesis. The motor imagery task consisted of imagined wrist movements (extension, pronation-supination) and mental simulations of reaching and object manipulation making use of a mirror box apparatus. One-hour sessions 3 times a week were given for 4 weeks to 2 MCA stroke patients with chronic hemiparesis. The outcome measures of grip strength, wrist functionality measures and timed performance measures improved following the intervention and at 3-month follow-up. The intervention targeted cognitive level of action processing, while its effects were realized in overt behavioral performance.[53] Internally simulating movements through motor imagery has shown promise to induce functional reorganization of the contralesional hemiplegic hand representation of a densely hemiplegic cerebral vascular accident patient.[54]

The acute rehabilitation setting involving a multidisciplinary rehabilitation team fosters better functional and cognitive outcome. Sixty patients aged between 43 and 80 years, were randomly divided into the inpatient rehabilitation group and the home based rehabilitation group. The inpatient group underwent therapeutic and neuromuscular exercises with occupational therapy with professional supervision. The home-based group underwent conventional rehabilitation with family caregiver and limited supervision. Significantly more favorable functional and cognitive outcomes with relatively low complications were associated with intense inpatient rehabilitation.[55]

The studies on cognitive retraining in stroke survivors are an emerging field. Research has indicated that cognitive remediation is promising in stroke patients. Research has to focus on the domains of cognition which are of importance in stroke such as neglect, apraxia. Significantly, the association of cognition with various parameters of functional outcome suggests that those areas of cognition, which influence global outcome, need to be improved in stroke survivors.

Conclusion

Cognitive deficits are varied and widely prevalent after stroke. Global functional outcome, specific functional outcome including motor, social, occupational, independence in living and instrumental activities of daily living is impacted by cognitive deficits. Improving cognitive functions through cognitive retraining would be a means of reducing the morbidity after stroke and improving the functional outcome. Cognitive retraining programs are available to improve specific cognitive functions. Many of the programs have been developed on head injured patients and their applicability to stroke patients needs to be examined as stroke causes discrete lesions, unlike traumatic brain injury with multiple deficits. A limited number of programs have been tried on stroke patients and these have shown promise. Research needs to develop and assess the efficacy of cognitive retraining programs, which would improve the global and specific functional outcomes in stroke patients.

References

1. Kandel ER, Schwartz JH, Jessell TM. Principles of Neural Science, 4th edn. New York: McGraw Hill; 2000.
2. Ozdemir F, Birtane M, Tabatabaei R, Ekuklu G, Kokino S. Cogntive evaluation and functional outcome after stroke. American Journal of Physical Medicine and Rehabilitation. 2001;80:410-15.
3. Weimar C, Kurth T, Kraywinkel K, Wagner M, Busse O, Haberl RL, et al. Assessment of functioning and disability after ischemic stroke. Stroke. 2002;33:2053-9.
4. Mok VC, Wong A, Lam WW, Fan YH, Tang WK, Kwok T, et al. Cognitive impairment and functional outcome after stroke associated with small vessel disease. Journal of Neurology, Neurosurgery and Psychiatry. 2004;75:560-66.
5. Van Zandvoort MJ, Kappelle LJ, Algra A, De Haan EH. Decreased capacity for mental effort after single supratentorial lacunar infarct may affect performance in everyday life. Journal of Neurology, Neurosurgery and Psychiatry. 1998;65: 697-702.
6. Rao SL, Subbakrishna DK, Gopukumar K. NIMHANS Neuropsychology Battery—2004 Manual. Bangalore National Institute of Mental Health and Neurosciences; 2004.
7. Zwecker M, Levenkrohn S, Fleisig Y, Zeilig G, Ohry A, Adunsky A. Mini-Mental State Examination, cognitive FIM instrument, and the Loewenstein Occupational Therapy Cognitive Assessment: relation to functional outcome of stroke patients. Archives Physical Medicine Rehabilitation. 2002;83:342-5.
8. Cavanagh SJ, Hogan K, Gordon V, Fairfax J. Stroke-specific models in an urban population. Journal of Neuroscience Nursing. 2000;32:17-21.
9. Martin C, Dellatolas G, Viguier D, Willadino-Braga L, Deloche G. Subjective experience after stroke. Applied Neuropsychology. 2002;9:148-58.
10. Visser-Keizer AC, Meyboom-de Jong B, Deelman BG, Berg IJ, Gerritsen MJ. Subjective changes in emotion, cognition and behaviour after stroke: factors affecting the perception of patients and partners. Journal of Clinical and Experimental Neuropsychology. 2002;24:1032-45.
11. Starr JM, Nicolson C, Anderson K, Dennis MS, Deary IJ. Correlates of informant—rated cognitive decline after stroke. Cerebrovascular Disease. 2000;10:214-20.
12. Azouvi P, Samuel C, Louis-Dreyfus A, Bernati T, Bartolomeo P, Beis JM, et al. Sensitivity of clinical and behavioral tests of spatial neglect after right hemisphere stroke. Journal of Neurology, Neurosurgery and Psychiatry. 2002;73:160-66.
13. Potter J, Deighton T, Patel M, Fairhurst M, Guest R, Donnelly N. Computer recording of standard tests of visual neglect in stroke patients. Clinical Rehabilitation. 2000;14:441-6.
14. Butler JA. How comparable are tests of apraxia? Clinical Rehabilitation. 2002;16:389-98.
15. Mazer BL, Sofer S, Korner-Bitensky N, Gelinas I. Use of the UFOV to evaluate and retrain visual attention skills in clients with stroke: a pilot study. American Journal of Occupational Therapy. 2001;55:552-7.
16. Bragoni M, Caltagirone C, Troisi E, Matteis M, Vernieri F, Silvestrini M. Correlation of cerebral hemodynamic changes during mental activity and recovery after stroke. Neurology. 2000;55:35-40.
17. D'Arcy RC, Marchand Y, Eskes GA, Harrison ER, Phillips SJ, Major A, Connolly JF. Electrophysiological assessment of language function following stroke. Clinical Neurophysiology. 2003;114:662-72.

18. Borgaro SR, Prigatano GP, Kwasnica C, Alcott S, Cutter N. Disturbances in affective communication following brain injury. Brain Injury. 2004;18:33-39.
19. Cockburn J, Haggard P, Cock J, Fordham C. Changing patterns of cognitive-motor interference (CMI) over time during recovery from stroke. Clinical Rehabilitation. 2003;17:167-73.
20. Wang SL, Pan WH, Lee MC, Cheng SP, Chang MC. Predictors of survival among elders suffering strokes in Taiwan: observation from a nationally representative sample. Stroke. 2000;31:2354-60.
21. Fong KN, Chan CC, Au DK. Relationship of motor and cognitive abilities to functional performance in stroke rehabilitation. Brain Injury. 2001;15:443-53.
22. Pohjasvaara T, Vataja R, Leppavuori A, kaste M, Erkinjuntti T. Cognitive functions and depression as predictors of poor outcome 15 months after stroke. Cerebrovascular Disease. 2002;14:228-33.
23. Vestling M, Tufvesson B, Iwarsson S. Indicators for return to work after stroke and the importance of work for subjective well-being and life satisfaction. Journal of Rehabilitation Medicine. 2003;35:127-31.
24. Liu C, McNeil JE, Greenwood R. Rehabilitation outcomes after brain injury: disability measures or goal achievement? Clinical Rehabilitation. 2004;18:398-404.
25. Gauggel S, Peleska B, Bode RK. Relationship between cognitive impairments and rated activity restrictions in stroke patients. Jouranl of Head Trauma Rehabilitation. 2000;15:710-23.
26. Haggard P, Cockburn J, Cock J, Fordham C, Wade D. Interference between gait and cognitive tasks in a rehabilitating neurological population. Journal of Neurology, Neurosurgery and Psychiatry. 2000;69:479-86.
27. Zinn S, Dudley TK, Bosworth HB, Hoenig HM, Duncan PW, Horner RD. The effect of post stroke cognitive impairment on rehabilitation process and functional outcome. Archives of Physical Medicine and Rehabilitation. 2004;85:1084-90.
28. Loranger M, lussier J, Pepin M, Hopps SL, Senecal B. Information-processing speed and assessment of early response latency among stroke patients. Psychological Reports. 2000;87:893-900.
29. Heruti RJ, Lusky A, Dankner R, Ring H, Dolgopiat M, Barell V, et al. Rehabilitation outcome of elderly patients after a first stroke: effect of cognitive status at admission on the functional outcome. Archives of Physical Medicine and Rehabilitation. 2002;83:742-49.
30. Thommessen B, Wyller TB, Bautz-Holter E, Laake K. Acute phase predictors of subsequent psychosocial burden in caregivers of elderly stroke patients. Cerebrovascular Disease. 2001;11:201-6.
31. Thommessen B, Aarsland D, Braekhus A, Oksengaard AR, Engedal K, Laake K. The psychosocial burden on spouses of the elderly with stroke, dementia and Parkinson's disease. International Journal of Geriatric Psychiatry. 2002;17:78-84.
32. Stapleton T, Ashburn A, Stack E. A pilot study of attention deficits, balance control and falls in the subacute stage following stroke. Clinical Rehabilitation. 2001;15:437-44.
33. McDowd JM, Filion DL, Pohl PS, Richards LG, Stiers W. Attentional abilities and functional outcomes following stroke. Journal of Gerontology B Psychological Sciences and Social Sciences. 2003;58:45-53.
34. Cherney LR, Halper AS, Kwasnica CM, Harvey RL, Zhang M. Recovery of functional status after right hemisphere stroke: relationship with unilateral neglect. Archives of Physical Medicine and Rehabilitation. 2001;82:322-8.

35. Paolucci S, Antonucci G, Grasso MG, Pizzamiglio L. The role of unilateral spatial neglect in rehabilitation of right brain-damaged ischemic stroke patients: a matched comparison. Archives of Physical Medicine and Rehabilitation. 2001;82:743-49.

36. Jackson D, Thornton H, Turner-Stokes L. Can young severely disabled stroke patients regain the ability to walk independently more than three months post stroke? Clinical Rehabilitation. 2000;14:538-47.

37. Hartman-Maeir A, Soroker N, Ring H, Katz N. Awareness of deficits in stroke rehabilitation. Journal of Rehabilitation Medicine. 2002;34:158-64.

38. Jehkonen M, Ahonen JP, Dastidar P, Koivisto AM, Laippala P, Vilkki J, Molnar G. Predictors of discharge to home during the first year after right hemisphere stroke. Acta Neurologica Scandinavica. 2001;104:136-41.

39. Hanna-Pladdy B, Heilman KM, Foundas AL. Ecological implications of ideomotor apraxia: evidence from physical activities of daily living. Neurology. 2003;60: 487-90.

40. Walker CM, Sunderland A, Sharma J, Walker MF. The impact of cognitive impairment on upper body dressing difficulties after stroke: a video analysis of patterns of recovery. Journal of Neurology, Neurosurgery and Psychiatry. 2004;75:43-8.

41. Teasell R, McRae M, foley N, Bhardwaj A. The incidence and consequences of fals in stroke patients during inpatient rehabilitation: factors associated with high risk. Archives of Physical Medicine and Rehabilitation. 2002;83:329-33.

42. Pohjasvaara T, Leskela M, Vataja R, kalska H, Ylikoski R, Hietanen M, et al. Post-stroke depression, executive dysfunction and functional outcome. European Journal of Neurology. 2002;9:269-75.

43. Stewart KJ, Gale SD, Diamond PT. Early assessment of post-stroke patients entering acute inpatient rehabilitation: utility of the WASI and HVLT-R. Archives of Physical Medicine and Rehabilitation. 2002;81:223-8.

44. Barreca SR, Finlayson MA, Gowland CA, Basmajian JV. Use of the Halsteahd Category Test as a cognitive predictor of functional recovery in the hemiplegic upper limb: a cross –validation study. Clinical Neuropsychology. 1999;13:171-81.

45. Gresham GE, Stason WB. Rehabilitation of the Stroke Survivor. In: Barnett HJM Mohr JP, Stein BM, Yatsu FM (Eds). Stroke: Pathophysiology, Diagnosis and Management, 3rd ed. Philadelphia: Churchill Livingstone. 1998;1389-401.

46. Ben Yishay Y, Piazetsky EB, Rattok J. A systematic model for ameliorating disorders in basic attention in neuropsychological rehabilitation. In: Meier M, Benton AC, Diller L (Eds). Neuropsychological Rehabilitation. New York: Churchill Livingstone.

47. Diamond PT. Rehabilitative management of post-stroke visuospatial inattention. Disability Rehabilitation. 2001;23:407-12.

48. Zeloni G, Farne A, Baccini M. Viewing less to see better. Journal of Neurology, Neurosurgery and Psychiatry. 2002;73:195-8.

49. Weiss PL, Naveh Y, Katz N. Design and testing of a virtual environment to train stroke patients with unilateral spatial neglect to cross a street safely. Occupational Therapy International. 2003;10:39-55.

50. Eskes GA, Butler B, McDonald A, Harrison ER, Philips SJ. Limb activation effects in hemispatial neglect. Archives of Physical Medicine and Rehabilitation. 2003;84:323-8.

51. Harvey M, Hood B, North A, Robertson IH. The effects of Visuomotor feedback training on the recovery of hemispatial neglect symptoms: assessment of a 2 week and follow-up intervention. Neuropsychologia. 2003;41:886-93.

52. Yoo E, park E, Chung B. Mental practice effect on line-tracing accuracy in persons with hemiparetic stroke: a preliminary study. Archives of Physical Medicine and Rehabilitation. 2001;82:1213-8.
53. Stevens JA, Stoykov ME. Using motor imagery in the rehabilitation of hemiparesis. Archives of Physical Medicine and Rehabilitation. 2003;84:1090-2.
54. Johnson-Frey SH. Stimulation through simulation? Motor imagery and functional reorganization in hemiplegic stroke patients. Brain and Cognition. 2004;55:328-31.
55. Ozdemir F, Birtane M, Tabatabaei R, Kokino S, Ekuklu G. Comparing stroke rehabilitation outcomes between acute inpatient and non intense home settings. Archives of Physical Medicine and Rehabilitation. 2001;82:1375-9.

13

Nutritional Management of Stroke

Shrabani Sanyal Bhattacharya

Stroke, a CNS vascular phenomenon, is directly or indirectly related to the nutritional and metabolic factors of an individual. Various nutritional areas which are related to the risk of developing vascular occlusion in brain are recently being focused in medical practice. The fatty deposits in vessels along with the other cardiovascular risk factors including smoking, sedentary life style, hypertension, type A personality, etc. increases the chances of cerebrovascular attacks. Moreover, various metabolic factors including diabetes mellitus, hyperlipidemia, high concentration of homocysteine, obesity, etc. are also risk factors for a stroke.

In rehab set-up, the stroke patients are admitted with varied metabolic abnormalities, and also having different food habits. Such patients require proper nutritional evaluation by identification of potential risk factors for stroke and are judged on the basis of various other disabilities and pathological factors including dysphagia, diabetes mellitus, anemia, hypothyroidism state, frequent urinary or other systemic infection, gastropathy, bowel disorders, obesity, hypertension, dyslipidemia, dyselectrolytemia, high homocysteine level, etc.

Moreover, during the rehab process of a stroke victim, it is essential to monitor the blood levels of possible abnormal parameters including, serum electrolytes, suger, glucose tolerance, liver enzymes, urea, creatinine, BUN, lipids, homocystine level at a regular interval and on that basis, the diatery regime should be recommended. It is also important to note the musculoskeletal disability and the requirement of protein, vitamin and minerals, which is of immense importance to improve the energy level of the patient, and this is a pillar of a successful rehab program.

In the dietary management of a poststroke individual one should also record the bowel dysfunction (neurogenic or pre-existing problem like habitual constipation) and recommendation should include the required fiber rich-menu.

In a case of gastrointestinal intolerance to certain foods, it is also important to consider withdrawing of particular foods. In the early phase of attack, the patient may exhibit hyponatremic state, the fall of sensorium may be mistakenly considered as a consequence of CVA itself and such states should be prevented and treated by increased salt intake either orally or parenterally. The fluid recommendation also requires close observation on urinary output, the ratio of amount of intake and output, any presence of cardiac failure or impaired renal function, etc.

Though it is established that low sodium (to prevent HTN) and high potassium intake reduces the chances of vaso-occlusive disorders; this idea may not be true after an acute attack, and in hyponatremia, high sodium is always recommended. However, in hypokalemic state extrasources of potassium (like fruits, potassium chloride) are essential.

So, it is clear that, after stroke the dietary management plays a big role in proper resettlement of an individual's disordered metabolic status, considering various factors. This not only saves the life of a patient but helps in quick return to a healthy life and thus, the domain of nutrition has proved itself as an essential and integral part of a successful rehabilitation process.

Oral feeding is the best choice for nourishment of a patient, but in most of the severely affected patients, with so many of limitations of oral feeding, tube feeding or parenteral feeding is restored. Dysphagia or difficulty in swallowing is a common consequence following stroke, which demands such ways of feeds.

After stroke nutrition may be maintained either enterally or parenterally:

1. *Enteral nutrition:* Enteral nutrition is achieved either by a nasogastric tube or directly by surgical intervention to the stomach (gastrostomy). A satisfactory tube feeding must be:
   a. Nutritionally adequate.
   b. Well tolerated by patient so that vomiting is not induced.
   c. Easily digested with no unfavorable reactions such as distension, diarrhea or constipation.
   d. Easily prepared.
   e. Inexpensive.

Types of foods supplied through the tube may be:
   a. Natural liquid foods.
   b. Blenderized to make liquid food.
   c. Commercially supplied polymeric mixtures or elemental diet (predigested diet).

The nature of food may be different for different individuals (according to the existing metabolic states) but a patient having no contraindication for all available dietary materials, natural liquid foods like whole or skim milk, egg white and some form of carbohydrate such as strained cooked cereals, sugar or molasses can be given. Vegetable oil or cream and non-fat dry milk are also incorporated to increase the calorie and protein levels respectively.

In blenderized feeding **(Table 13.1)**, the ordinary food items which cannot be swallowed, are blended to make thin liquid which can pass through naso-gastric tube. Food is cooked before putting in an electric mixer **(Table 13.2)**.

Table 13.1: Composition of blenderized food for tube feeding for hospital practice (for standard weight adult stroke patient)	
Ingredient	Amount (g)
Rice	75
Green gram *dal*	40
Bread	20
Milk	200
Skimmed milk powder	60
Spinach	50
Pumpkin	50
Carrots	50
Banana	70
Sugar	60
Refined oil	20
Butter	7

In this regime:
- Water is added to make the volume 1500 mL
- 1500 kilocalories, is supplied
- Each mL provides one kilocalorie
- 50 g protein, is supplied
- Cost is no more than an average meal in hospital.

A concentration of about 1 kcal per mL is satisfactory. The feeding is started through a continuous drip at a rate of 50 mL per hour. The rate is increased by 20 mL every 24 hours until the required volume is achieved, usually with 100–120 mL per hour. The concentration or rate of flow may have to be decreased, if there is vomiting, abdominal cramps or diarrhea. The feeding is gradually shifted to a timed frame.

Feeding solutions have to be treated with full hygenic precautions during the preparation, storage and administration. Feeds should be stored in a refrigerator to avoid bacterial growth and taken out before administration in time to reach room temperature; very cold feeds are not tolerated. A feed should be discarded when it has been more than 24 hours out of storage.

Table 13.2: Feeding requirements in tube feeding	
Nutrient	Amount
Fluids	30 mL/kg
Energy	32 kcal/kg
Protein	1 g/kg body weight
Sodium	30–40 mMol (provided, there are no external losses)
Potassium	1 m Mol/g of protein

Vitamins and minerals supplementation should be given.

2. *Parenteral nutrition:* Here the nutrient is supplied intravenously to a stroke patient. This method may be used to supplement normal feeding by mouth and provides all the nutrients necessary to meet a patient's requirements. It is called total parenteral nutrition (TPN).

Total parenteral nutrition is defined as provision of all nutrients for normal homeostasis and growth in the required amounts through parenteral route. The same process is called hyperalimentation when at least 150% of daily requirements are provided to produce a positive nitrogen balance for gaining weight. Partial parenteral nutrition provides 30–50% of daily nutrients while the rest is provided thorough enteral route.

The daily requirements which have to be mandatorily provided in any TPN programs are:

a. Glucose.
b. Emulsified fat.
c. Crystalline amino acids.
d. Vitamins including B_{12}, folic acid and vitamin K.
e. Electrolytes—sodium, chlorine, phosphorous, potassium, calcium and magnesium.
f. Trace elements—zinc, copper, chromium, manganese and iodine.
g. Water.

Total parenteral nutrition provides all nutrients in a concentrated form to avoid fluid overload. Adequate nonprotein calories are provided in the program so that amino acids are used only for protein synthesis (150 NPC/g of nitrogen). TPN is given to patients who cannot eat, should not eat, or will not eat soon and who are not having the contraindications for recommendation of such food materials.

Nutrition-related Risks and Preventive Diets for Stroke

1. *Obesity:* If men have a body mass index of more than 27.8 and women have more than 27.3, they are susceptible to stroke. Grade I obesity in combination with hypertension increases the risk. Obese patients have too much body stores of fat and may have high blood cholesterol levels.

2. *Diet and food habits*
   a. *Excess sugars:* They promote triglyceride production in the liver and intestine. They also promote production of VLDL without the increases in cholesterol or protein changes. Fructose and sucrose are more triglyceridemia than glucose and starch. Large amounts of sugar stimulate the production of insulin which is lipogenic.
   b. *Excess fat:* High intake of saturated fatty acid increase plasma cholesterol and so promotes formation of plaque. Saturated fats reduce the formation of LDL receptors or VLDL receptors. A raised level of triglycerides are associated with increased risk of stroke only in the presence of reduced HDL cholesterol. Animal fat like egg yolk, butter, meat fat have a high amount of saturated fatty acid. Margarine, ghee, hydrogenated fat and

coconut oil also contain high amount of saturated fat. Diets deficient in polyunsaturated fatty acids are associated with increased risk of stroke.

   c. *Antioxidants:* Studies shown that a dietary intake of antioxidants including flavonoids (polyphenolic antioxidants) naturally present in colored vegetables and fruits, tea, wine and vitamin E is associated with a decline in stroke event. Low levels of beta carotene are seen in patients of stroke especially among smokers.

3. *Drinking water:* There is a negative association between hardness of drinking water and mortality from stroke. The harder the drinking water, the lower the death rate from stroke. Calcium and magnesium or other trace elements in hard water may be beneficial. Studies shown that large amounts of calcium lower cholesterol and triglyceride levels.

4. *Alcohol:* Several studies have indicated that a moderate alcohol intake raises HDL cholesterol levels which in turn reduce the risk of developing plaque. Too much alcohol increases the risk of stroke. The recommended limits for alcohol consumption are 21 units each week for women and 28 units each week for men. People who drink more than this run a higher risk of stroke, liver disease and dementia.

5. *Homocysteine:* Elevated levels of homocysteine are seen in stroke patients and homocysteinemia has been established as an independent risk factor for stroke. Deficiency of vitamin B_6, B_{12} and folic acid can cause elevated plasma homocysteine and supplementation with these vitamins can reduce plasma homocysteine.

6. *Hypertension:* As the blood pressure increases, the incidence of stroke also increases.

Blood pressure (mm Hg)	% of persons developing stroke
140/90 or less	35
140/90 to 160/100	50
160/100 and above	65

7. *Diabetes mellitus:* The incidence of stroke is doubled in diabetics because it affects the blood vessels and the blood.

8. *Hyperlipidemia:* High concentration of cholesterol, triglycerides or LDL in the blood indicate hyperlipidemia which increases the incidence of stroke.

Dietary Management

Low calorie, low fat particularly low saturated fat, low cholesterol, high in PUFA, low carbohydrate and normal protein, minerals and vitamins are suggested.

   Those patients whose weight is at a desirable level are permitted a maintenance level of calories during convalescence and their return to activity. The total calories should be restricted so as to reduce the weight to the expected normal for the height, age and sex.

Mild degree of weight loss for the cardiac patient of normal weight is recommended. Usually, a 1000 to 1200 kilocalorie (kcal) diet is suitable for an obese patient in bed.

Fat

The first step involves restriction of fats to no more than 20% of the total calories consumed. Levels as low as 20% are tolerated without side effects. It is not desirable to restrict all forms of fat, as severe restrictions result in mental and physical depression. In the diet the proportion of saturated to monounsaturated to polyunsaturated fat should be 1:1:1.

The important polyunsaturated fatty acids in foods are linoleic acid (n-6), alpha-linolenic acid (n-3), arachidonic acid (n-6), eicosapentaenoic acid (n-3), docosahexaenoic acid (n-3). PUFA promote esterification of cholesterol and put it into easily utilizable form. The ratio of PUFA to saturated fats is known as P/S ratio. The ratio of 0.5 or over is satisfactory. PUFA decrease the synthesis of the precursor of VLDL which are associated with an increased incidence of stroke. It also decreases the production of LDL and triglycerides and also help in the clearance of LDL. Linoleic acid prevents accumulation of cholesterol in blood serum and walls of blood vessels and plays a key role in transport of cholesterol.

The monounsaturated fatty acids are oleic acid and erucic acid. Monounsaturated fats are present in vegetable sources such as olive oil and groundnut oil. They lower LDL without lowering HDL cholesterol. The trans isomers of oleic acid (present in margarine) raise LDL to the same extent as saturated fatty acid **(Table 13.3)**.

Table 13.3: Polyunsaturated/saturated fatty acid ratio of some common fats (Desirable > 1.0)	
Fats	*P/S ratio*
Safflower oil	8.2
Sunflower oil	6.4
Corn oil	4.46
Soybean oil	4.07
Cotton seed oil	1.96
Sesame oil	2.66
Soybean (hydrogenated)	2.46
Peanut oil	1.82
Coconut oil	0.04
Butter	0.06

Fish are good sources of n-3 fatty acids. Consumption of 100–200 g of fish two to three times a week helps prevent stroke, the daily consumption of 10–15 g of fish oil extract representing 3–5 g n-3 fatty acid is probably adequate to control moderate hypertriglyceridemia.

Cholesterol

Cholesterol level in the diet should not exceed 300 mg. Liver synthesizes as much as 2 g of cholesterol per day. If cholesterol levels are above 260 mg/dL, it is almost impossible to bring about a drop by diet alone.

The advantage of a vegetarian diet are that it is low in calories, fat and cholesterol and that it has a high p/s ratio and it has adequate fiber which helps in binding cholesterol and increase the excretion of cholesterol. Vegetable oils diminish the plasma cholesterol not only due to polyunsaturated fatty acids but also because the plant sterol inhibits cholesterol absorption. Cholesterol rich and poor foods are given below:

Rich	Poor
Butter, cheese, cream, eggyolk, kidney, liver, red meat, brain.	Cottage cheese, egg white, fish, all vegetable oils, milk, skim milk, vegetables, fruits.

Cholesterol rich foods should be limited in the diet. To prevent stroke, one can use ground nut oil or gingelly seed oil. One can also use sunflower or safflower oil with low levels of palm oil for cooking.

Recent studies have shown that nuts are useful in protecting against stroke and diabetes. It is advised to have a handful (9–15 nuts) of a variety of plain unroasted nuts daily especially walnuts and almonds instead of having biscuit or piece of cake. Nuts can reduce the risk of stroke; it contains monounsaturated, polyunsaturated fats and other compounds that influence blood cholesterol. Nuts seem to help lower blood lipids, reduce the oxidation of LDL and maintain blood vessel health.

Hypocholesterolemic Agents

High fiber in the diet reduces cholesterol. Pectin (apples, guavas) lowers the level of serum cholesterol and enhances the excretion of fecal steroids. It has no effect on serum triglycerides and HDL cholesterol. Guar gum (excracted from seeds of cluster beans) has hypocholesterolemic effect. Legumes, vegetables and fruits can lower the level of serum cholesterol but the effect is usually small compared with the well known effect on HDL and serum triglycerides.

Studies shown that blood pressure can be reduced by using fiber-rich diets. Dietary fiber also reduces serum fibrinogen levels, which in turn lower the risk of blood clot formation and myocardial infarction. Oat products which contain high amount of betaglucan content has hypocholesterolemic effect. Turmeric, bengal gram, onion and garlic have cholesterol lowering effects.

Tea helps in protecting against stroke, osteoporosis, cancer and even skin cancer if it is drunk with lemon. One recent study has shown that drinking of tea can reduce the risk of death after a stroke by 44% and may also help maintain total bone mineral density, thus, reducing the risk of developing osteoporosis. It is better to consume tea daily (green, black or oolong) may be taken with a twist of lemon. Since, total calories are restricted, carbohydrate intake should be reduced by reducing sugar intake. Regarding proteins, vitamins and minerals, normal allowances are recommended. Since, total fat, animal fat, organ meats, eggs and sea food are restricted; vitamin A deficiency may occur. Therefore, supplement of vitamin A is essential.

Sodium

It is restricted when there is hypertension. Usually restriction of sodium of 1600–2300 mg is satisfactory in patients with stroke. When sodium is restricted, other sources of iodine should be prescribed. A severe restriction of sodium also reduces the intake of vitamin A because egg and green leafy vegetables that are high in sodium are restricted.

The restriction of fluid is not required as long as sodium is not restricted.

Table 13.4: Substitution food for a stroke patient	
Instead of these	*Choose these*
1. *Palak* paneer	Greens dal
2. Whole milk	Skim milk
3. Fruit juice with milk	Whole raw fruit
4. Potato chips	Papad (grilled)
5. French toast	Vegetable sandwich
6. Omelette	Poached egg
7. Cake	Bread
8. Carrot *halwa*	Raw carrot salad or carrot milk shake without sugar
9. Rice	Wheat or *ragi*
10. *Ghee* or vanaspati, butter	Oil
11. Ice cream	Cut fruits
12. *Paratha*	*Phulka*
13. Dosa	*Idli*

Conclusion

Stroke can be prevented by keeping plasma LDL cholesterol as low as possible throughout the life and since, the beginning in early childhood. This involves lifelong dietary restriction and the use of drugs. The diet should be low in saturated fats and cholesterol but polyunsaturated fats from vegetable oils and in other foods are permitted.

Diet is clearly a cause of hyperlipidemia but is not the only one. To reduce the risk of stroke, a healthy diet containing variety of foods with adequate starch and fiber are advised, limitation of saturated fat, cholesterol, too much of sugar and salt are recommended to lower the hazard of stroke, however, consumption of alcohol in a moderate way may be permitted. Nutritional intervention does not always indicate the quantity of food intake but the quality of the same. It can not be standarized for the population at large, rather it needs to be recommended according to the basic disorders and maladopted nutritional and metabolic problems of the individual having cerebrovascular accident.

Bibliography

1. Axelsson, et al. Nutritional status in patients with acute stroke. Acta Med Scand. 1988;224(3):217-24.
2. Choi-Kwon, et al. Nutritional status in acute stroke: Undernutrition versus overnutrition in different stroke subtypes. Acta Neurologica Scandinavica. 1998;98(3):187-92.
3. Dávalos, et al. Effect of Malnutrition after Acute Stroke on Clinical Outcome Stroke. 1996;27:1028-32.
4. Gariballa SE, Sinclair AJ. Assessment and treatment of nutritional status in stroke patients. Postgraduate Medical Journal. 1998;74:395-9.
5. Gariballa, et al. Influence of nutritional status on clinical outcome after acute stroke. American Journal of Clinical Nutrition. 1998;68:275-81.
6. Perry Lin, Mclaren Susan. Nutritional support in acute stroke: The impact of evidence-based guideline. Clinical Nutrition. 2003;22(3):283-93.
7. Martin Dennis. Nutrition after stroke. British Medical Bulletin. 2000;56:466-75.
8. Salah, et al. Nutritional status of hospitalized acute stroke patients. British Journal of Nutrition. 1998;79:481-7.
9. Weekes, et al. Resting energy expenditure and body composition following cerebro-vascular accident. Clinical Nutrition. 1992;11:18-22.
10. Wilmore, et al. Catabolic illness: Strategies for enhancing recovery. New England Journal of Medicine. 1991;325:695-702.

Section 2

Spinal Cord Injury Rehabilitation

Spinal cord injury rehabilitation is a medical process for re-establishing the patient to his or her highest level of functional independence by a continuous and scientific intervention. It aims for the recovery of the lost neuromuscular status or promote substitution of the lost function. The medical complications of the injury are also controlled in the process of SCI rehabilitation, to lengthen the patient's life span.

14

Anatomy of Spinal Cord

Syed Ali Asad

The spinal cord is a pliable and almost cylindrical cord of nervous tissue, about 18 inches long and just thicker than a pencil. It lies in the upper two thirds of vertebral canal in adult and is continuous with medulla oblongata at the emergence of first pair of spinal nerve just below foramen magnum and above the upper border of atlas. It ends at the lower border of first lumbar vertebra in adult and lower border of L3 in infant, at which it rapidly tapers to a cone, the conus medullaris. Spinal cord is present throughout the vertebral canal up to 3rd month of fetal life and then recede back to the levels mentioned due to disproportionate growth of vertebral column and the cord.

Enlargements: Two swellings—but for the most part it is circular in section and regular in outline.

Cervical enlargement: Oval in section. There are aggregations of large nerve cells that supply the upper limb structures. This enlargement with the mass of the gray matter is destined to form the brachial plexus. Cervical enlargement is the larger of the two.

Extention: C4 to T2 vertebra, opposite to the attachments of roots of brachial plexus (C5 to T1).

Thickest opposite 6th cervical segment and narrows away opposite 2nd thoracic vertebra.

Lumbar enlargement: Slightly smaller and affords origin to the nerves of the lower limbs, forming lumbar plexus of nerves.

Extent: T10 to L1 vertebra, reaches maximum breadth opposite twelfth thoracic vertebra; opposite the roots of lumbar plexus (L2 to S3 cord segments).

Weight: About 25–30 g.

Laminar Concept of Spinal Gray Matter

B Rexed mapped out the arrangements of spinal gray matter according to the architectural pattern of cells and their packing materials into ten laminae. This classification is also based on neuronal links of the gray matter of the spinal cord.

Laminae I to VI lie in the posterior gray column. Lamina I lies in lamina marginalis.

Lamina II corresponds with SG (substantia gelatinosa).

Laminae III to VI corresponds with nucleus (N) proprius.

Lamina VII occupies intermediate region of gray matter and extends into the anterior gray column. It includes N dorsalis, intermediolateral columns of autonomic system. Predominantly, it is made up of interneurons.

Lamina VIII lies at medial part of anterior gray column in the cervical and lumbosacral enlargement of the cord and in the base of the anterior column in other cord segments.

Lamina IX lies at lateral part of the anterior gray column of enlarged cord segments for the limbs. Some neurons of lamina VII however, invaginate in the gray column between laminae VIII to IX.

Lamina X: The zone around central canal. It contains less cells and more neuroglial cells.

Functional Aspect of these Laminae

Lamina I to IV (a) Receive cutaneous sensations carried through dorsal nerve roots. (b) Tract cells of lamina IV (and V and VI?) give rise to ascending pathways mostly spinothalamic. These pathways arouse consciousness to cutaneous sensations or produce reflexes at the brainstem level. (c) Concerned with spinal reflexes.

Laminae V to VI

a. Receive mostly proprioceptive senses from dorsal roots and collaterals of ascending tracts of dorsal funiculi.
b. Receive the termination of the pyramidal and rubrospinal tracts at pre-or postsynaptic level and modulate the sensory input, which controls the type of movements.

Lamina VII

a. Has got connection with ipsilateral cerebellum and brainstem by afferent and efferent fibers—helps to control posture and movement.
b. Preganglionic neurons of autonomic system are lodged here.
c. Origin of Renshaw cells, which inhibit excessive firing of alpha neurons.

Lamina VIII

a. Vestibulospinal and reticulospinal tracts are received here and then their efferents projected to the lamina IX.

b. Some neurons send commissural fibers to the opposite side.

Lamina IX

It contains alpha and gamma motor neurons (and beta neurons), and many interneurons.

Alpha motor neurons supply extrafusal fibers of skeletal muscles.

Gamma neurons supply intrafusal fibers of muscle spindle.

Beta neurons supply both extra- and intrafusal muscle fibers.

Alpha and Gamma neurons receive synaptic terminals directly of through interneurons from corticospinal, rubrospinal, vestibulospinal and reticulospinal tracts.

Alpha neurons receive sensory input through the dorsal nerve roots. It forms monosynaptic reflex arc from Ia fibers of muscle spindle. This reflex arc is absent in gamma neurons.

It is observed that alpha and gamma neurons are excited simultaneously by the pyramidal tract; others propose that alpha neurons being fast conductors initiate muscle contraction without limit of shortening; the gamma neurons through the reflex loop of servo-mechanism maintain muscle contraction with a desired length.

This is the possible explanation of why muscle contraction is clumsy in early phase of voluntary movement and very precise contraction in later part of the movement.

White Matter of Spinal Cord

The white matter of each side is divided into three main columns or funiculi by the anterior horn with emerging anterior roots, posterior horn with entering dorsal roots.

- Anterior white column lies between the anterior horn and anterior median fissure.
- Lateral white column lies between the anterior and posterior horns.
- Posterior white column lies between the posterior horn and posterior median septum.

Arrangements of Tracts

Anterior Funiculus or Column

Descending tracts are:

a. Anterior corticospinal (controls skilled voluntary movements).

b. Olivospinal.

   c. Vestibulospinal (concerned with the balance reflex).

   d. Tectospinal (concerned with visual and auditory reflexes).

   e. Ventral reticulospinal (controls muscle tone and ordinary activities that do not require constant conscious effort. It has a facilitatory effect on the motor activity of anterior horn cells).

Ascending tracts:

Ventral spinothalamic (conveys touch and pressure impulses; the touch is lateral to pressure fibers).

Anterolateral Funiculus

Descending tracts:

   a. Lateral corticospinal (controls skilled voluntary movement).

   b. Rubrospinal (controls muscle tone—stimulates the flexor tone and inhibits extensor tone).

   c. Lateral reticulospinal (inhibits extensor motor neurons and facilitates the flexors).

   d. Spinal sympathetic.

Ascending tracts:

   a. Lateral spinothalamic (transmits fast pain and temperature sensations – pain fibers are lateral to temperature fibers).

   b. Spinotectal (controls reflex movements of head required for fixation of gaze).

   c. Anterior spinocerebellar (concerned with general posture and movements of the whole lower limb).

   d. Posterior spinocerebellar (conveys unconscious proprioceptive, touch and pressure sensations from the lower limb and lower half of body to ipsilateral cerebellum).

Posterior Funiculus

Descending tracts:

   a. Fasciculus septomarginalis in the lower half of the cord adjacent to the posterior septum.

   b. Fasciculus interfascicularis in the upper half of the cord between the fasciculus gracilis and cuneatus.

These are concerned with association and integration.

Ascending tracts:

   a. Fasciculus gracilis medially.

   b. Fasciculus cuneatus laterally.

    Carry informations of discriminative touch and pressure, conscious sense of position, movements and stereognosis. The proprioceptive fibers from muscle spindle (Ia fibers) and from Golgi tendon (Ib fibers) pass through this column.

Descriptions of Few Tracts

Descending Tracts

These tracts influence the activities at lower motor neurons from different functional levels of the brain. They arise from cerebral cortex (corticospinal or corticonuclear) or from the nuclei of gray matter between cortex and spinal cord (extrapyramidal).

Corticospinal Tract and Corticonuclear Tracts (Pyramidal Tract)

Fibers of the corticospinal tract arise as axons of giant pyramidal cells (upper motor neurons) (Betz cells) situated in the fifth layer of cerebral cortex from areas 4, 6, 3, 1, 2 and probably from other areas of the cortex. Axons of these neurons descent successively through the corona radiata, posterior limb of internal capsule, middle two thirds of basis pedunculi of midbrain, pons and pyramid of the medulla oblongata. Some fibers also arise from the postcentral gyrus which do not control motor activity but influences sensory input to the nervous system.

In the lower medulla, about 70–80% fibers decussate and descend on the contralateral lateral funiculus of the cord as lateral corticospinal tract (crossed)—8–10% fibers pass uncrossed in the anterior funiculus as the anterior (ventral) corticospinal tract. This tract however, ultimately crosses through anterior white commissure to the opposite anterior gray matter and terminate; it is still about 20% fibers which descend ipsilaterally to terminate uncrossed in the lateral corticospinal tract. Myelination starts about 3 years after birth and is completed by puberty.

a. *Lateral corticospinal tract:*
   - It is situated in the lateral funiculus lateral to posterior gray column, in front of the dorso lateral tract and deep to the posterior spino cerebellar tract and behind rubrospinal tract.
   - It appears at the surface below the second lumbar segment due to absence of posterior spinocerebellar tract at the lower level. Externally, it is present behind the attachment of ligamentum denticulatum.
   - These fibers are somatotopically arranged. In cervical segment longer fibers for lower limb are superficial, intermediate fibers for trunk occupy middle part and shorter fibers from upper limb lie in the deeper plane.
   - These fibers extend whole length of the spinal cord.
   - In its course through the brain stem, the pyramidal tract gives off corticonuclear fibers, which give synaptic connections with the motor nuclei of all the cranial nerves, which has voluntary muscle innervations. These are bilaterally connected; thus, the lesions of the pyramidal system of one side above the level of the brain stem affect only to a slight extent the voluntary movements of the muscles supplied by the cranial nerves.

b. *Anterior corticospinal tract:*
   - It is located in the anterior funiculus alongwith tectospinal tract ventrally.

- It extends only up to the mid thoracic region. These fibers eventually cross the midline and terminate in the anterior gray column of spinal cord segments in the cervical and upper thoracic regions.

Mode of Termination of these Fibers

Most of the corticospinal fibers end in the laminae IV to VII of spinal gray and are connected to the alpha and gamma motor neurons via interneurons of lamina IX, barring few which directly synapse with alpha and gamma neurons of lamina IX.

They provide excitatory fibers to the flexor muscles and inhibitory fibers to the extensor muscles of the trunk.

It is important to note that CS tract fibers are not the sole pathway for serving voluntary movement. Rather they form the pathway that confers speed and agility to voluntary movements and is responsible to modulate the sensory input of spinal cord and brain stem.

Functions

- Essentially, it is concerned with the skillful, nonpostural, volitional movements of the flexor muscles of the trunk and distal parts of the limbs.
- The sensory inputs are modulated for smooth performance of movements.
- As the pyramidal tract contains some ascending spinocortical fibers, it conveys the exteroceptive sensations.
- The pyramidal tract contains some descending autonomic fibers as could be evidenced by some vasomotor disturbance in its lesion.
- The brisk and purposeless movements of the newborn are found to be partly reflex in origin and partly motivated by the extrapyramidal pathways. Thus "Babinski's extensor response" is observed in new born. Volitional control of micturition appear usually after 3 years with the onset of myelination of pyramidal tract.

Extrapyramidal Tracts

This motor system simply represents all motor pathways that do not pass through the pyramids of the medulla. Rubrospinal, vestibulospinal, reticulospinal, tectospinal and olivospinal form this extrapyramidal system. It needs a short description.

Rubrospinal Tract

Origin: From the parvocellular and magnocellular parts of the red nucleus in the midbrain tegmentum.

Course: The axons of the neurons in this nucleus cross the midline decussating with opposite side fibers and descend in the rubrospinal tract through the pons and medulla to enter in the lateral white column of the spinal cord. The fibers then terminate in laminae V to VII of spinal gray.

This tract influence alpha and gamma motor neurons of lamina IX through interneurons. Some ipsilateral corticorubral fibers are received from the motor cortex by the red N. The corticorubrospinal tract thus formed may act as an alternate route of pyramidal system to exert influence on lower motor neurons.

This tract is somatotopically arranged. Fibers are dorsal in cervicothoracic region and ventral in lumbosacral region of the cord.

It facilitates the flexor muscles and inhibits the extensor muscles or antigravity muscles of the body.

The red N, in addition, receives also the input from cerebellum and globus pallidus, so this tract stimulates flexor and inhibit extensor tone.

Vestibulospinal Tract

It originates from the lateral vestibular nucleus situated in the pons and medulla. It descends through the medulla, dorsal to the olivary nucleus. The afferent fibers from the internal ear are received by the vestibular nuclei. The axons from them form the vestibulospinal tract.

The tract descends uncrossed through the length of the spinal cord in the anterior white column and terminate by synapsing with internuncial neurons of the anterior gray column. The cerebellum and inner ear through this tract facilitate the activity of the extensor muscles and inhibit the activity of the flexor muscles in association with the maintenance of the balance.

Olivospinal Tract

It arises from the inferior olivary N and to descend in the internal white column of the spinal cord. It is ipsilaterally present up to the cervical segments.

It influences the activity of the motor neurons in the anterior gray column.

Tectospinal Tract

It arises from the nucleus of the superior colliculus of the midbrain. Most of the fibers cross the midline soon after their origin, descend through brain stem close to the medial longitudinal fasciculus. It is present up to the cervical segment of the cord. The fiber terminals reach the laminae VI to VIII. This tract is believed to be responsible for reflex postural movements in response to visual and hearing stimuli. It forms part of reflex pathway for rotating head and moving the arms in response to visual, hearing and other exteroceptive stimuli.

Reticulospinal Tracts

Groups of scattered nerve cells and nerve fibers exist throughout the midbrain, pons and medulla that are collectively known as reticular formation. They extend throughout the cord.

There are two reticulospinal tracts—medial and lateral.

Medial Reticulospinal

Arise from medial part of pontine reticular formation:
- Descend uncrossed in anterior funiculus and terminate in laminae VII and VIII of spinal gray.
- And it influence facilitates extensor motor neurons and inhibits the flexors.

Lateral Reticulospinal

Originates from gigantocellular component of medullary reticular formation.

- Descend in lateral funiculus of spinal cord medial to pyramidal tract, a rubrospinal tracts.
- Few cross and most fibers are uncrossed.
- Make synapses at all spinal cord levels with laminae VII, VIII and IX by interneurons.

This tract inhibits extensor motor neurons and facilitates the flexors. So, it is opponent to the medial one.

The reticular formation of the brain stem gets input mainly from the motor cortex through the corticoreticular fibers that accompany the corticospinal tracts. This tract thus provides a pathway by which the hypothalamus can control the sympathetic outflow and the sacral parasympathetic outflow.

Medial Longitudinal Fasciculus

It is present ventral to aqueduct of midbrain, which is continuous throughout the length of the brainstem, near midline of the floor of the 4th ventricle. It can be traced caudally into the spinal cord as the anterior inter segmental tract. This new tract is connected to the ventral gray column of the cervical segments of the spinal cord.

Functionally

- A pathway for communication between the cranial nerve nuclei in brain stem and for transmission of fibers from the vestibular nuclei to brainstem and spinal cord.
- It coordinates the activities of the various motor nuclei of cranial nerves by connecting them together, e.g. 3rd, 4th and 6th cranial nerves are interconnected for associated movements of eyes.
- Fibers from both the ipsilateral and contralateral vestibular nuclei send impulses to various cranial nerve nuclei through it. These connections provide for certain postural reflexes, which occur in response to labyrinthine stimuli.
- Some of its fibers relay in medial geniculate body and thereafter are projected to the head region of postcentral gyrus.

Ascending Tracts

Lateral Spinothalamic

It is the main pathway for fast pain and temperature sensations. The pain impulses are transmitted to the spinal cord in fast conducting delta A type fibers and slow conducting C type fibers. The fast conducting fibers alert the individual to initial sharp pain, and the slow conducting fibers are responsible for prolonged burning aching pain. The sensations of heat and cold also travel via delta A and C fibers. The axons entering the spinal cord from the posterior

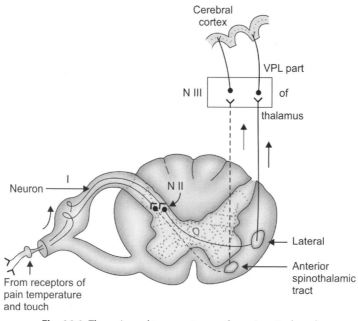

Fig. 14.1: The pain and temperature pathway in spinal cord
Abbreviation: VPL, ventral posterolateral

root ganglion proceed to the tip of the posterior gray column and divide into ascending and descending branches. These branches travel for a distance of one or two segments of spinal cord and form the *posterolateral tract of Lissauer.* These fibers form the first order neuron, terminate by synapsing with cells in the posterior gray column (laminae IV to VII), N proprius, including cells in substances gelatinos. Substance P, a peptide, is thought to be the neurotransmitter at these synapses **(Fig. 14.1).**

The second order fibers arising from the tract cells (nucleus proprius) cross to the opposite side in front of the central canal in the anterior white commissures and ascend through the opposite lateral funiculus to form the lateral spinothalamic tract. Pain fibers in it cross immediately in the same cord segment and temperature fibers a bit obliquely in rostral direction.

This tract lies deep to anterior spinocerebellar tract. It extends along the entire length of the cord. Its position externally is represented by a narrow strip ventral (anterior) to the attachment of ligamentum denticulatum. This position is important to the neurosurgeons while doing tractotomy operation for relieving intractable pain.

The fibers are somatotopically arranged; in upper cervical segment, the arrangement of fibers from superficial to deep are sacral, lumbar, thoracic and cervical. In brain stem superficial fibers go to dorsal aspect.

Temperature fibers are dorsal and pain fibers lie ventral. A few uncrossed fibers of spinothalamic tract arise from the tract cells of same side posterior gray column. Its deeper fibers possibly carry visceral pain sensations.

Further tracing of the fibers above the spinothalamic tract ascends through the medulla oblongata lies between interior olivary nucleus and the nucleus of spinal tract of the trigeminal nerve. It is now accompanied by the anterior spinothalamic tract and the spinotectal tract; they together form the spinal lemniscus. This lemniscus runs cranially lateral to the medial lemniscus in the upper part of brain stem. Ultimately it terminates in the posterolateral part of the ventral (VPL) nucleus of thalamus as well as intralaminar nuclei.

Lesion of this tract produces contralateral loss of pain and temperature of the body below the level of lesion. The third order neuron from the thalamus pass through the posterior limb of the internal capsule and corona radiata to reach the somesthetic area in the post central gyrus of the cerebral cortex.

The cerebral cortex is interpreting the quality of the sensory informations at the level of consciousness.

Anterior Spinothalamic Tract

- Situated in the anterior white funiculus dorsal to the vestibulospinal tract. Spinotectal tract stands between it and lateral spinothalamic tract.
- Fibers of the tract are crossed fibers, which arise from the cells in the laminae IV to VII of the opposite spinal gray column. Discriminative touch and pressure sensations ascend ipsilaterally in posterior funiculus and relays in the N gracilis and cuneatus.
- The tract cells receive afferents of simple touch and pressure from first neurons, through the medial division of dorsal nerve roots and the collaterals of ascending pathways of posterior white funiculi. Therefore, the touch and pressure fibers spread over number of cord segments before entering the spinal gray.
- Second neurons (commences as internal arcuate fibers) cross the middle line and travel via anterior white commissure and proceed above as anterior spinothalamic tract. It joins with lateral spinothalamic tract and forms medial lemniscus.
- Then reaches posterolateral part of ventral N of thalamus.
- So, touch possesses double pathways in the cord and this sensation is rarely lost in any cord lesion.

Spinocerebellar Tracts

Anterior Spinocerebellar

- It lies superficially in the lateral white column infront of posterior spinocerebellar tract.
- It arises in the thoracic and lumbar levels mostly from opposite tract cells of laminae V to VII and partly from the corresponding neurons of the same side.
- It receives afferents through the collaterals of posterior funiculi, wide area of golgi tendon organs and from flexor tendon receptors in the lower half of the body and lower limbs.

- Crossed and uncrossed fibers from the tract cells ascend in the anterior spinocerebellar tract, reach up to midbrain and makes a sharp turn caudally into superior cerebellar peduncle.
- It terminates in the lower limb area of cerebellar cortex.
- It carries unconscious proprioceptive and exteroceptive informations from the lower limbs and lower part of the body. The informations from muscle spindles, tendon organs and joint receptors of the trunk and lower limbs are carried via this tract.
- Upper limb equivalent of the anterior spinocerebellar tract is represented by the rostral spinocerebellar tract which travesl close to anterior spinocerebellar tract.

Posterior Spinocerebellar Tract

- It is located in the posterior part of superficial surface of the lateral funiculus—extends above the level of second or third lumbar segment.
- Cells of origin are at the base of posterior gray column, Clarke's column (lamina VII) which extends from T1 to L2 segments of the cord.
- Fibers (axons) of Clarke's column ascend on the same side as posterior spinocerebellar tract, enter through the inferior cerebellar peduncle and terminate in the limb areas of the anterior and posterior lobes of the cerebellum. This tract is somatotopically arranged.
- It carries unconscious proprioceptive and touch and pressure sensations from lower limbs and lower half of the body to the cerebellum. It is also concerned with fine coordination of individual lower limb muscles during posture and movement.
- It is said collateral branches of some of the axons of this tract are given off in the lower medulla where they terminate in the Z-nucleus of Brodal and Pompeiano. It lies cranial to nucleus gracilis.
- It forms part of the pathway for the conscious proprioception from the lower limb.

The proprioceptive and touch and pressure afferents from the upper limb and upper half of the body ascend through ipsilateral fasciculus cuneatus and terminate in the accessory cuneate nucleus of lower medulla. Axons from the latter from cuneocerebellar tract and reach cerebellum through inferior cerebellar peduncle. Accessory cuneate nucleus corresponds with the nucleus dorsalis and cuneocerebellar tract is the counterpart of posterior spinocerebellar tract.

Pain Control Mechanism

It is believed that fibers of the cells concerned with pain sensation pass through posterior gray column. The analgesic system can suppress both sharp pricking pain and burning pain sensations. Two compounds, enkephalins and endorphins in CNS are neurotransmitters in the analgesic system of the brain and they inhibit the release of polypeptide substance P in the posterior gray column. Substantia gelatinosa cells (SG cells) (lamina II) act as inhibitory neurons and inhibit the T-cells (Tract cells) of lamina IV, which is the chief source of origin of lateral spinothalamic tract.

- Large diameter afferent fibers for touch excite both SG cells and T-cells. Therefore, the incoming signals of pain sensation from T-cells is blocked by simultaneous stimulation of inhibitory SG cells.
- Small diameter afferent fibers excite the T-cells but inhibit the SG cells. Therefore, the gate of pain signal is kept open since the SG cells cannot exert its inhibitory influence.

Thus gentle rubbing (say ointment) over the painful skin area lessens the pain and acts as counterirritant.

Corticospinal tract modify the sensory input of the dorsal root by providing terminals in the interneurons of the posterior gray column.

Biochemical Theory of Pain

It is postulated that fast pricking pain is transmitted by delta type of A-fibers and slow pain of burning and aching is transmitted by unmyelinated C-fibers. Both varieties of pain enter the spinal cord via lateral division of dorsal nerve root and make synapses with neurons of laminae I to IV. To repeat, P substance is liberated at this site, a neurotransmitter.

The ultimate effect of activating neurons around the periaqueductal gray matter is to stimulate serotonergic neurons in the nucleus raphe magnus.

The serotonergic neurons project to the SG neurons of the spinal cord via raphespinal tract, situated lateral to the posterior horn.

The serotonin stimulates the release of enkephalin from the SG cells and this neurotransmitter in its turn blocks and action of substance P.

When the P substance is insufficiently inhibited by the descending pain control mechanism, the T-cell neurons send signals to the lateral spinothalamic tract.

Collaterals from this tract activate periaqueductal grey matter and the medullary raphe nucleus in medulla. This produces an activation of feed-back loop, which enhances activity in the descending pain control system.

Blood Supply of Spinal Cord

- The spinal cord receives its arterial supply from the following arteries:
  - Anterior spinal branches of vertebral artery
  - Posterior spinal branches from deep cervical, ascending cervical, intercostal and lumbar arteries. These branches form three longitudinal arterial trunks, anterior median and two posterior. The fourth part of the vertebral artery gives two spinal branches, anterior and posterior.
- Each anterior spinal artery joins with its opposite fellow and forms an anterior arterial trunk. It descends along with anterior median fissure. It supplies anterior two thirds of the spinal cord (includes anterior gray

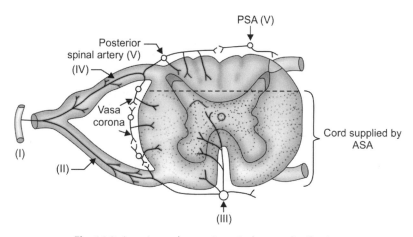

Fig. 14.2: Anterior and posterior spinal artery distribution
Abbreviations: PSA, posterior spinal artery; ASA, anterior spinal artery

columns, bases of posterior gray columns and adjoining parts of white matter). Anterior radicular arteries join with this trunk **(Fig. 14.2)**.

- This anterior trunk supplies the ventral two-thirds of the cross-section of spinal cord.
- Posterior spinal artery—two in number, are derived directly or indirectly from the vertebral artery. They divide to form two descending branches on either sides, one behind and the other in front of the dorsal spinal nerve root. They supply the white matter of the cord. They join with the posterior radicular arteries.
- The spinal branches of the rest of the arteries mentioned above reach the cord as the anterior and posterior radicular arteries along the corresponding roots of the spinal nerves. The three arterial trunks anastomose around the cord and the pial arterial plexus is formed, known as vasa corona **(Fig. 14.3)**.
- A quarter of anterior radicular arteries (about 8 in number) are enlarged in lower cervical, lower thoracic and upper lumbar regions. These enlarged arteries join with anterior spinal artery and anterior arterial trunk is formed.
- The largest of the great radicular arteries is known as the arteria radicularis magna (artery of Adamkiewicz). It varies in position; but usually arises from lower thoracic or upper lumbar branches of aorta. Lower two-thirds of the spinal cord are supplied by the arteria magna through its anterior and posterior branches to the anterior and posterior trunks respectively.
- The posterior one-third of the cord is supplied by a pair of posterior arterial trunks and by the vasa corona **(Fig. 14.4)**.
- Certain zones of the spinal cord where different major arteries meet are vulnerable to ischemic necrosis due to vascular injury. The zones are T1 to T4 and L1 segments.

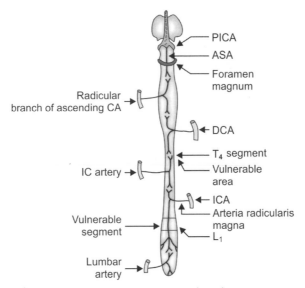

Fig. 14.3: Anterior arterial trunk

Abbreviations: PICA, posterior inferior cerebellar artery; ASA, anterior spinal artery; DCA, deep cervical artery; ICA, internal carotid artery

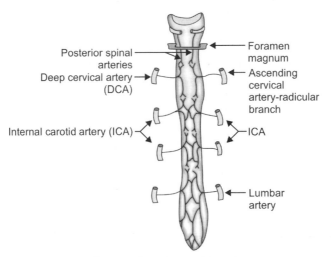

Fig. 14.4: Posterior arterial trunk

Applied Anatomy on Spinal Cord

The cord may be injured from trauma, impairment of blood supply, infection, degenerative and demyelinating disorders and from extramedullary tumors.

1. *Lesion of dorsal root:* Due to slipped disk or extramedullary tumor:
   - Sharp pain felt over affected dermatomes.
   - Occasional paresthesia such as numbness and prickling.

- Segmental cutaneous vasodilatation due to reflex of autonomic system.

Such irritative features of severe root pain is found in degenerative disease like tabes dorsalis (neurosyphilis) or in herpes zoster (viral infection). Cell bodies, in both diseases, of dorsal root ganglion are affected.

2. Complete destruction of dorsal root fibers; ipsilateral and segmental loss of all sensations.
   - Anesthesia and analgesia.
   - Loss of conscious muscle sense, producing ataxia.
   - Loss of unconscious muscle sense from stretch receptors of muscle spindle with hypotonia or atonia.
   - Trophic ulcers due to loss of sensations.
   - Loss of reflex functions.

3. *Complete destruction of posterior white funiculus:* Loss of position sense, vibratory sense, sense of stereognosis and discriminative touch on the same side at and below the level of cord lesion.

4. *Spinothalamic tract lesion:*
   - *If lateral spinothalamic tract is injured:* There is loss of pain and temperature on the opposite side below the level of lesion.
   - *If anterior spinothalamic tract is injured:* Touch and pressure senses on the opposite side are not much affected as these senses are also being carried by uncrossed fibers of posterior funiculi.

5. *Syringomyelia:* Damage to the decussating lateral spinothalamic fibers due to cavitation near the central canal produces syringomyelia. It causes bilateral and segmental loss of pain and temperature of both upper limbs as the cavitation affects the central canal destroys the decussating spinothalamic fibers in anterior funiculi in cervical region; the touch escapes. It is known as "dissociated sensory loss".

6. Combined upper and lower motor neuron disease is caused by bilateral damage to the corticospinal tract and motor neurons in the anterior horn. This may be caused by degenerative disease like amyotrophic lateral sclerosis. The disease is manifested with weakness, atrophy and fasciculation of the muscles of hands and arms; it is followed by spastic paralysis of lower limbs.

7. *Thrombosis of the anterior spinal artery:* It involves anterior gray columns, spinothalamic and corticospinal tracts of both sides.
   - If thrombosis be in the upper thoracic segments, it produces flaccid paralysis and atrophy at the level of lesion due to loss of lower motor neurons of the anterior gray column.
   - It will be associated with spastic paraplegia (due to pyramidal tract involvement) and loss of pain and temperature sense below the level of lesion due to loss of lateral spinothalamic tracts. The onset must be sudden. Conscious proprioceptive sensations are preserved as the posterior funiculi are supplied by posterior spinal arteries.

8. *Hemisection of the cord:* (Brown–Sequard syndrome)—(due to bullet or knife injury). Clinically, it is a rare.

   i. *On the same side of the lesion:*
- Involvement of lateral corticospinal tract (produces spastic paralysis, tendon reflexes exaggerated and Babinski sign positive. Ipsilateral UMN paralysis. Ataxia is not demonstrated due to paralysis.
- *Involvement of posterior funiculus:* Produces loss of position and vibration senses, disturbances of stereognosis and tactile discrimination. (Ipsilateral loss).
- *Involvement of hypothalamospinal tract:* Produces Horner's syndrome.

   ii. *On the opposite side of the lesion:*
- Involvement of lateral spinothalamic tract produces loss of pain and temperature, one or two segments below the level of lesion.
- Contralateral little or no loss in sense of touch due to injury of anterior spinothalamic tract. Tactile impulses ascend on both sides of the cord.

   From injury of local cord segments and nerve root:
- Same side anesthesia over the dermatome innervated by the segment of lesion due to damage of dorsal nerve roots.
- Same side hyperesthesia or radicular pain above the level of lesion: Due to irritation of dorsal nerve roots.
- Same side LMN paralysis in the segment of lesion due to injury to ventral nerve roots.

9. *Destruction of ventral root produces:* [LMN paralysis] Flaccid paralysis of the muscle occur with loss of reflexes. Poliomyelitis results from damage to motor neurons in the anterior horn.

10. The tracts of posterior column and lateral corticospinal tracts undergo bilateral degeneration in pernicious anemia (vitamin B_{12} neuropathy). Loss of position sense and vibration sensations and tactile discrimination (posterior column lesion) and bilateral spasticity, tendon reflexes exaggerated and Babinski sign positive occur.

11. *Direct injury to conus medullaris destroys segmental neurons (conus syndrome):* It produces
- Weakness of movement in the feet and loss of sensation in the buttocks (due to involvement anterior and posterior gray horns), paralysis of urinary bladder and rectum (due to involvement of intermediolateral cell column—S2. S3. S4 segments).
- It may be caused by injury to vertebra L1 or prolapse IVD between L1 and L2 since the sacral segments of nerves lie against these vertebrae.
- Saddle shaped anesthesia in buttock.
- Knee and ankle jerks normal.

12. *Lesion in sensory tract:* Tabes dorsalis—it is caused by syphilis (bilateral involvement of dorsal root and fasciculus cuneatus and gracilis). Affection usually takes place in lower thoracic and lumbosacral regions.
The following signs and symptoms may be exhibited:
- Stabbing pains in the lower limbs.

- Hypersensitivity of skin to touch, heat and cold.
- Loss of sensation in the skin of the trunk and lower limbs and numbness in lower limbs.
- Loss of awareness about the fullness of the urinary bladder.
- Loss of appreciation of posture or passive movements of the lower limbs especially the legs. Romberg's sign is positive.
- Loss of pain sensation in the skin, e.g. side of the nose or the medial border of the forearm or the thoracic wall between the nipples.
- Locomotor ataxia, corrected by vision (unlike cerebellum).
- Loss of tendon reflexes due to degeneration of the afferent fibers of the reflex arc (the knee and ankle tendon jerks are lost early in the disease).
- Hypotonia, as the result of loss of proprioceptive information that arises from muscles and joints.
- Intractable pain can be treated in selected cases by cutting the appropriate posterior nerve roots (posterior rhizotomy) or by division of the spinothalamic tract on the side opposite the pain sensation felt (tractotomy or cordotomy). A needle passed 3 mm into the cord (lateral column) anterior to the ligamentum denticulatum and then swept anteriorly from this point will sever the spinothalamic tract but preserve the pyramidal tract lying immediately posterior to it. In upper limb involvement with pain, the tract is often cut in the midbrain. In cases of involuntary tremor or movements, the anterior white columns or the lateral white columns posterior to ligamentum denticulatum have been sectioned to interrupt various motor paths. The pain fibers in lateral spinothalamic tract is superficial to temperature fiber which is deep.

13. Complete transection of the cord is followed by total loss of sensation in the region (supplied by the cord segments) below the level of injury together with flaccid muscle paralysis (injury to corticospinal tracts). Voluntary sphincter control is lost but reflex emptying of bladder and rectum subsequently return, provided that the cord centers situated in the sacral zone of the cord are not injured.

    If the transection occurs above fifth cervical cord segment, the patient succumbs due to paralysis of respiratory muscles following involvement of phrenic nucleus.

14. There is an area in the spinal cord between L4 and S2 spinal segment, known as Epiconus. Its syndrome is rare. In the injury of this segment of the cord produces:

    i. Reduced or loss of lateral rotation (L4 to S1) and extension (L4 and L5) of hip joint.
    ii. Reduced of loss of flexion of the knee (L5 to S1).
    iii. Reduced or loss of flexion and extension in the joints of foot and toes (L4 to S2).
    iv. Tendo Achilles reflexes is absent (L5. S1. S2).
    v. Knee jerk (reflex) is preserved (L2,3,4).

vi. Sensory disturbances in L4 to S2 dermatomes.

vii. *Emptying of urinary bladder and rectum:* Preserved (L12 to L2 and S3 to S5).

viii. Absence of sweat secretion.

15. The cauda equina is conglomeration of ten pairs of nerves disposed around filum terminale. It includes four lumber (except L1), five sacral and one coccygeal nerves in pairs. It may be injured by its compression within the vertebral canal or inadvertent puncture of the cauda during lumbar puncture. The regeneration is possible.

    Features of injury:
    a. LMN type of paralysis.
    b. Sensory loss in root distribution.
    c. Severe root pain.
    d. Knee and ankle jerks absent.
    e. Late urinary bladder and rectum symptoms.

16. When the fasciculi gracilis and fasciculus. cuneatus are selectively sectioned the following effects are observed: As these two tracts carry conscious proprioceptive and deep sensations from muscles, joints, tendons and ligaments, some degenerative diseases like tabes dorsalis destroy them. Sense of position, pressure movement and tactile discrimination also are being carried by these tracts.

Effects

- Impairment of proprioceptive sense, i.e. sense of tactile discrimination, vibration and posture.
- The patient cannot maintain balance with eyes closed—Romberg's sign.
- Touch—light and crude—is preserved as it is being carried by spinothalamic tract.

Bibliography

1. Engler, Cole and Merton. Spinal cord diseases: Diagnosis and treatment. Informa Health Care; 1989. pp. 1-14.
2. Frederick M Maynard. Functional Classification of Spinal Cord Injury. Spinal Cord. 1997;35:266-74.
3. Gelfan, et al. Physiology of Spinal Cord, Nerve Root and Peripheral Nerve Compression. American Journal of Physiology. 1956;185:217-29.
4. Govender, et al. Congenital Cervical Spinal Cord Lesions: Pathogenesis, Management, and Outcome. Journal of Child Neurology. 2007;22:874-9.
5. Greathouse, et al. Blood Supply to the Spinal Cord. Physical Therapy. 2001;81: 1264-5.
6. Hiersemenzel, et al. From spinal shock to spasticity: Neuronal adaptations to a spinal cord injury. Neurology. 2000;54:1574-82.
7. Hughes JT. Pathology of the spinal cord. Major Problems in Pathology. 1978;6: 1-257.
8. Kakulas BA. Pathology of spinal injuries. Central Nervous System Trauma. 1984;2:117-29.

9. Laising Yen, Robert G. Kalb. Review: Recovery from Spinal Cord Injury: New Approaches. Neuroscientist. 1995;1:321-7.
10. Laslett EE, Warrington WB. Observations on the ascending tracts in the spinal cord of the human subject. Brain. 1999;22:586-92.
11. Lois A Gillilan. Veins of the spinal cord: Anatomic details; suggested clinical applications. Neurology. 1970;20:860.
12. Marion, et al. Topographical anatomy of the posterior columns of the spinal cord in man: The long ascending fibers. Brain. 1984;107:671-98.
13. Morishita, et al. Anatomical study of blood supply to the spinal cord. Annals of Thoracic Surgery. 2003;76:1967-71.
14. Ove Hassler. Blood Supply to Human Spinal Cord: A Microangiographic Study. Archive of Neurology. 1966;15:302-7.
15. Robert F Spetzlerj. Modified classification of spinal cord vascular lesions. Neurosurgery. 2002;96:145-56.
16. Roth EJ. Traumatic central cord syndrome: Clinical features and functional outcomes. Archive of Physical Medicine and Rehabilitation. 1990;71(1):18-23.
17. Schiff and Neill. Intramedullary spinal cord metastases: Clinical features and treatment outcome. Neurology. 1996;47:906-12.
18. Solsberg, et al. High-resolution MR imaging of the cadaveric human spinal cord: Normal anatomy. American Journal of Neuroradiology. 1990;11:3-7.
19. Wall PD, Werman R. The physiology and anatomy of long ranging afferent fibers within the spinal cord. Journal of Physiology. 1976;255:321-34.
20. William P, et al. Spinal cord infarction: Etiology and outcome. Neurology. 1996;47:321-30.
21. Williamson RT. The Direct Pyramidal Tracts of the Spinal Cord. British Medical Journal. 1993;1:946-7.

15

Pathophysiology of Spinal Injury

Milind Deogaonkar

Introduction

Understanding pathophysiology of spinal injury involves unfolding two entirely separate but equally important processes that run hand in hand. The phenomenon of spinal cord injury evolves simultaneously along with the biomechanics of spinal column injury. Though entirely different in the nature of progression, timing of treatment and outcomes, these two phenomena form two wheels of the dynamics of progression of spinal injuries. Treating physician has to be aware of the intricacies and nuances of molecular changes occurring in the spinal cord parenchyma as well as the biomechanics of an unstable spine for successfully treating a spinal injury.

Biomechanics of an injured spinal column is decided by the nature of traumatic forces, direction of injury and pre-existing spinal diseases. Since the spinal cord is covered on all sides by the bony spinal canal, cord injury is in almost all cases accompanied by and usually a consequence of vertebral injury. The vertebral column itself consisting of 33 separate bony elements does not move as a single piece but rather movement occurs to varying degrees between separate elements, the culmination of which helps to achieve the whole range of motion. In some places, e.g. the cervical spine, stability has been sacrificed for increasing mobility. The reverse occurs in the thoracic spine.

Spinal Column Injury: Traumatic Forces

In a dynamic and multisegmented structure such as spinal column, different traumatic forces produce different types of injuries. The direction and nature of traumatic force decides the type of injury.[1] The traumatic forces can be broadly grouped as follows (**Figs 15.1A and B**):

Axial Loading Force

- Fibers are pushed together in a crushing manner
- Tends to fracture vertebrae in multiple pieces
- Usually associated with flexion, extension, or rotational injuries.

Distraction Force

- Bony, disk, or soft tissue elements are pulled apart
- Usually associated with flexion or extension injuries.

Shear Force

- Force parallel to the surface on which it acts; results in a translation or subluxation movement
- Usually results in anterior or lateral displacement of affected elements.

Rotational Force

- Torsional force that creates a rotational tension on tissue fibers
- Often associated with axial forces.

The nature of injury a spinal column sustains is directly proportional to the force of impact and so does the injury to spinal cord.

Spinal Column Injury: Mechanism of Injury

Knowing the mechanism of spinal injury can also assist in proper diagnosis. When the patient has suffered an injury that involves fall from height it results in axial loading type of injury. In a vehicular accident it could be multiple types of traumatic forces but the most common are flexion-extension injuries that are commonly called as whiplash injuries.[2] Allen, in 1982 developed a classification system for cervical spine injuries that takes into account the mechanisms of injury.[3] He grouped injuries to lower cervical spine into six categories, based on the position of the cervical spine at the time of impact and on the predominant area of damage. The six categories were compressive flexion, vertical compression, distractive flexion, compressive extension, distractive extension, and lateral flexion. Of these, the distractive flexion injuries were the most common, followed by the compressive extension injuries and the compressive flexion injuries. The characteristics of the commonest, i.e. flexion and extension injuries are as follows (**Figs 15.1A and B**):

Flexion

- Severe forward bending of the neck or trunk
- Causes compressive force on the anterior vertebral column; teardrop or wedge type fracture to vertebral body.

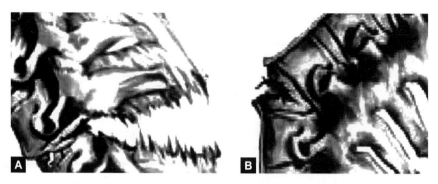

Figs 15.1A and B: Flexion and extension injuries of cervical spine

Extension

- Severe backward bending of the neck or trunk
- Axial loads often also associated
- Causes fractures to the spinous process and lamina.

Spinal Column Injury: Concept of Stability

A major question that decides nature, urgency and method of treatment in all spinal injuries is whether the injured spine is stable or not? As a 'safe assumption' all injured spinal columns should be considered unstable unless proven otherwise before the full clinical and radiological evaluation is carried out. The concept of spinal stability has undergone a vast change in last three decades due to work of some dedicated investigators like Dennis, White and Panjabi.

Holdsworth in 1970, advocated the concept of the two-column spinal stability.[4] According to him the anterior column had the vertebral body, disk, and anterior and posterior longitudinal ligaments; and the posterior column consisted of the posterior bony arch, interspinous and intertransverse ligaments, and facet joints. He called a spine unstable when both these columns were injured.

In 1983, Denis changed it to a three-column concept of spinal stability[5] **(Fig. 15.2)**. He described the three-column spine, in which the middle column comprised of the posterior half of the vertebral body and disk as well as the posterior longitudinal ligament. According to Denis, if two columns are injured then the spine is unstable. Though this was a concept originally devised for thoracolumbar spine, it is presently applied to the whole spinal column.

Panjabi has further validated and refined this concept of three-column spinal stability.[6] Punjabi and White[7] have enumerated criteria of spinal stability through detailed study of spinal biomechanics and have proven that an unstable spine entails the risk of furthering neurological injury.

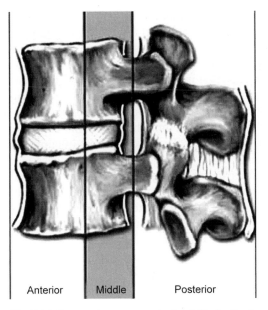

Anterior   Middle   Posterior

Fig. 15.2: Three-column concept of stability by Denis

Spinal Cord Injury: Pathophysiology

Experimental and clinical studies on spinal cord injury noted that there is a spectrum of pathologic appearances that evolve over the initial days following injury. This led to the concept that the injury process was a result of both primary and secondary insults. While the primary injury was not amenable to any pharmacological intervention, the effects of secondary insult could be mitigated if treatment was started early enough. 'Primary' spinal cord injury generally causes a temporary loss of function with pathologic change caused by the direct impact. However, the initial trauma initiates a cascade of downstream injury mechanisms that include accumulation of excitatory amino acids, neurotransmitters, vasoactive eicosanoids, oxygen free radicals, by-products of lipid peroxidation and activation of programmed cell death pathways. Loss of the "blood-cord barrier" causes edema and increased tissue pressure that, along with cord hemorrhage, limit the blood supply, with the result that cell ischemia may further damage the cord. This is the 'secondary' cord injury, which generally is preventable if proper and early treatment is ensued. Initial spinal cord injury initiates a variety of complex systemic and local responses. Ischemia is a prominent feature of events occurring after spinal cord injury.[8] Within the first two hours of a spinal cord injury, there is a significant reduction in spinal cord blood flow. It is not clear as for the reasons of this reduction in the local blood flow. The spinal cord also possesses autoregulatory capacity like elsewhere in the nervous system. Any fall in systemic blood pressure can reduce the spinal cord blood flow as the loss of autoregulation at the injured segment makes local blood flow solely dependent on the systemic blood pressure. In a patient with other systemic injuries and hypotension, there can be exacerbation of the primary injury. Another complicating factor is edema. It develops first in the injured segments but then rapidly spreads to many segments below and above. Cord hypoxia further aggravates edema. The role of edema in causing neurological worsening is not fully understood. In a compressed spinal cord though, the edema can further increase the neurological injury. There is also an immediate inflammatory response as a response to injury. This is accompanied by the release of toxic substances, which cause further tissue damage, or secondary injury. As already stated, processes resulting in secondary injury involve generation of free radicals, excessive calcium influx and excitotoxicity, the release of eicosanoids and cytokines, and programmed cell death.

The important part to understand here is, all these secondary injury pathways can be stopped with early intervention. Avoiding systemic hypotension is a key issue. As shown by the NASCIS 2 and NASCIS 3 studies, use of methylprednisolone within 3–8 hours of injury prevents part of the secondary injury and improves neurologic recovery.

References

1. Allen BL, et al. A mechanistic classification of closed, indirect fractures and dislocations of the lower cervical spine. Spine. 1982;7:1.
2. Macnabb I. The "whiplash syndrome." Orthop Clin North Am. 1971;2:389.
3. Allen BL, et al. A mechanistic classification of closed, indirect fractures and dislocations of the lower cervical spine. Spine. 1982;7:1.
4. Holdsworth F. Fractures, dislocations, and fracture dislocations of the spine. J Bone Joint Surg Am. 1970;52:1534.
5. Denis F. The three-column spine and its significance in the classification of acute thoracolumbar spine injuries. Spine. 1983;8:817.
6. Panjabi MM, et al. Validity of the three-column theory of thoracolumbar fractures. Spine. 1995;20:1122.
7. White AA III, Panjabi MM. Update on the evaluation of instability of the lower cervical spine. Instr Course Lect. 1987;36:513.
8. Sandler A, Tator C. Review of the effects of spinal trauma on vessels and blood flow in the spinal cord. J Neurosurg. 1972;45:638.

16

Evaluation of Spinal Cord Injury

HS Chhabra

Introduction

A proficient and accurate clinical evaluation is the most vital component of therapeutic intervention and effective management of a disease. This forms the foundation of all therapeutic programs in clinical practice, be it surgical or conservative.

The clinical evaluation holds special relevance in the management of spinal cord injuries, as it is a continuous process and involves multi-dimensional aspects for the complete and comprehensive management of spinal cord injuries.

The initial evaluation permits the development of a rational plan of treatment and determination of the likely prognosis. As the functional consequences of an acute spinal cord injury are variable, consistent and reproducible, neurological assessment scales are required to define the patient's neurological deficits and to facilitate communication about the patient's status to the agonized and apprehensive family members. It also helps in estimating the prognosis on the basis of outcomes of earlier patients with a similar neurological deficit.

The baseline evaluation of patient documents the initial status, which can be used as a comparative parameter for detecting the later improvement or deterioration in patient's condition.

The evaluation process continues throughout the program allowing the team to evaluate progress, reassess goals, and update the program, so that any blocks to progress can be identified and solved accordingly. It also helps in planning a smooth transition of patient from the hospital setup into the community, with suitable vocational and social modifications.

An evaluation at discharge helps in determining the outcomes accurately. It also helps to evaluate the effectiveness of the therapeutic program.

It forms the basis of future evaluation/management of the patient by his family physician and for a lifelong follow-up.

A thorough assessment on the basis of accurate, reproducible neurological assessment scales and reliable functional outcome measurement tools is vital for the evaluation of new therapies proposed for the management of spinal cord injuries.

A comprehensive evaluation of the spinal cord injured includes emergency room assessment, detailed history including clinical, social, sexual and vocational issues, general medical evaluation, neurological assessment, determination of functional ability status, assessment for potential complications which may or may not be directly related to trauma, psychological assessment and assessment with regard to requirement for equipment, aids and appliances and home, workplace and environment modifications. Emergency room assessment is vital but outside the scope of the book and hence will not be discussed.

History

The history should include date, level and mode of the injury. It should also mention any associated trauma or complications, any change in neurological status since the time of injury and any other medical condition which could affect the functional outcome. The history should also include information about first-aid received at the site of accident, mode of transport to the hospital, number of institutional transfers before reaching definitive hospital and a summary of the treatment received at the initial hospital.

Any relevant past history related to patients physical or psychosocial status should also be elicited. A detailed history of social issues should be taken at an appropriate time. These issues include the marital status, details of family members and children, kind of family (nuclear or joint), family support, educational level, individual and family income, financial issues, kind of lifestyle, hobbies and recreational activities. All relevant details should be taken regarding the nature of previous vocation especially with regard to the feasibility of pursuing it from the wheelchair. This knowledge along with that of the educational and social background is useful in planning for a suitable vocation for the patient.

The history with regard to sexuality issues would help in working out a plan for sexual rehabilitation. A detailed history should also be taken with regard to access at home, neighborhood and workplace.

Impairment, Disability and Handicap

Impairment is the lack of normal anatomical or psychological function. Disability is the inability to perform functional tasks as a result of the impairment. Handicap is the social disadvantage secondary to a disability. Neurological examination scales are used to assess the impairment. Functional ability assessment would document the resultant disability. Handicap is partly determined by the premorbid social, financial and vocational status.

Neurological Assessment

Frankel et al. were the first to report a stratified neurological scale for patients with acute traumatic spinal injuries in 1969. A five grade (A to E) scale was used to define spinal cord injuries in 682 patients managed at Stoke Mandeville hospital between 1951 and 1968. Grade A patients had complete motor and sensory impairment, Grade B patients had only sensory function below the level of injury, Grade C patients had motor and sensory function below the level of injury but the motor function was useless, Grade D patients had useful but not normal motor function below the level of injury and Grade E patients had no motor, sensory or sphincter disturbance. The Frankel scale was widely used in the 1970s and 1980s. It was easy to use, was based solely upon motor and sensory functions and required very little patient assessment for classification. However, differentiation between patients classified into Grades C and D was imprecise. They were broad groups with considerable range within each grade. The sensibility of the Frankel scale to change in serial measurements, particularly among patients in grades C and D was poor. Significant improvements in patient function could occur over time without the patient advancing a Frankel grade. The use of Frankel scale as either an acute assessment tool or an outcome measure has largely been abandoned due to its lack of sensitivity.

Various other neurological assessment scales were introduced like University of Miami Neurospinal Index (UMNI), Yale Scale, Sunnybrook Cord Injury Scale, National Acute Spinal Cord Injury Study Scale (NASCIS Scale). However, the American Spinal Injury Association (ASIA) standard for neurological classification of spinal injury patients first generated in 1984 has been the most accepted one. The neurological assessment used a ten muscle group motor index score (zero to five points scale) and incorporated the Frankel classification as the functional abilities assessment tool. The sensory examination was not scored but the most cephalad of normal sensation was noted. These standards were revised in 1989 to provide better, more specific sensory level determination. However, studies showed that the inter-observer reliability was "less than optimal".

Some studies showed that one classification system or scale alone does not adequately describe SCI patients in both the acute and follow-up settings. They favored a combination of two scales to characterize acute spinal cord injury patients, one based on neurological impairment and the other on functional disability.

The study by Lazor et al. in 1989 concluded that the motor index score is a useful tool in predicting function during rehabilitation, although individual differences in ambulation, particularly for patients with paraplegia, limit the predictive utility of this index.

In 1992, ASIA generated new standards for neurological and functional classification of spinal cord injury in conjunction with the International Medical Society of Paraplegia (IMSOP). These standards replaced the revised 1989 version. The new assessment recommendations included motor index scores, sensory examination scores (zero to two point scale), the ASIA impairment scale (modified Frankel classification) and incorporated the Functional Independence Measure (FIM). FIM is a functional assessment tool and is used to assess the impact of SCI on the patient's functional abilities. It quantifies the extent of individual disability and complements the neurological assessment by providing scoring for activities of eating, grooming, bathing, dressing upper body, dressing lower body and toileting. Improvements in neurological function over time or with treatment (as documented by neurological examination scales) can be measured in terms of functional or meaningful improvement to the patients with the addition of FIM in the assessment battery. However, Jonson et al found weak inter-rater reliability for scoring patients with incomplete spinal cord injuries.

In 1996, ASIA/IMSOP provided a revised version of the international standards for neurological and functional classification of spinal injury (an update of their 1992 recommendations). Further refined by input from numerous international organizations, the combination of the ASIA impairment scale, the ASIA motor index score, the ASIA sensory scale and FIM is considered to be the most representative assessment and classification tool for patients with acute spinal cord injuries. It was felt to be an improvement on the pre-existing 1992 standards, which were subject to criticism.

ASIA Scoring

American Spinal Injury Association scoring system classifies patients on the basis of their clinical examination, and not by radiological or anatomical abnormalities. The essential elements include the bilateral assessment of 10 index muscles and 28 dermatomes. Rectal sensation and voluntary sphincteric contraction are also evaluated.

The index muscles are assessed in the supine position **(Table 16.1)**. Each index muscle receives a score from 0 to 5. The motor level is the lowest index muscle with at least grade 13 strength; all cephalad muscles must have grade 15 strength. Thus, a left and right motor level can be obtained. The motor level is deemed the most caudal segment with normal motor function. The "final" motor level is the higher of the left and right motor levels. The motor score is the sum of the individual motor assessment from each index muscle. This value ranges from 0 to 100.

Table 16.1: Index muscles examined for ASIA scoring system		
Myotomes	Index muscle	Action
C5	Biceps, brachialis	Elbow flexors
C6	Extensor carpi radialis	Wrist extensors
C7	Triceps	Elbow extensors
C8	Flexor digitorum profundus	Finger flexors
T1	Abductor digiti minimi	Small finger abductors
L2	Iliopsoas	Hip flexors

Contd...

Contd...

Myotomes	Index muscle	Action
L3	Quadriceps	Knee extensors
L5	Tibialis anterior	Ankle dorsiflexors
L5	Extensor hallucis longus	Long toe extensors
S1	Gastrocnemius	Ankle plantar flexors

Assessment of Strength

0. Total paralysis
1. Palpable or visible contraction
2. Active movement, full range of movement with gravity eliminated
3. Active movement, full range of movement against gravity
4. Active movement, full range of movement against moderate resistance
5. Normal active movement, full range of movement against full resistance.

Light touch and pinprick are assessed from 28 dermatomes bilaterally. For every segment, a score of 0 (absent), 1 (impaired), and 2 (normal) is determined for each modality. Four different scores are generated: left light touch, right light touch, left pinprick, and right pinprick. The sensory score is the sum of the dermatomal sensory scores for each modality and ranges from 0 to 112. Based on this clinical assessment, a sensory level can be determined for the left and right sides of the body. The sensory level is defined as the highest level with entirely normal sensory function (i.e. both pinprick and light touch). The "final" sensory level is the higher of the left and right sensory levels.

The rectal exam is an essential element of the ASIA scoring system. The examiner's finger must be placed in the rectum, and the patient must be asked if he perceives any sensation. The patient is also asked to "bear down" on the examiner's finger to determine if volitional contraction of the sphincter exists.

The neurological level is the most caudal spinal segment with entirely normal function. Evaluation of the C5 to T1 and L4 to S1 segments involves the assessment of a motor and sensory function. However, all other segments (C2 to C4, T2 to T12 and S2 to S4/5) require only an assessment of sensory function. To determine the neurological level, it is helpful to review the left and right motor and sensory levels. For example, a patient with a left and right C7 motor level and a left and right C6 sensory level would be assigned a C6 neurological level. However, motor function in the thoracic spinal segments below the T1 level are not scored with the ASIA paradigm. Sensation (pinprick and light touch) is the only function that is scored between the T2 and T12 segments. Consider the case where an individual had a grade 5 power in all the index muscles of the upper extremity (i.e. left and right T1 motor level) and grade 10 power in the lower extremities. In addition, this person had a left and right T8 sensory level. In this example, the neurological level assigned would be T8.

In summary, four different levels are obtained: left motor, right motor, left sensory and right sensory. On occasion, the process of assigning a neurological level results in misrepresentation of patient's true impairment. This is particularly evident when there is a marked discrepancy between the motor and sensory levels, or in a lesion with asymmetrical motor and sensory findings. It is advisable to document all four levels, in addition to the final neurological level. The ASIA impairment rating provides a framework to classify injuries as complete or incomplete. To categorize an injury as incomplete, there must be some intact sensory or motor function in the S4/5 segments; this is manifested by some sensation at the anal musculocutaneous junction, deep anal sensation on rectal examination, or voluntary contraction of the anal sphincter.

The zone of partial preservation (ZPP) refers to the number of partially intact dermatomes and myotomes caudal to the neurological level. By ASIA directive, the ZPP should only be calculated in complete lesions.

Steps in Assigning an ASIA Level

1. Examine 10 index muscles bilaterally
2. Examine 28 dermatomes bilaterally for pinprick and light touch
3. Complete rectal exam to assess sensation and volitional sphincteric contraction
4. Determine left and right motor levels
5. Determine left and right sensory levels
6. Assign "final" motor and sensory levels
7. Determine neurological level, which is the most caudal segment with normal motor and sensory function
8. Categorize injury as complete or incomplete by ASIA impairment scale **(Table 16.2)**
9. Calculate motor and sensory score
10. Determine zone of partial preservation in complete injury ("A" on ASIA impairment scale) **(Fig. 16.1)**

Table 16.2: ASIA impairment scale		
☐	A	*Complete:* No sensory or motor function is preserved in the sacral segments S4/5.
☐	B	*Sensory incomplete:* Sensory but no motor function is preserved below the neurological level and includes the sacral segments S4/5.
☐	C	*Motor incomplete:* Motor function is preserved below the neurological level, and more than half of the key muscles below the neurological level have a muscle grade less than 3. There must be some sparing of sensory and/or motor function in the sacral segments S4/5.
☐	D	*Motor incomplete:* Motor function is preserved below the neurological level, and at least half of the key muscles below the neurological level have a muscle grade greater than or equal to 3. There must be some sparing of sensory and/or motor function in the sacral segments S4/5.
☐	E	*Normal:* Sensory and motor functions are normal. Patient may have abnormalities on reflex examination.

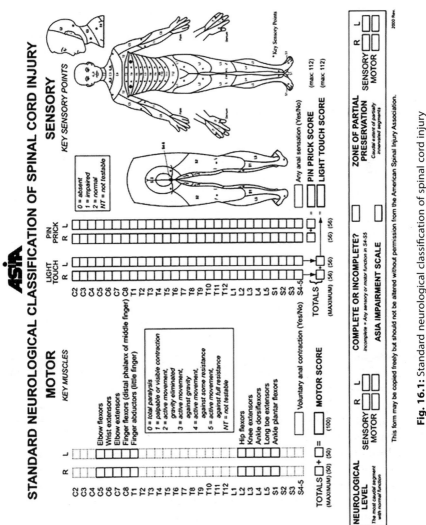

Fig. 16.1: Standard neurological classification of spinal cord injury

Clinical Syndromes

	☐	Central cord
	☐	Brown-Sequard
	☐	Anterior cord
	☐	Conus medullaris
	☐	Cauda equina

Functional Outcome Scales

Functional outcome scales are nonspecific measures of human performance ability relevant to medical rehabilitation, that is, how a person functions with activities of everyday life. Several scales have been developed in an effort to accurately characterize an injured victim's functional skills and disabilities in order to quantify his or her functional independence. They attempt to determine a patient's ability or inability to live independently. The functional evaluation provides a starting point for goal setting and program development. The areas commonly covered in a functional evaluation include mat and bed abilities, transfers, wheelchair skills, ambulation and the ability to instruct others in dependent activities.

Mat and bed abilities: The therapist should evaluate the patient's capabilities in rolling, coming to sitting, and gross mobility (moving to the right or left, forward or backward) on an exercise mat. These activities should also be evaluated on a bed because functioning on beds is much more difficult.

Transfers: The evaluation should address even and uneven transfers. Even transfers involve moving between the wheelchair and a surface that is level with the wheelchair seat. An uneven transfer involves moving between the wheelchair and a higher or lower surface such as a bathtub, toilet, couch, truck, car, plinth, or the floor.

To be independent in a transfer from a wheelchair, a person must be able to set up for the transfer. This includes positioning the wheelchair, locking the brakes, removing or repositioning an armrest, positioning the leg and footrests, and positioning the sliding board, if one is used. The person must be able to move his/her entire body onto the surface, including his/her legs. To be independent in a transfer to the wheelchair, he/she must be able to prepare to leave the area following the transfer. This involves positioning his/her body appropriately on the wheelchair seat, removing the sliding board (if used), positioning his/her footrests and armrests, placing his/her feet on the footrests, and unlocking the brakes.

To transfer safely, a cord-injured person must move from one surface to another without falling and without traumatizing his/her skin.

Wheelchair: The therapist should check the person's capabilities in wheelchair propulsion and obstacle negotiation. Propulsion over even surfaces, distance that he is able to travel and the time required to propel this distance should be recorded. Evaluation of obstacle negotiation should cover the ability to maneuver over uneven terrain (grass, dirt, gravel, sidewalk), curbs (the therapist should specify the height that can be managed independently), inclined surfaces, doorways, and stairs. Any special equipment that is required for propulsion, such as pegs or surgical tubing on the wheelchair hand rims should be noted.

Pressure relief in a wheelchair are critical to a spinal cord-injured person's health. The evaluation should determine both whether the person is capable of performing pressure relief and whether he/her assumes the responsibility to get the relief at appropriate intervals.

Ambulation: If a cord-injured person is ambulatory, the therapist should determine how far he/her can walk, the time required to walk this distance, the gait pattern used, and the level of assistance required. Capabilities in obstacle negotiation (obstacles listed above in wheelchair skills section) should also be assessed. Additional ambulatory skills that should be addressed included donning and doffing the orthoses, walking backward and to the side, safe falling techniques, coming to stand from the floor, coming to stand from sitting, and returning to sitting from a standing position.

Scales for functional rating include, the Barthel Index (BI), Modified Barthel Index (MBI), the Functional Independence Measure (FIM), the Quadriplegic Index of Function (QIF), the Spinal Cord Independence Measure (SCIM), the Walking Index for Spinal Cord Injury (WISCI), and the Spinal Cord Injury Functional Ambulation Inventory (SCI-FAI). They are applicable to wide range of nervous system disorders, however the QIF, the SCI-FAI and the SCIM are more specific for patients with SCI. All of these scales have been successfully used to characterize SCI patients.

Among many available functional assessment scales, the BI has been one of the most popular. It has been utilized for both the characterization of individual patients, and in the evaluation of the efficacy of various rehabilitation programs. The BI has ten ratable patient skill items. Values are assigned to each item (zero, five points or ten points) based on the amount of physical assistance required to perform each task. A BI total score ranges from zero to 100 points (0: fully dependent; 100: fully independent).

In the original version, (MBI) each item is scored in three steps. The Modified Barthel Index (MBI) with a five-step scoring system appears to have greater sensitivity and improved reliability than the original version, without examination difficulty or an increase in implementation time.

The FIM was developed to provide uniform assessment of severity of patient disability and medical rehabilitation outcome. It is an 18-item, 7-level scale designed to assess severity of patient disability, estimate burden of care and determine medical rehabilitation functional outcome. The FIM has emerged as a standard assessment instrument for use in rehabilitation programs for disabled persons. FIM as a functional outcome tool has been studied extensively. It is easy to administer and is valid and reliable. Inter-rater agreement with FIM has been high in several studies. Various studies have shown that FIM had high internal consistency, adequate discriminative capabilities and was a good indicator of burden of care. However, other studies have suggested that this instrument may not be sensitive or appropriate for functional assessment in SCI patients. Younz et al recommended that additions to FIM may be useful, especially in feeding, dressing and bed activity category in order to improve sensitivity **(Table 16.3)**.

The Quadriplegia Index of Function (QIF) was developed in 1980 because the Barthel Index was deemed too insensitive to document the small but significant functional gains made by quadriplegics (tetraplegics) during medical rehabilitation. The QIF is comprised of variables that are each weighted and scored (transfers, grooming, bathing, feeding, dressing, wheelchair mobility, bed activities, bladder and bowel program and understanding of personal care). A final score ranging from zero to 100 points is derived that characterizes each patient's functional abilities and serves as a reference for future assessment.

The study by Younz et al. concluded that the percentage of recovery on ASIA motor scores was significantly correlated only to gain in QIF scores, not FIM.

Catz et al. developed a new disability scale specific for patients with spinal cord pathology, SCIM and compared it to FIM in the assessment and characterization of 30 patients. The authors found the SCIM more sensitive than FIM to changes in function of spinal cord lesion patients. SCIM detected all functional changes detected by FIM, but FIM missed 26% of changes detected by SCIM scoring. The authors concluded that SCIM may be a useful instrument for assessing functional changes in patients with lesions of the spinal cord.

The Walking Index for SCI (WISCI) was proposed as a scale to measure functional limitations in walking of patients following SCI. It incorporates gradations of physical assistance and devices required for walking following paralysis of the lower extremities secondary to SCI. The purpose of the WISCI is to document changes in functional capacity with respect to ambulation in a rehabilitation setting.

The SCI-FAI is a functional observational gait assessment instrument developed at the University of Miami by Field Fote EC et al. that addresses three key domains of walking function in individuals with SCI: gait parameters/symmetry, assistive device use and temporal distance measures. The authors concluded that the SCI-FAI is a reliable, valid and relatively sensitive measure of walking ability in individuals with SCI.

Table 16.3: Functional Independence Measure (FIM™) Instrument			
	Admission	*Discharge*	*Follow-up*
Self-care			
A. Eating			
B. Grooming			

Contd...

Contd…

	Admission	Discharge	Follow-up
C. Bathing			
D. Dressing—Upper Body			
E. Dressing—Lower Body			
F. Toileting			
Sphincter Control			
G. Bladder Management			
H. Bowel Management			
Transfers			
I. Bed, Chair, Wheelchair			
J. Toilet			
K. Tub, Shower			
Locomotion			
L. Walk/Wheelchair			
M. Stairs			
Motor Subtotal Score			
Communication			
N. Comprehension			
O. Expression			
Social Cognition			
P. Social Interaction			
Q. Problem Solving			
R. Memory			
Cognitive Subtotal Score			
Total FIM Score			
	Independent			
L	7	Complete Independence (Timely, Safely)			
E	6	Modified Independence (Device)			No Helper
V	**Modified Dependence**			
E	5	Supervision (Subject = 100%+)			
L	4	Minimal Assist (Subject = 75%+)			
S	3	Moderate Assist (Subject = 50%+)			Helper
	Complete Dependence			
	2	Maximal Assist (Subject = 25%+)			
	1	Total Assist (Subject = less than 25%)			

Note: Leave no blanks. Enter 1 if patient is not testable due to risk.

Assessment/Evaluation for Complications

Since the spinal injured could have other associated trauma such as neurosurgical, orthopedic, general surgical, cardiothoracic, and faciomaxillary trauma, the patient should be evaluated properly in this regard. The neurological deficit in the area complicates the matter since the patient may have no symptoms associated with it and the trauma is likely to be missed unless there is a proper assessment.

The patient needs to be evaluated periodically for complications associated with spinal injuries like pressure sore, deep vein thrombosis, pain, spasticity, respiratory, gastrointestinal, cardiovascular, metabolic and other complications. This evaluation may need to be more frequent during the acute and subacute phase.

Psychological Assessment

Spinal injury is a malady, which has far reaching consequences on the individual's psyche since it is an ailment that leaves his/her world topsy-turvy. The spinal injured goes through an entire spectrum of emotions ranging from shock, denial, anger, sadness, anxiety, depression, agitation, restlessness, loss of self-confidence, self-criticalness, guilt, a feeling of failure, pessimism about his future, lethargy and fatigue, loss of interest—a whole gamut of emotions which can be seen and understood as a reaction to his loss.

If we look at the rehabilitation of the spinal injured individual then the psychological intervention becomes one of the most important parts of rehabilitation since it is a cathartic space meant for the individual to vent out his/her sorrows, to break down and not maintain a brave front all the time, to be held and heard, to be motivated and guided, to be understood.

We have also to keep in mind that injury not only affects the individual himself/herself but also undermines the family's emotional/financial resources, often debilitating and incapacitating them in many ways.

To reiterate, different people react differently to this crisis. In such a situation it becomes important to assess variables like depression and anxiety in order to get an accurate idea of their inner reality and how far the injury has affected them emotionally. Additionally, at this point such measures also provide us with an idea as to the need for any pharmacological intervention with the help of the psychiatrist since spinal injury might be seen as a precipitating factor for many emotional disorders, which would need the necessary intervention.

Another relevant measure is a scale for measuring their coping skills since it would not only provide an insight into the person's coping repertoire such that one can draw from his premorbid skills/belief systems which helped him deal with other losses but also could possibly use them to help the person come to terms with this loss by putting things in the right perspective.

As mentioned earlier, a spinal injured person's social support system forms a very crucial part of his progression to recovery; a social support measure becomes a very useful tool to gauge the familial-relational resources at his disposal as well as his own perception of the same.

Different people react differently to this malady. While some still retain their sense of control and believe that they are active participants and agents in their own course of recovery, there are still others who see themselves after the injury as passive receivers, with their recovery not being in their hands but determined by external factors like fate/luck, contribution of other people such as doctors, family members, etc. A tool, which measures their locus of control gives an idea into this very crucial aspect.

A tool measuring quality of life or another measuring their global adjustment gives a fair insight into the actual reality after rehabilitation informing us about his/her adjustment in various spheres such as familial, emotional, occupational, and sexual.

To summarize, from the psychological vantage point, it is imperative to start from each individual's own set of experiences and to return to them their own individuality and uniqueness, instilling a sense of hope and urgency such that they are in a position to face life's hardships and challenges.

Some of the instruments that can throw light on the psychological condition of the spinal injured individual, providing important and relevant information in this context are:

1. *Beck Depression Inventory (BDI):* This questionnaire was introduced by Beck, Ward, Mandelson, Mock and Erbaugh in 1961 and later on revised in 1971. BDI contains 21 items measuring different aspects, symptoms, and manifestations of depression. It is a self-report scale, which has been found to have high reliability and validity. It includes questions relating to various categories and validity. The various categories are sadness, pessimism, sense of failure, dissatisfaction, guilt, expectation of punishment, dislike of self, self-accusation, suicidal ideation, episodes of crying, agitation, social withdrawal, indecisiveness, feeling of worthlessness, loss of energy, insomnia, irritability, loss of appetite, difficulty in concentration, fatigability and loss of interest in sex. It has been widely used with SCI patients.

2. *State Trait Anxiety Inventory (STAI):* The State Trait Inventory was developed by Charles D Spiel Berger and is one of the most extensively used instruments to measure anxiety whether for the purposes of research or for clinical practice. It contains two self-report scales, with 20 statements each. Two scores are obtained on the two categories of State Anxiety and Trait Anxiety. To elaborate, State Anxiety measures the person's feeling state at that very moment whereas the Trait Anxiety measures 'how people generally feel'. This instrument has been used widely in medical, surgical, psychosomatic and psychiatric patients and adapted in many languages. The original form X was revised in 1979 and Form Y was developed. This instrument has been used successfully with SCI patients in many studies.

3. *Multidimensional Health Locus of Control Scale (MHLC):* This scale was developed by Kenneth A Wallston, measuring peoples' general health locus of control beliefs without giving one total score. Rather with the help of its 18 items it assesses individuals on different dimensions like internality, chance, powerful others, doctors and other people to be

answered on a 6 point Likert Scale ranging from strongly disagree to strongly agree. Different people react differently to this malady. While some still retain their sense of control and believe that they are active participants and agents in their own course of recovery, there are still others who see themselves after the injury as passive receivers, with their recovery not being in their hands but determined by external factors like fate/luck, contribution of other people such as doctors, family members, etc. A tool, which measures their Locus of Control gives an idea into this very crucial aspect which can guide the intervention to be held with the patient with the SCI.

4. *Temperament and Character Inventory (TCI):* This is a personality inventory, which assesses individuals on their relatively stable and moderately inherited temperament as well as their character. The temperament dimensions are Novelty Seeking, Harm Avoidance, Reward Dependence and Persistence and the character dimensions are Self-Directedness, Cooperativeness and Self-Transcendence. It can be seen as providing an in-depth description of an individual's characteristic way of thinking, feeling and reacting to life's experience.

5. *SCL-related coping scale:* Developed by Elfstrom, Ryden, Kreuter, Persson and Sullivan. It is a tool, measuring coping through three valid and reliable coping factors which are Acceptance (four items), Fighting spirit (five items) and Social reliance (three items). Another relevant measure is a scale for measuring their coping skills since it would not only provide an insight into the person's coping repertoire such that one can draw from his/her premorbid skills/belief systems which helped him deal with other losses but also use them to help him/her come to terms with this loss by putting things in the right perspective.

6. Instruments such as social support scale, quality of life scale could also provide very useful information for SCI-related patients.

Evaluation for Requirement of Equipment, Aids and Appliances

Equipment, aids and appliances are vital to augment the functional independence of spinal injured. They are all the more important for tetraplegics. Such equipment, aids and appliances include wheelchairs, standing frame, environment control systems, suitable orthosis, various splints, etc. An evaluation for patient requirements in this regard should be performed at an appropriate time so that they can be arranged. A pre-discharge rush to procure them should be avoided since it gives suboptimal results.

Evaluation of Home, Workplace and Environment

A detailed evaluation of patient's home, workplace and environment is of crucial importance in order to rehabilitate the individual according to the environment he/she would go back into and also to suggest appropriate modifications in order to make it free of architectonical barriers.

During the initial evaluation, the therapist should find out what environment the patient would return to after discharge and then plan goals accordingly. For example, if the patient has to return to rural areas, his physical rehabilitation may differ substantially from an individual who has to settle in an urban area. Subsequently a more detailed assessment of the home should be done through a visit by a team of occupational therapist and social worker in order to study the home, workplace and environment with regard to access and suggest modifications as required.

Summary

Evaluation provides an opportunity to learn about the patient's physical and functional status and to investigate other areas of concern. The information gathered during initial and subsequent evaluations is the basis for goal setting and for the design, evaluation, and revision of the therapeutic program.

Bibliography

1. Aaron T Beck. Psychometric properties of the Beck Depression Inventory: Twenty-five years of evaluation. Clinical Psychology Review. 1988;8(1):77-100.
2. American Spinal Injury Association/International Medical Society of Paraplegia: Standards for Neurological and Functional Classification of Spinal Cord Injury, Revised. Chicago: American Spinal Injury Association, 1992.
3. Bednarczyk, et al. Comparison of functional and medical assessment in the classification of persons with spinal cord injury. Journal of Rehabilitation Research Development. 1993;30:405-11.
4. Bieling, et al. The State-Trait Anxiety Inventory, Trait version: structure and content re-examined. Behaviour Research and Therapy. 1998;36:17-8, 777-88.
5. Botsford DJ, Esses SI. A new scale for the clinical assessment of spinal cord function. Orthopedics. 1992;15:1309-13.
6. Bracken MB, Webb SB Jr, Wagner FC. Classification of the severity of acute spinal cord injury: Implications for management. Paraplegia. 1978;15:319-26.
7. Catz, et al. SCIM: Spinal Cord Independence Measure—A new disability scale for patients with spinal cord lesions. Spinal Cord. 1997;35:850-6.
8. Cohen ME, et al. A test of the 1992 International Standards for Neurological and Functional Classification of Spinal Cord Injury. Spinal Cord. 1998;36:554-60.
9. Ditunno JF Jr. American spinal injury standards for neurological and functional classification of spinal cord injury: Past, present and future—1992 Heiner Sell Lecture of the American Spinal Injury Association. Journal of American Paraplegia Society. 1994;17:7-11.
10. EI Masry, et al. Validation of the American Spinal Injury Association (ASIA) Motor Score and the National Acute Spinal Cord Injury Study (NASCIS) Motor Score. Spine. 1996;21(5):614-9.
11. Harvey, et al. The Walking Index for Spinal Cord Injury. Australian Journal of Physiotherapy. 2009;55(1):66.
12. Hobart and Thompson. The five item Barthel index. Journal of Neurology, Neurosurgery and Psychiatry. 2001;71(2):225-30.
13. Ota, et al. Functional assessment of patients with spinal cord injury: Measured by the motor score and the Functional Independence Measure. Spinal Cord. 1995;34:531-5.
14. Waters, et al. Definition of complete spinal cord injury. Paraplegia. 1991;9:573-81.

17

Role of Electrodiagnostics in Spinal Cord Injury and Stroke Rehabilitation

Arun B Taly, KPS Nair

Introduction

The degree of recovery following spinal cord disorder, often depends on the severity and extent of the lesion. Currently, the rehabilitation assessment of spinal cord injuries is predominately clinical, the examination is influenced and restricted by the cooperation of the subject and experience of the clinician. Associated peripheral nerve lesions are often masked, especially during the phase of spinal shock. Advances in biomedical engineering have widened the vista of investigations of spinal cord injury and today, electrodiagnosis stands as an extension of the bedside examination of the spinal cord injury patient for the precise localization of the lesion **(Fig. 17.1)**.

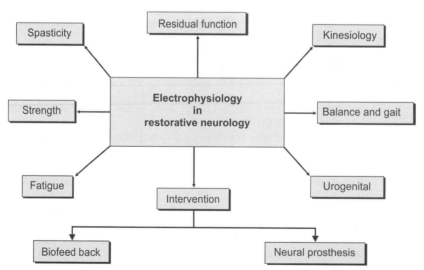

Fig. 17.1: Specific uses of clinical neurophysiology in restorative neurology

Clinical electrophysiology is the best means for objective evaluation of the functional integrity of the nervous system and therefore, it has tremendous potential in the practice of spinal injury rehabilitation. A wide variety of neurophysiological tests applicable to different parts of the nervous system are now available. Some of these are qualitative while others are quantitative. Majority of them are routinely practiced in most clinical neurophysiological laboratories.[1,2] These techniques can be used to establish the diagnosis, localize the precise site of lesion, understand the mechanism of impaired function, quantify the deficit responsible for disability, record the residual function, plan the appropriate therapies and monitor the effect of various therapeutic interventions in patients with spinal cord disorder **(Table 17.1)**.[3-5]

Table 17.1: Electrophysiological tests—nervous system	
Part of the nervous system tested	*Test*
Cerebral cortex	EEG and quantitative EEG • Functional brain imaging • Cortical stimulation • Sensory evoked potentials • Long loop reflexes (LLR) • Bereitschaftspotential • Movement related potential
Descending tracts	Cortical and spinal stimulation • Central EMG • Long loop reflexes (LLR) • Audiospinal facilitation
Ascending tracts	Somatosensory evoked potential (SSEP) • Long loop reflexes (LLR)
Motor neurons	M, F and H study Electromyography
Interneurons	Vibration inhibition • "H" reflex recovery curve • Silent period
Others	Sympathetic skin response (SSR)
Nerve roots • Anterior • Posterior	'F' Wave H Reflex SSEP
Peripheral nerves	Motor conduction • Sensory conduction • F, H and SSEP • Sympathetic skin response (SSR) • Refractory • Microneurography

Evoked Potentials

The evoked potentials record activity from specific neuronal pathways of the brain in response to stimulation of specific sensory modalities. Visual evoked potential (VEP), Brainstem auditory evoked response (BAER) and

Somatosensory evoked potentials (SSEP) are some of the most commonly used techniques. Besides objective documentations of abnormal functions, these are employed in the detection of lesions of the respective pathways (active/quiescent, clinical/subclinical) as well as prognostication. Patients with nontraumatic and noncompressive myelopathies may have multiple sclerosis, acute disseminated encephalomyelitis, and subacute combined degeneration and multimodality evoked potentials often assist in establishing the diagnosis and designing management protocol. Somatosensory evoked potentials are also useful in ascertaining the functional integrity of ascending tract in patients with spinal cord disorders and perioperative monitoring during surgery. It must be realized that the abnormalities of evoked potentials imply involvement of these neuronal systems by the disease but may provide no clue to the etiology of the illness. Thus, they are no substitute for a careful history, clinical examination and imaging techniques.[1]

Electromyography

Electromyography (EMG) is the study of the electrical activity of resting muscle and muscle in action. Conventional EMG involves introduction of a concentric needle electrode into a muscle near its motor point under aseptic conditions. The muscle is sampled at multiple sites and the activity is recorded while the needle is introduced (insertional activity), at resting state of muscle (spontaneous activity) and with varying degree of contraction (recruitment). These activities can be stored, displayed on a video, heard with audio and can also be recorded on a paper. EMG examination helps in identifying associated anterior horn cell involvement at the level of the spinal cord lesion as also lesions of motor roots and peripheral nerves.

The technique of kinesiologic EMG (KEMG) is a window through which muscle can be seen alive and in action. It enables one to assess the pattern of muscle response, onset and cessation of activity, involvement of different muscles in complex and coordinated movements and level of muscle response in relation to effort, type of muscle contraction and position of joint. Recording of conventional EMG alone does not give information concerning the strength and type of contraction. Force transducers, goniometers, photographic precision, accelerometers and microswitches are needed for simultaneous documentation of other data. Instrumentation for KEMG includes surface or wire electrodes, multichannel amplification and recording system for simultaneous muscle and other physiologic data.[2,6] Surface electrodes are more commonly used. Skin is abraded and cleaned to maximize signal transfer and electrodes are placed using coupling electrode gel, close together on the muscle to be studied and parallel to the direction of muscle fibers. When small deep or weak muscles need to be examined, flexible wire electrodes are used. They are also used as a preliminary to research when surface electrodes have to be applied. Using sterile technique the wire electrodes are inserted through a hypodermic needle. When the electrodes are appropriately fixed the subject can move freely without discomfort.

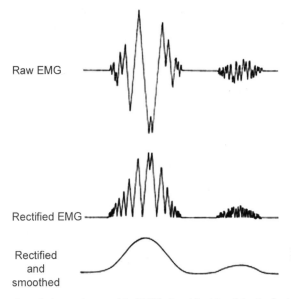

Fig. 17.2: Processing of electromyographic (EMG) signal for kinesiologic electromyography. The area under the rectified and smoothened curve gives a measure of overall muscle activity

During conventional EMG, a raw signal is displayed for visual analysis. However, in KEMG overall activity of muscle during specific action or task is important and therefore, EMG signal needs special processing by microcomputers **(Fig. 17.2)**. Through a process called "rectification" both the positive and negative components of the signal appear above the base line. Another type of circuit provides "integration" of EMG signal through accumulation of energy on a capacitor. Integrated EMG results from summation of the area under the curve and can be expressed in units. The signal can also be analyzed for spectral frequency and displayed in various forms. Because of the variability of the EMG procedure and anatomy and movements characteristics of muscle, it is important to "normalize" the data for validation of comparison. EMG is initially recorded at maximum voluntary contraction or at defined submaximal level of contraction. All subsequent values are then expressed as percentage of this "control" value.[2]

Due consideration should be given to instrumentation, equipment and supplies required and physical set-up of the study. Subject's comfort and safety should be ensured. Recording techniques should be standardized by repeated trials. Raw data should always be stored for review before rectification, integration or alteration by computers. This prevents wrong interpretation of artifacts caused by motion, cable artefact, poor electrode contact, wire sway, electrode failure or extraneous electrical signal.

When multichannel KEMG data are recorded with electrogoniometer, pressure transducer, microswitches, accelerometers and other equipments, it has several applications in rehabilitation, e.g. determining pattern or sequence of EMG activity in normal and abnormal motion, documentation of altered muscle function in spastic or weak muscles, evaluation of gait, measurement of strength, endurance and fatigue, selection of most efficient exercise therapy or biofeedback training, establishment of the effectiveness of orthotic/prosthetic devices, drugs, restorative strategies and other therapeutic measures and conducting research in rehabilitation.

Nerve Conduction Studies

While EMG evaluates the function of motor unit and muscle, the nerve conduction studies are carried out to assess functional status of nerves. These studies are used to identify and quantify the associated peripheral nerve involvement in spinal cord lesions (e.g. Cauda equina injuries associated with spinal cord injury, pressure palsies). Conduction studies are performed by stimulating the nerve at one site and recording the evoked motor or sensory potential at another. The median, ulnar and radial nerves are commonly studied in the upper limbs while the common peroneal, posterior tibial and sural nerves are sampled in the lower limbs. For motor conduction studies, the nerve is stimulated by using "supramaximal" current strength at two points along its course. The latency, amplitude, duration and area of the evoked motor response are measured from corresponding muscle. Motor conduction velocity is calculated by dividing the distance (in mm) by the difference in latencies (in msec) from proximal and distal sites. Similarly latency, amplitude and duration of the sensory nerve action potential (SNAP) evoked by antidromic or orthodromic stimulation of peripheral sensory nerves are also measured and sensory conduction velocity is calculated, e.g. for median nerve, digit II is stimulated with ring electrode and recording is done at the wrist (orthodromic) while sural nerve is stimulated at midcalf and recording is done at the ankle (antidromic recording). Recording of sensory conduction in peripheral nerves enables the localization of sensory loss to pre- or postganglionic segment. For example, despite sensory impairment due to preganglionic lesion, the sensory conduction parameters remain unchanged. Nerve conduction velocity depends on the age of the patient, temperature of limb and height of individual and has a wide range even in healthy people. A number of newer techniques namely study of late response (F and H), sympathetic skin response (SSR), refractory period (RP) and collision technique are used for assessing spinal roots and nerve fiber of different diameters, to improve the yield of electrodiagnostic tests.

Evaluation of Autonomic Function

Spinal cord is an integral part of autonomic nervous system and an autonomic dysfunction contributes significantly to disability following spinal cord lesions.[6] Conventional nerve conduction studies essentially evaluate large diameter fast conducting fibers, while autonomic functions are mediated through unmyelinated very slow conducting fibers. Two new tests, the sympathetic skin response (SSR) and R-R internal variability recording help in assessing sympathetic sudomotor fibers and cardiovagal function respectively. SSR is recorded using standard EMG disk electrodes placed over the palm and dorsum of hand in upper limb and sole and dorsum of foot in the lower limb. A change in skin conductance can be produced by biological (deep inspiration cough, sound stimuli) or electrical stimuli. A biphasic response of varied morphology and fairly consistent latency can be obtained from foot and hand. Absent response suggests impaired sympathetic function.[7] The heart rate (R-R interval) varies at rest and the variation increases on deep inspiration. This variability can be recorded through EMG systems. Absent or reduced variability of R-R interval during respiration as compared to age matched control is one of the most sensitive indicators of cardiovagal, i.e. parasympathetic function. Evaluation of vasomotor functions and cardiovascular responsers can be done in autonomic laboratory using Valsalva maneuver and tilt table test in controlled conditions. These tests are now routinely carried out along with other bedside tests for the evaluation of dysautonomia following spinal cord injury.[6]

Muscle Strength Testing

Quantification of neuromuscular function through measurement of muscle strength is necessary for maintaining uniformity of data collection, understanding pathophysiology of disease, proper comparison of various studies and monitoring natural history of the disease and effect of therapeutic exercises, drugs and rehabilitation measures. Most clinical studies include manual muscle testing, recording of range of movement at different joints, documentation of activities of daily living and timed motor function measures. While these data provide adequate information for clinical use, they do not give objective measure of muscle strength. Electromyographic techniques such as single fiber EMG, concentric needle EMG and macro-EMG are useful means of assessing only the function of individual motor units and total electrical strength of muscle.[8] Quantification of muscle strength thus requires mechanical devices.[9] Many instruments are now available which can measure muscle strength during isometric (force at constant length) and isokinetic (force at constant velocity) muscle contractions. An ideal equipment should be economic, simple to use, adopted for patients with different disabilities and not time consuming. It should measure maximal and submaximal strength with precision and have test-retest reliability. Regular calibration of equipment is necessary for obtaining correct values. Some of the commonly used equipment are spring balance, cable tensiometer, hand held dynamometer, myometer and newer dynamometers such as Cybex, Lido and Kin-com.[10] Each of these systems has certain advantages and limitations and attempts are being made to improve these techniques for accurate measurements and standardized body positions are described. Patient should be comfortable and have adequate fixation of body segments. Patient needs to understand the technique and should be encouraged throughout the procedure so as to optimize motivation. Test trials are usually necessary before the measurements. Due consideration should be given to factors like age, gender, anthropometric data and physiological and psychological status of the patient.

Quantification of muscle strength has become an integral part of rehabilitation and research in the field of disorders of motor neuron, peripheral nerve and muscle. However, it is important to have adequate knowledge of the equipment and the system used, technical standards and biological variables for proper interpretation of the results.[10]

Evaluation of Fatigue

Fatigue is an important limiting factor in rehabilitation. It is defined as a failure of muscle to produce or maintain initial peak force or torque. It could be due to failure at one or more sites between the motor cortex and the muscle fibers, e.g. there may be failure of descending voluntary drive to motor neuron pool resulting in "central fatigue", abnormality of excitation contraction coupling in muscle fibers, inhibitions from periphery or inefficiency of contractile apparatus. The traditional method of testing fatigue is an incremental exercise using bicycle ergometry or treadmill. Clinical electrophysiological techniques like frequency analysis, acoustic myography, vibromyography and repetitive electrical stimulation can help in documentation and understanding of fatigue. Fatigue is complex and still incompletely understood phenomenon and its measurement is in the phase of evolution. Studies involving NMR spectroscopy, EMG and force measurement may improve our knowledge. Currently, available techniques are, however, helpful in optimizing therapeutic exercises and serve as a guide for preventing over-work phenomenon.

Posturography

Human balance is a sensitive and complex process involving detection of body position, integration of sensory—motor information and execution of skeletal muscle response. Sensory input chiefly comes from visual, vestibular and somatosensory systems. Any mismatch of information causes disturbance of balance and interferes with stance and mobility. Abnormalities of balance pose significant problems in rehabilitation and therefore, quantitation of balance and understandings of compensatory strategies are vital in management. The technique of recording balance is referred to as posturography. There are two types of posturographic recordings: (1) "static" which records swaying during quiet stance and (2) "dynamic" which assesses sensory control of balance and coordinated reflex motor responses after platform perturbations.[11] While posturography is an integral component of evaluation in rehabilitation practice, it falls outside the scope of electrophysiology technology and therefore is not covered in this chapter.

Gait Analysis

Human walking is the most common of all the movements and locomotor disability is a universal phenomenon in physical rehabilitation. Analysis and understanding of normal and abnormal gait thus becomes very important. There are two methods of gait analysis: (1) Observational and (2) Quantitative.[10] Observational gait analysis was developed at Rancho Los Amigos Hospital, Los Angeles for achieving greater precision of gait description and consists of recording events occurring at joints and adjacent sections. The procedure requires several hours, causes inconvenience to the patient and is unreliable for quantitation. Therefore, most laboratories now use commercially available instruments for quantitative analysis. Walking, being a complex motion needs analysis of several factors. Essential components of quantitative analysis are: (1) time distance measurement, (2) kinematic factors, (3) kinetic factors, (4) electromyography and (5) metabolic factors[10] analyzed for oxygen and carbon dioxide content to determine metabolic energy factor.

For clinicians, the complexity, the technical difficulties and the expertise required for these methods are prohibitive. However, like many other techniques, gait analysis has advanced and now become an integral part of gait laboratories. It has been used for pre- and postoperative evaluation of patients for cerebral palsy, selection of orthotic and prosthetic devices, understanding the pathophysiology of gait abnormalities in various neurological disorders, planning treatment and monitoring of therapeutic techniques and biofeedback.

Quantification of Spasticity

Spasticity is defined as a velocity dependent increase in the tonic stretch reflex ("muscle tone") with exaggerated tendon jerks. It is very common and disabling residual problem following spinal injury and myelopathies. Whenever a patient requires evaluation of spasticity the following question arise: (1) Is spasticity present? (2) Is it tonic, phasic or combined? (3) What is the contribution of segmental hyperexcitability? (4) What supraspinal mechanism(s) are involved? (5) How severe is spasticity, and (6) What therapy will be most suitable for the patient? Neurophysiological methods can partly answer these questions.

Spasticity evaluation techniques can be broadly classified into two groups: (1) mechanical methods and (2) electrophysiological methods. Mechanical techniques rely on motion applied to a joint and involve gravitational, manual, controlled displacement and controlled torque methods.[12] The most easily performed mechanical technique among these is "pendulum test".

Pendulum Test

For assessing the spasticity of quadriceps muscle, the patient is made to sit and the leg is raised to horizontal level at knee and dropped. The leg oscillates for a few seconds before acquiring static position. Knee movement is assessed by electrogoniometer and rate of movement by tachometer. In view of increased resistance to passive stretch the amplitude and the number of oscillations are reduced in patients with spasticity. Further, it takes longer time for the leg to acquire position of rest. It is now possible to study this phenomenon by using isokinetic systems. These instruments can be used for different muscles in upper and lower extremities and allow application of passive stretch at varied rate and force. Spastic limbs demonstrate resistance to joint movements, which is augmented by increasing the angle of movement and rate at which it is moved.[10,12]

Electrophysiological Methods

Clinical neurophysiological techniques are useful in documentation and quantification of spasticity. These help in objective recording of clinically observed phenomenon, e.g. hyperactive stretch reflex, clonus **(Fig. 17.3)**, lack of reciprocal inhibition during voluntary movements **(Fig. 17.4)**, etc. In addition, these are also useful in revealing the underlying pathophysiological mechanism of spasticity.[13,14] Some of these methods are described here.

Tendon Jerk

In spasticity, tendon jerks have lower threshold and higher amplitude and are followed by after discharge of motor units. Surface electrodes are placed over the muscle belly and stretch reflex is elicited by electrodynamic hammer. Threshold force required, maximum amplitude of tendon jerk ("T" wave) and ratio of "T" wave to "M" wave (direct muscle response to supramaximal nerve stimulation) are recorded. Similar to "H" max/"M" max ratio, the "T" max/"M" max ratio also provides information about spasticity. "T" wave can be recorded from many muscles as compared to "H" reflex.[10]

"H" Reflex

Hoffman reflex is the electrical equivalent of tendon jerk **(Fig. 17.5)**. Using low intensity and long duration electrical stimulus spindle afferents can be stimulated to activate alpha motor neurons. In normal individuals, "H" reflex is restricted to soleus and flexor carpi radialis muscles but in patients with

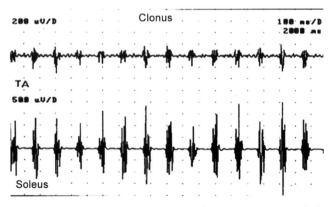

Fig. 17.3: Electromyographic evidence of clonus (7.0 Hz) recorded by using surface electrodes from tibialis anterior and soleus

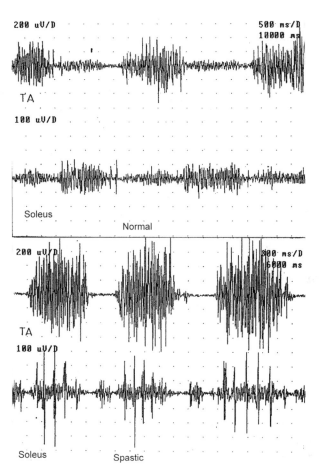

Fig. 17.4: Electromyographic recording from tibialis anterior and soleus muscle during alternate voluntary dorsiflexion and plantar flexion of foot. Normal subject (Top) show smooth EMG bursts alternately in TA and soleus while spastic subject shows intermittent brief EMG bursts in soleus during dorsiflexion of foot

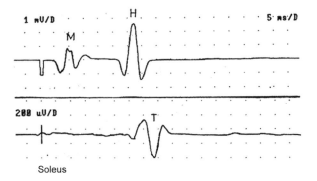

Fig. 17.5: Recording of electrical "H" and tendon reflex by electrodynamic hammer ("T") from soleus muscle. Note the slightly prolonged latency and lower amplitude of tendon reflex

spasticity, "H" reflex can be obtained from other muscles as well, e.g. tibialis anterior and intrinsic hand muscles of hand **(Fig. 17.6)**.

The amplitude of "H" denotes the availability of excitable motor neuron pool in the spinal cord. The ratio of "H" max to "M" max is normally less than 0.5 but due to increased excitability of alpha motor neurons, the "H" max/"M" max ratio exceeds 0.5 in spasticity **(Fig. 17.7)**. This parameter is very useful in patients with unilateral lesions as the unaffected side of the subject can serve as a "control".

As "H" reflex bypasses muscle spindle, a dissociation in tendon reflex ("T") and electrical "H" ("T" being more than electrical "H") is believed to suggest increased sensitivity of muscle spindles and increased gamma motor neuron activity. However, this concept is now debated in light of recent microneurographic studies.

"H" reflex excitability/recovery curve also show changes in pyramidal lesion. This is studied by giving a second stimulus at various intervals from the test stimuli. In normal individuals, a second "H" reflex of identical amplitude is noted only when the stimuli are separated by 100–150 msec interval.

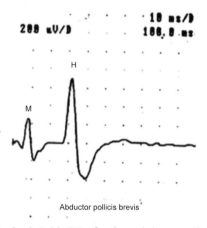

Fig. 17.6: Easily elicitable "H" reflex from abductor pollicis brevis muscle in a subject with high cervical myelopathy

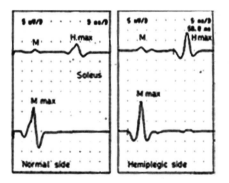

Fig. 17.7: "H" max/"M" max ratio in a subject with stroke. Note the ratio is higher (0.63) on the hemiplegic side than the normal side (0.3)

However, in spastic condition recovery period is shorter and the amplitude of second "H" is higher. This depends on the influence of descending tracts on motor neuron.

In normal individuals, voluntary contraction of tibialis anterior or stimulation of peroneal nerve has inhibitory effect on "H" reflex due to reciprocal inhibitory mechanism by descending tracts. This may be lost in spasticity and can be demonstrated electrophysiologically.

When a vibrator (100 Hz) is applied over the muscle during elicitation of stretch reflex, there occurs an inhibition, which remains constant throughout the period of vibration. This is due to presynaptic inhibition on Ia terminals. The same phenomenon can be demonstrated on "H" reflex also. The index so obtained (H max vibrated/"H" max X 100) is often consistent for a given individual but varies among different people. Vibration inhibition index is reduced in chronic spasticity but not in patients of Parkinsonism or hyperreflexia of other origin, and therefore is considered specific. However, this index does not correlate with the severity of spasticity. It is symmetrical on both sides in healthy subjects and therefore, this test is very useful in unilateral lesion. Diazepam enhances the vibration inhibition index in spasticity while baclofen does not. Selection of antispastic drug can thus be based on this therapeutic test.[10]

"F" Wave

"F" response (wave) is obtained from muscle by supramaximal stimulation of its motor nerve and is believed to be due to antidromic activation of alpha motor neurons. Following recovery from acute state patient with hemiplegia and patients with chronic spasticity show increased amplitude and persistence of F wave and reflect hyperexcitability of alpha motor neuron.

Plantar Withdrawal Reflex

Stroking, the plantar surface of foot electrically results in flexion of great toe and adduction of other toes. In patients with spasticity, there occurs an extension of great toe and abduction of other toes. This is believed to reflect global interneuron activities. In some patients, excessive muscle contractions of other muscles and withdrawal of extremities is noted. This phenomenon can be recorded by polyelectromyography and the threshold, pattern and size of elicited plantar response can be observed. EMG activity can help in differentiating voluntary withdrawal and genuine abnormal plantar response. A reduced threshold and increased size of response are characteristic feature of spasticity and can be quantified.

Thus, electrophysiological methods can help detection and quantification of spasticity (Pendulum test, "H"max/"M" max ratio), understanding of pathophysiological mechanism (abnormal "F" and "H" suggest alpha motor neuron hyperexcitability, "H" reflex recovery curve provides evidence of descending influences and vibration induced alteration in "H" reflex indicates presynaptic inhibition) as also selection of therapy (Diazepam for patients with presynaptic mechanism and baclofen for patients with abnormal "H" reflex recovery) and long-term monitoring of patients.[10]

Urogenital Dysfunction

A number of patients develop bowel, bladder and sexual dysfunction due to spinal cord disorders and require interventions. When combined with clinical and urological tests, electrophysiological techniques provide useful information about the underlying mechanism for the dysfunction. Commonly used methods are: (1) sphincter electromyography, (2) study of sacral reflexes, (3) evoked potential studies and (4) pudendal motor nerve latency.[15,16]

Sphincter EMG: This has been in use since the early days of clinical EMG and has two main applications: (1) to record activity of urethral sphincter during urodynamic studies and (2) to assess the innervation of pelvic floor muscles. The striated muscle is active tonically to maintain continence all the time. Its activity increases abruptly whenever there is a rise in intra-abdominal pressure and it becomes silent during detrusor contraction when voluntary voiding is performed. As urethral sphincter is not easily accessible, EMG is performed on the anal sphincter on the presumption that both the sphincters behave in similar manner. Various electrodes used are: surface electrodes on either side of anal region, anal plug electrodes to be put into the anal canal, electrodes mounted on catheters and sponge mounted vaginal electrodes to be placed behind the urethral sphincter. Detailed EMG analysis of motor units of anal or urethral sphincter can be done by direct insertion of concentric needle or single fiber EMG needle. In males, urethral sphincter needle is inserted in the left lateral position through perineum, 4 cm in front of the anus and being guided through the finger in rectum towards the apex of prostate. In females, it is passed through using the transvaginal approach. In patients with spinal cord injuries, sphincter EMG studies assist in identifying detrusor sphincter dyssynergia, which if left untreated may result in hydroureteronephrosis and chronic renal failure. The studies also help in identifying lower motor neuron lesions causing incontinence due to sphincter incompetence.[15]

Sacral Reflex

Erectile dysfunction is frequent following spinal cord disorders (Ashraff). These may be due to disruption of the local reflex arc or interruption of the autonomic and somatosensory pathways within the cord. Reflex erections are often preserved among subjects with lesions of spinal cord. Identification of associated sacral root involvement is important during selection of the management options. Latency and type of reflex contractions of the pelvic floor muscles in response to stimulation of genitalia or perineum have been studied by electrical stimulation and measure functional integrity of sacral reflex arc. Bulbocavernosus reflex can be recorded using concentric needle inserted into the bulbocavernosus muscle or surface electrodes placed over the same muscles. Stimulation of penis is done through ring or hand held bipolar stimulator. A consistent response has two components: An early response with a latency of 24–45 msec and late response with a latency of 60–70 msec. Vesicourethral and vesicoanal reflex can be elicited from respective sphincter muscles by stimulation of catheter mounted ring electrode. These studies are useful in the evaluation of patients with erectile dysfunction due to spinal cord injury and when abnormal, suggests involvement of peripheral nerves or roots.[15,17]

Evoked Potentials

Somatosensory pathways from genitalia to cortex can be evaluated by stimulating dorsal nerve of penis or clitoris and recording potentials from scalp, two centimeters behind CZ. Pudendal evoked potential have latency and configuration, similar to posterior tibial nerve potential.[15,17] Stimulation of bladder and urethra also evoke cortical response. However, these are of lower amplitude and longer latency, because the afferents involved are probably small unmyelinated fibers. Motor evoked potential from pelvic floor muscles, anal and urethral sphincter can be obtained by electrical or magnetic stimulation of cortex and spinal cord.[10,17]

Pudendal Nerve Latency

To date, study of conduction in pudendal nerve is difficult secondary to the inaccessibility of the nerve. A newer system consisting of stimulating electrode fixed at the tip of finger and recording electrode at the base of index finger has made it possible. Finger is introduced into anus and the pudendal nerve is stimulated at the site it crosses ischial spine. EMG response can be recorded from anal and from urethral sphincter.[15]

The EMG from smooth muscle of corpus cavernosum (CCEMG) can be recorded using concentric needle electrodes. Rhythmic bursts of activity is seen when penis is flaccid. Penile tumescence is accompanied by silent CCEMG. In subjects with neurogenic impotence, CCEMG activity persists during sexual stimulation preventing erections.[15]

Sympathetic skin response is a simple, noninvasive electrophysiological test for sudomotor function. SSR from perineum and sole is a potentially useful test for evaluation of erectile dysfunction and incontinence.[16,17]

These techniques in varying combination have been widely used to investigate patients of fecal and urinary incontinence, monitor children with spina bifida and neurogenic impotence.[10,15]

Assessment of Residual Function

Recovery of patients following spinal cord injury depends on the severity and extent of neurological lesion. Accurate prognostication, selection of restorative procedures and critical evaluation of therapeutic interventions need documentation of the integrity of the descending influence and residual function.[18-22] Electrophysiological methods being highly objective have played an important role in assessing residual function of the descending tracts and final motor out put. Many techniques have been used for this by Dimitrijevic and his colleague to assess residual upper and lower motor neuron control, following a protocol known as "Brain motor control assessment" (BMCA), in subjects with spinal injury.[18]

The surface electrodes are applied over the muscle belly of quadriceps, adductor, hamstring, triceps surae, tibialis anterior bilaterally and lower abdominal and lumbar paraspinal muscles. Myoelectric signals are recorded from these muscles with a high sensitivity using a number of maneuvers and data obtained from the polyelectromyography are analyzed. EMG activity is recorded from the muscles after asking the patient to contract the muscles at multiple joint on three trials. Presence of EMG activity in clinically "paralyzed" muscles suggests preservation of motor control. After a relaxation for 10 minutes in supine position patient is required to perform reinforcement maneuvers consisting of forceful closure of eyes, clinching of jaws, forceful shrugging of shoulder against resistance, neck flexion against resistance, deep inspiration, clinching of fist, etc. These maneuvers are repeated on three occasions. A dissociation between EMG activity during voluntary activity and reinforcement maneuvers provide information regarding integrity of upper motor neuron.

Recording of tendon reflexes, vibration reflex and plantar reflex also form part of the study. After baseline study, the subject is asked to augment or suppress the response. Demonstration of patient's ability to modify the response indicates residual descending influence. Further, the effect of Jandressistet maneuver, caloric stimulation and audiospinal facilitation has also been studied on tendon and "H" reflex **(Fig. 17.8)**.[21,22] Audiospinal and

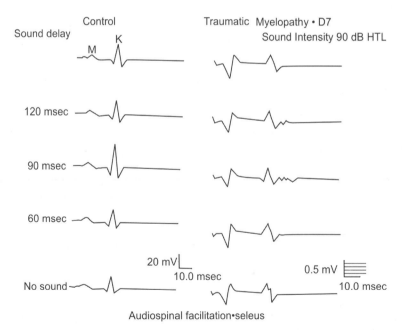

Fig. 17.8: Audiospinal facilitation of "H" reflex from soleus muscle in normal subject and patient with complete spinal cord transection at D7 level. Note the absence of facilitation in the latter

caloric stimulation facilitation of stretch and "H" reflex help in evaluating reticulospinal tracts.

Magnetic and electrical stimulation of cortex and spinal cord can evoke motor response from muscle and provide indication about the functional integrity of pyramidal tracts. Sherwood et al[20] using brain motor control assessment protocol analyzed data of the patients with spinal cord injury referee for rehabilitation. They observed that of the 88 patients with clinically "complete" lesion, 74 (84%) were "incomplete" lesion, i.e. had evidence of residual brain influence. These tests are now routinely used prior to therapeutic intervention, e.g. gait training using body weight support system for spinal injury patients, functional electrical stimulation, etc. However, these tests are time consuming, require patient's cooperation, accurate application of electrodes and precise documentation of data.

Conclusion

Disorders of spinal cord cause impairment of sensory, motor and autonomic dysfunctions. Clinical neurophysiology help in identification and quantification of sensory, motor and autonomic involvement. They help in identification of associated peripheral nerve and root lesions. They permit assessment of impairment in physiologic terms and allow development of therapeutic strategies, which can correct this dysfunction among people with disorders of spinal cord. However, these techniques do not measure disabilities and may not be applicable in all circumstances. Further, some of these techniques need mechanical devices and other methods for comprehensive evaluation. Nevertheless, these techniques are complementary to clinical evaluation and to a certain extent therapeutic interventions.

Acknowledgments

The secretarial assistance of Mr MV Srinivasan, Mr K Bhaskar and Ms Manjula Sharman and help of the staffs of the departments of medical illustration and clinical electrophysiology section of neurology are gratefully acknowledged.

References

1. Taly AB, Anisya V. Electrodiagnosis in neurology. In: Sainani GS (Ed). API Text Book of Medicine, 5th edn. API, Bombay; 1994. pp. 800-06.
2. Portney LG. Electromyography and nerve conduction tests. In: O'Sullivan SB, Schmitz TJ (Eds). Physical Rehabilitation: Assessment and Treatment, 3rd edn. FA Davis, Philadelphia; 1994. pp. 133-65.
3. Delwaide PJ, Pennisi G. Quantitative evaluation of the results of restorative neurology. In: Young RR, Delwaide PJ (Eds). Principles and Practice of Restorative Neurology. Butterworth Heinemann, Oxford; 1992. pp. 16-31.
4. Sedgwick EM. Clinical neurophysiology in rehabilitation. In: Illis LS, Sedgwick EM, Glanville HJ (Eds). Rehabilitation of the Neurological Patient. Blackwell Scientific, Oxford; 1982. pp. 85-120.
5. Hook O. Neurophysiological methods in rehabilitation medicine. Scand J Rehab Med. 1994;30(Supple):1-182.

6. Kamath V. Dysautonomias in spinal cord disorders: Clinical and electro-physiological profile. Thesis submitted to NIMHANS, Deemed University, Bangalore, 2000.

7. Nair KPS, Taly AB, Arunodaya GR, Rao S, Murali T. Sympathetic skin response in myelopathies. Clin Auton Res. 1998;8:207-11.

8. Desmedt JE (Ed). New Developments in Electromyography and Clinical Neurophysiology (Vol. I)—Karger, Basel, 1973.

9. Bengt N. Mechanical evaluation of muscle power in clinical practice with some aspects on training. Scand J Rehab Med. 1994;30(Supple):45-52.

10. Taly AB. Electrophysiology in resistive neurology. In: Taly AB, Nair KPS, Murali T (Eds). Neurorehabilitation: Principles and Practice. Ahuja Book Company, Bangalore; 2001. pp. 56-76.

11. Sharma R, Singh R, Guruprasad HV. Balance rehabilitation. In: Taly AB, Nair KPS, Murali (Eds). Neurorehabilitation: Principles and Practice. Ahuja Book Company, Bangalore; 2001. pp. 196-202.

12. Price R. Mechanical spasticity evaluation techniques. Critical Reviews in Physical Medicine and Rehabilitation. 1990;2:65-73.

13. Zider J, Dimitrijevic MR. Clinical neurophysiological assessment of spasticity. In: Sidou M, Abott R, Keravel Y (Eds). Neurosurgery for Spasticity: A Multi disciplinary Approach. Springer Verlag, New York; 1991. pp. 39-46.

14. Katz RT, Rovai GP, Brait C, Rymer Z. Objective quantification of spastic hypertonia: Correlation with clinical findings. Arch Phy Med Rehabil. 1992;73:339-47.

15. Vodusek DB, Fowler CJ. Neurology of bladder, bowel and sexual dysfunction. J Clin Neuromuscul Dis. 1999;1(2):112.

16. Beck R, Fowler CJ. Clinical neurophysiology in the investigation of genitourinary tract dysfunction. In: Rushton DN (Ed). Handbook of Neuro Urology. Marcel Dekker. New York; 1994. pp. 151-80.

17. Ashraff VV. Erectile dysfunction in myelopathies: A clinical and electrophysio-logical studies. Thesis submitted to NIMHANS, Deemed University, Bangalore, 2002.

18. Dimitrijevic MR. Motor control in chronic spinal cord injury patients. Scand J Rehab Med. 1994;30(Supple):53-62.

19. Dobkin BH, Taly AB, George SU. Use of the audiospinal response to test for completeness of spinal cord injury. J Neuro Rehab. 1994;8:187-91.

20. Sherwood AM, Dimitrijevic MR, McKay WB. Evidence of subclinical brain influence in clinically complete spinal cord injury: Discomplete SCI. J Neurol Sci. 1992;110:90-8.

21. Taly AB, Dobkin BH, George SU. Audiospinal reflex. A novel method of assessing reticulospinal tracts in man. Neurology India. 1994;42:196-201.

22. Taly AB, Dobkin BH. Motor recovery and therapeutic intervention. Neurology India. 1995;43:1-10.

18

Acute Care and Surgical Aspects of Spinal Injuries

Milind Deogaonkar

> *"One having a dislocation in the vertebra of his neck while he is unconscious of his two legs and two arms, and his urine dribbles. An ailment not to be treated."*
>
> **Case 31.** The Edwin Smith Surgical Papyrus, c.3000-2500 B.C.

The nihilistic approach to the treatment and outcome of spinal cord injury that is apparent in this document dating back 5000 years, written at the time of the building of the Great Pyramids of Egypt, prevailed for many centuries amongst physicians treating spinal cord injuries. The acute care and surgical treatment of spinal cord injuries (SCIs) has definitely changed radically since that time.

Historical Aspects

Many physicians and surgeons have tried to improve the treatment of SCI since antiquities and Middle Ages through the emergence and advancement of modern medicine. Some of the techniques that were used have stood the test of time and proved useful till today. Hippocrates in 400 B.C. used a traction apparatus for the first time. Modification of this apparatus was used for centuries as the only form of treatment and a modern version is still used in unstable cervical spine injuries. In 1824, Charles Bell first suggested the use of decompressive laminectomy in SCI. Alfred Allen in 1911 first created an experimental model of spinal injury and established the correlation between impact and extent of injury and neurological outcome. He along with Frazier in 1914 advocated longitudinal myelotomies for the treatment of SCI. Riddoch in 1930s first advocated special care of bladder, skin and nutrition in SCI patients, which dramatically improved the survival rates in these patients. Sir Ludwig Guttman's work in 1930s and 40s had a major impact on how the SCI are treated. He advised great gentleness and avoidance of hasty laminectomies or forceful manipulations in SCI and strongly advocated planned rehabilitation.

Epidemiology

Accident is the fourth most common cause of death in the USA after heart disease, cancer and stroke. The incidence accounts for 50 deaths per 1,00,000 population each year. Three percent of these are a direct result of spinal cord injury from trauma. SCI affects 1 in 40 patients presenting at major trauma centers. SCI alone has an annual incidence of 1–5 per 1,000,000 populations in developed countries. The incidence is 5 times greater in males than in females. While in the absence of a national spinal cord injury registry in India, the exact incidence is not known, it is estimated that 20,000 new cases of SCI are added every year, 60–70% of which are poor or illiterate villagers who fall from height. In developed countries, most common cause of SCI is traffic accidents (50%) while in India and other developing countries fall from height is the commonest (44.5%). The cervical cord remains the most common site of involvement (55%). Young adults account for half of all SCI.

Clinical Picture

Outcome in SCI primarily depends upon high degree of clinical suspicion, accurate clinical localization and assessment of spinal injury and detailed and proper radiological assessment of vertebral injury. While encountering initially a trauma victim, following 'Safe Assumptions' help in avoiding misdiagnosis or secondary injury:

1. Every unconscious patient with head injury has a SCI.
2. Every patient with polytrauma has a SCI.
3. Every fall, vehicular accident, workplace accident or sports injury has a SCI.
4. Every SCI is unstable and any rotation, movement or weight bearing on the spinal column will worsen the injury.

Following these assumptions in an emergency department helps in avoiding further complications or missing a SCI all together. While examining a polytrauma victim, when the history is inadequate, following 'Spinal Clues' can aid in diagnosis of SCI:

1. Hypotension and bradycardia in absence of major intra-abdominal or intrathoracic injury
2. Paradoxical respiration
3. Bilateral paralysis of all four limbs or only legs or arms more than legs, especially flaccid
4. Lack of response to peripheral pain
5. Response to pain only by head turning or grimacing
6. Sweating level
7. Priapism
8. Horner's syndrome
9. Brown-Séquard syndrome

American Spinal Injury Association (ASIA) along with the International Medical Society of Paraplegia (IMSOP) has classified neurological impairment following SCI into five grades:

Grade A	Complete	No motor or sensory functions preserved in the sacral segments S4-5
Grade B	Incomplete	Sensory but not motor function preserved below the neurologic level of injury through S4-5
Grade C	Incomplete	Motor functions preserved below the level of injury but the power is below muscle grade 3 in all muscle groups
Grade D	Incomplete	Same as Grade C, but power in muscle groups is 3 or greater than 3
Grade E	Normal	Normal

The prognosis and neurologic outcomes are vastly better in incomplete injuries especially grades C and D. In all these grades it is very important to localize the level of injury. The level of spinal injury can be localized clinically while the location of corresponding vertebral injury can be further confirmed using imaging. The localization of SCI is further compounded by presence of 'spinal shock'. Spinal shock is the loss of motor, sensory and autonomic functions due to SCI below the level of injury. The motor and sensory components of spinal shock recover as early as 4 hours after injury, though it may take days before all the components recover.

Several acute syndromes of incomplete SCI have been described and aid in diagnosis of extent of the injury. Some important syndromes are:

a. *Brown-Séquard syndrome:* Presentation of ipsilateral pyramidal and posterior column impairment and contralateral hemisensory loss—a manifestation of cord hemisection.

b. *Central cord syndrome:* Weakness of upper limb more than lower limbs with or without suspended, disseminated sensory loss—a manifestation of damage to the central areas of the cervical cord common in whiplash injuries.

c. *Cervicomedullary syndrome or syndrome of cruciate paralysis:* This resembles the central cord syndrome but has additional cranial nerve dysfunction and trigeminal sensory deficit—a manifestation of upper cervical and lower medullary dysfunction.

d. *Anterior cord syndrome:* Complete paralysis below the level of lesion with sparing of touch and vibration—a manifestation of damage to the anterior part of the spinal cord.

e. *Conus medullaris syndrome:* Loss of perineal sensation with varying degrees of sphincter dysfunction—a manifestation of damage to the terminal cord common in thoracolumbar fracture dislocations.

f. *Reversible syndromes:* These are neuropraxias commonly seen in athletes and variously called as 'burning hand syndrome' or 'stingers'.

g. *SCI without obvious radiological abnormality (SCIWORA):* SCI without obvious radiological abnormality either on X-rays or CT scan is commonly seen in children and form 14% of all SCIs.

Prehospital Management

While rescuing a victim from the scene of injury, anticipating a SCI and assuming that the patient has a SCI unless proven otherwise is very important. Once the primary survey and ABC (airway, breathing and respiration) are completed, immobilization of the spine is very important. The neck should be immobilized with a hard collar after achieving a gentle manual neutral 'eye forward' position of the head without applying any force. This maneuver should be abandoned if patient complains of pain or airway becomes compromised, in that case patient should be immobilized in the deformed position. Then the patient should be 'log-rolled' on a 'spinal board' or long backboard. Before the patient is transferred to a trauma center, intravenous fluids should be given to correct hypotension as hypotension during the transportation can further increase the spinal damage.

Acute in-hospital Care

The cornerstones of early in-hospital care comprise of airway and ventilation, traction and immobilization, methylprednisolone and imaging.

1. *Airway and ventilation:* After completing the secondary survey in the hospital a detailed respiratory assessment should be carried out (clinical and radiological) to rule out flail chest, tension pneumothorax and hemopnumothorax. Once the airway is cleared of all the secretion and any major intrathoracic injury is ruled out, if the respiration is still inadequate, endotracheal intubation or ventilatory support should be considered. General guidelines for intubation or ventilatory support are:
   - Rapid, shallow respiration with rate < 30–35 per minute
   - Labored paradoxical breathing
   - Inability to clear secretions
   - Progressive neurological deterioration
   - PaO_2 less than 60 mm Hg and SaO_2 less than 40%
   - $PaCO_2$ over 40 mm Hg
   - pH less than 7.3.

   Intubation in SCI patients should be carried out with care and gentleness without moving the neck too much. Nasal intubation or fiberoptic bronchoscope assisted intubation is sometimes necessary. If intubation is difficult, urgent tracheostomy, tracheotomy or percutaneous mini-tracheostomy is often necessary.

2. *Methylprednisolone:* Methylprednisolone has been shown to prevent secondary injury to the injured spinal cord due to lipid peroxidation. The National Acute Spinal Cord Injury Study (NASCIS-2) has shown that when given within 8 hours of injury methylprednisolone improves neurological recovery without adding to morbidity or mortality. It is recommended that the initial loading dose of 30 mg/kg should be given within the first 8 hours of injury followed by a continuous infusion of 5.4 mg/kg/hour for 23 hours. After NASCIS-3 study though the recommendations have

changed on the duration of the continuous infusion. Those patients that received the initial bolus of methylprednisolone between 3 and 8 hours after injury should receive a 48-hour infusion instead of the standard 24-hour regimen used for patients treated within 3 hours.

3. *Imaging:* A full series of initial radiographic study of spine should include
   a. *Cervical spine films:*
      - A cross table lateral view with all 7 vertebrae **(Fig. 18.1)**
      - If C7-T1 is not visualized then hands should be pulled down or a 'swimmers view' should be taken through axilla with arms abducted
      - Anteroposterior (AP) view to see rotational injury
      - Open mouth view for odontoid **(Fig. 18.2)**

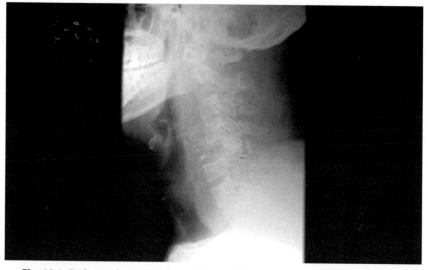

Fig. 18.1: Radiograph showing lateral view of all 7 vertebrae with injury at C4 level

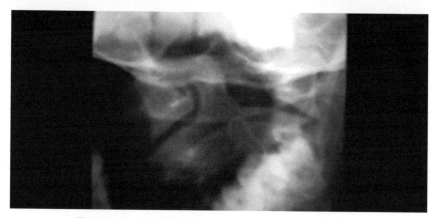

Fig. 18.2: Radiograph showing open mouth view of odontoid

  b. *Thoracic spine films:* Lateral and AP views of all 12 vertebrae

  c. *Lumbosacral spine films:* Lateral and AP views of all 12 vertebrae.

  All the radiographs should be properly examined for alignment, bony injury, cartilaginous or disk space injury and soft tissue changes (ABCS). Alignment could be distorted producing loss of lordosis, focal kyphosis, facet locking, listhesis or widened interpeduncular distance. Bony injuries may be evident as fractures, chip fractures or wedging. Cartilage and joint space could be widened or narrowed. Soft tissues in pre or paravertebral regions could be widened.

  Computerized tomography (CT) scan could be used to further delineate the extent of bony injury in preselected areas. Magnetic Resonance Imaging (MRI) scan further enhances the visualization of spinal cord parenchymal injury. It also gives excellent anatomic definition of soft tissue injury and the type of injury to spinal cord (hematoma, edema, etc.) and accurately defines the extent of compression on the spinal cord **(Fig. 18.3)**.

4. *Traction immobilization:* Goals in treatment of SCI is maximal neurologic recovery and spinal stabilization. Before any surgical intervention is carried out skeletal traction is used in cervical SCI to immobilize the spine. It helps realigning the spinal canal and prevents any further injury to spinal cord and nerve roots due to compression and movement at the unstable level. Various devices are used for skeletal traction but the most common once are Crutchfield tongs and Gardner-Wells tongs. Halo tractions are also used for traction-immobilization where available. Following guiding principles should be followed while applying the traction:

  • Maintain a constant traction force at all times. Do not allow the weights to touch ground especially during the postural drainage

  • Clean insertion site regularly every 8 hours using antiseptic solutions

  • Turn and position the patient at least every 2 hrs

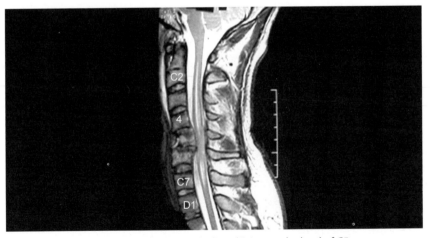

Fig. 18.3: MRI showing spinal cord injury at the level of C5

- Generally use maximum of 5 lbs of weight per level of injury (e.g. C5 fracture= 25 lbs of weight)
- Repeat lateral X-ray after every increase in weight
- Avoid over distraction.

Surgery for Spinal Cord Injury

Surgery for SCI is discussed based on two important aspects, timing of surgery and indications of surgery. Occasionally early surgery is used if the spinal cord appears to be compressed by a herniated disk, blood clot, or a bone fragment. This is most commonly done for patients with an incomplete spinal cord injury or with progressive neurological deterioration. The entire issue of the timing of surgical decompression of an acutely injured spinal cord is currently under intense debate. Traditionally, surgeons have felt that waiting for several days was the safest course of action, since there was some evidence that operating immediately may actually worsen outcome. However, more recently, some surgeons have begun advocating immediate early surgery, but this hypothesis has never been scientifically tested. A clinical trial to test this is currently in the planning stage. This trial is being organized by the Joint Sections on Neurotrauma and Critical Care and on Spine and Peripheral Nerves of the American Association of Neurological Surgeons and the Congress of Neurological Surgeons.

Surgery in SCI cannot reverse damage to the spinal cord but still surgery may be needed to decompress and stabilize the spine to prevent further injury to spinal cord and future pain or deformity. The goals of surgery include dural decompression, prevention of tethering and spinal stabilization. The type of surgery performed (anterior vs posterior), distraction forces during surgery, preoperative grade all influence the outcome. While anterior decompression has proven to be better than a posterior approach and stabilization with fusion gives definite benefits in an unstable spine, till now no clear consensus on timing of surgery has emerged with proponents of both early and late intervention claiming advantages. Surgical technique of spinal stabilization though has exploded over recent years giving a variety of options to the surgeons. In cervical SCI, anterior plating **(Fig. 18.4)** can be used to stabilize a spine alone or can be aided by posterior fusion using lateral mass screws and rods. In thoracolumbar spine anterior and posterior instrumentation and fusion can be used similarly alone or complementing each other **(Fig. 18.5)**. Endoscopic minimally invasive spinal fixations are also practiced. Recently surgeries to repair the damaged spinal cord are also carried out in patients as well as experimental animals. In one study, rats with completely severed spinal cords apparently showed limited functional improvement with multiple peripheral nerve section implants. The cells in the grafts initially include supporting cells, and cut axons. These axons degenerate, however, leaving behind a natural tube for the CNS axons to regrow through. In the study, the CNS axons grew across the grafts and apparently made connections with the neurons that move the legs. Postsurgical management also encompasses

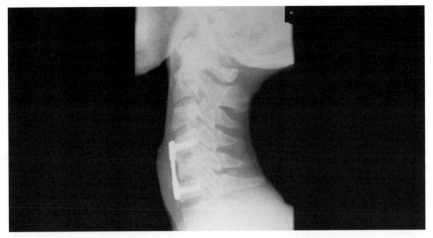

Fig. 18.4: Cervical spine stabilization through anterior plating

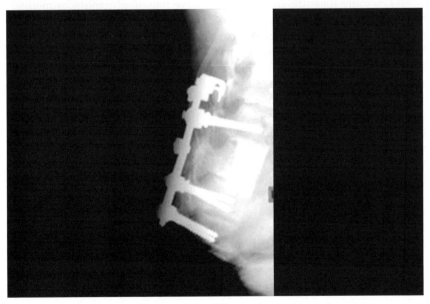

Fig. 18.5: Thoracolumbar spine stabilization by anterior and posterior instrumentation and fusion

aggressive nursing programs including turning (to prevent decubitus ulcers), pulmonary care, deep venous thrombosis prophylaxis, management of orthostatic hypotension, limb edema and nutrition supplementation. Regular physiotherapy instituted early in the course of illness keeps muscles supple, delays wasting, prevents contractures and allows for better functional recovery should reinnveration occur.

Functional restoration is also achieved by life techniques like bio-feedback, instructions regarding ambulation and transfer, wheelchair considerations (including altering the environment to suit the patient), braces and reconstructive surgery. Devices like implantable pumps (to reduce spasticity), diaphragmatic pacers (to render a patient ventilator free) are also a part of a comprehensive rehabilitation programme.

Outcome of Patients with Spinal Cord Injury

The main determinant of outcome is the patient's neurological grade at the time of admission with patients having complete motor and sensory myelopathy showing the worst prognosis. Other predictive factors include rectal tone status, admission blood pressure and pulse status, reflexes, and medical and surgical management since injury. The time course of recovery is also prolonged and recovery itself often incomplete. Taking all grades and locations into considerations a study concluded that while the majority of cases improved within a year, even at 3 years post injury 23.3% continue to improve whereas 7.1% deteriorated. The trend continued in the 5th year post-injury also with 12.5% and 5.5% respectively showing further improvement and late deterioration.

Bibliography

1. American Spinal Injury Association, International Medical Society of Paraplegia. 'International Standards for Neurological and Functional Classification of Spinal Cord Injury' Revised, 1992. Chicago, IL: ASIA/IMSOP 1992.
2. Bracken MB, Shepard MJ, Collins WF et al. 'A randomized, controlled trial of methylprdnisolone or nalaxone in the treatment of acute spinal cord injury'. Results of the second National Acute Spinal Cord Injury Study. N Engl J Med. 1990;322:1405-11.
3. Breasted JH. 'The Edwin Smith Surgical Papyrus', Univ of Chicago press, Chicago. 1930;1:327.
4. Guttman L. 'Spinal Cord Injuries: Comprehensive management and research' Blackwell Scientific, Oxford, England, 2nd edn., 1976.
5. Priestley JV, Ramer MS, King VR, McMahon SB, Brown RA. 'Stimulating regeneration in the damaged spinal cord'. J Physiol Paris. 2002.
6. Sonntag VK, Francis PM. 'Patient selection and timing of surgery'. In: Benzel EC and Tator CH (Eds). 'Contemporary management of spinal cord injury'. AANS, Park Ridge, IL, USA; 1995.pp.97-107.
7. Tator CH. 'Clinical manifestations of acute spinal cord injury'. In: Benzel EC and Tator CH (Eds). 'Contemporary management of spinal cord injury'. AANS, Park Ridge, IL, USA; 1995.pp.15-26.
8. Tator CH. 'Epidemiology and general characteristics of spinal cord injury patient'. In: Benzel EC and Tator CH (Eds). 'Contemporary management of spinal cord injury'. AANS, Park Ridge, IL, USA; 1995.pp.9-13.
9. Wilberger JE. 'Immobilisation and traction'. In: Benzel EC and Tator CH (Eds). 'Contemporary management of spinal cord injury'. AANS, Park Ridge, IL, USA; 1995.pp.79-85.

19

Concepts in Spinal Cord Injury Rehabilitation

Mouli Madhab Ghatak

Injury to the spinal cord is not restricted to any community or race and it has been a serious medical problem since, the beginning of mankind. The ancient document of Edwin Smith during 2500–3000 BC has clear descriptions of spinal cord injury (SCI) with successive commentaries like 'a condition not to be treated' as even after the all available (limited) treatment options, possibility of cure was not there.[1]

Even today medical professionals in many areas of the world, provide suboptimal treatment for such patients and in some areas it is treated as because it looks to be a serious problem following an accident but often with poor results. The survival and quality of life largely depends on meticulous scientific steps being followed from the time of injury. The modern management of SCI treatment with surgery, medical care and rehabilitation was largely developed by Dr. Ludwig Guttman at Stroke Mandeville Hospital in England and Donald Munro at Boston City Hospital of USA both of whom observed and treated numerous war affected SCI patients with various successive complications and mortality.[2] It was evident that 80% of such patients died either of urinary sepsis, or of bedsore. They understood the crisis and developed a specialized center for treatment and rehabilitation center to provide proper surgical intervention, acute and long-term medical care and a comprehensive rehabilitation facility. Subsequently, Dr. Geisler and coworkers studied 1510 SCI patients in Canada (during 1973–1980)[3] and recorded 194 deaths arising from cardiovascular, renal, respiratory, hepatic, neoplastic diseases and sepsis or suicides. There is a marked decrease in death rates in recent years with an advanced bladder management and bedsore prevention and treatment measures. On the other hand the mortality rate from suicide and liver diseases are becoming higher in such patients.

The latest US statistics estimated that there are approximately 40 SCI cases per million of people and about 11,000 new cases every year. NCISC (National Spinal Cord Injury Statistical Center) data of June 2005 shows about 2,50,000

alive SCI patients in US having an average age of 28.7 years, the most common ages affected range from 16 to 30 years. About 80% of SCI patients are male.[4]
Among all SCI, the eventual results of paralytic distribution are per below.[5]
Incomplete tetraplegics – 34%.
Complete paraplegic – 23.1%.
Complete tetraplegic – 18.4%.
Incomplete paraplegic – 17.5%.

The long-term complications of seg patients will be cared, managed and guided mostly by the rehabilitation professionals. The prevention of death as a result of different complications is to be properly monitored, handled with clinical anticipation. A long-term survival in spinal cord injury depends on the level of neurological injury, degree of injury, age at injury and the events in the earlier years of injury (Frankel et al 1998).[5,6] Therefore, the management of urinary system, the cardiovascular system and the respiratory system in early decades is of immense importance over a period of 10 years. Middleton et al (2004)[7] found that 58.6% of patients required one or more rehospitalization because of complications. The causes of such repeated hospitalizations are shown to be genitourinary (24%), gastrointestinal (11%), further rehabilitation (11%), skin related problem (8.9%), psychiatric illness (6.8%), musculoskeletal complications (8.6%). A long-term rehabilitation at home or any care center should have proper medical coverage to address all these problems.

A Comprehensive SCI Rehabilitation

A comprehensive SCI rehabilitation is an integrated multidisciplinary approach with a multi faceted management protocol comprising of:
1. The early stage management.
2. Surgical procedures when and if required.
3. General and nursing care.
4. Medical care and medicinal treatment.
5. Therapeutic and orthotic intervention.
6. Long-term rehabilitation measures with vocational and social guidelines.
1. *The early stage:* Proper resuscitation of the patient, immobilization of the injured part, identifying additional injuries and treating those and surgical intervention as early as possible are important. Physical therapy including passive ROM exercises of limbs, chest physiotherapy and assurance are also to be applied in this stage.[8,9]
2. *Surgical intervention:* In a grossly damaged spinal column with instability or alignment disorder, stability of the spine is assured by spinal stabilization operation and in milder cases the cord may be saved by release of compression of the cord (discussed already in another chapter).
3. *Nursing care:* Meticulous nursing care which plays the greatest role in prevention of so many of complications including bedsore, recurrent infections, urinary sepsis, spasticity development, etc. In a patient with associated vertebral fracture or multiple site musculoskeletal injuries, a round the clock supervision and care including frequent turning in the bed, antiseptic dressing of wound, care of the limbs having poor sensory

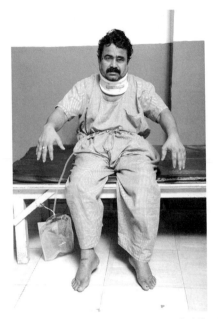

Fig. 19.1: A quadriplegic on acute care rehabilitation
(For color version, see Plate 6)

inputs (protecting the limb from any further injury), cautious handling of the spinal column (maintaining the integrity and stability of the fractured spine), etc. are vital to patient care. Moreover, the nursing personnel also address the various medical problems and notes the complaints and preferences of the patient and inform the physiatrist and therapists. Proper positioning of the limbs instructed by the physicians and the therapists are to be maintained and supervised by the nurses. The feeding process as per the recommendation of the nutritionist is also supervised by the rehabilitation nurse. Any sort of physical and mental deterioration, any special behavioral pattern and any other day-to-day happenings of the patient are noted and reported to the doctor or responsible person **(Fig. 19.1)**.[10-12]

4. *Medical care and medicinal treatment:* Medicine cannot cure a spinal injury patient but the patient having cervical, dorsal or lumber spine injury requires a series of investigations, medical checkup and medicinal interventions in order to maintain the health status and to combat different complications that may arise out of such injury. The prime medical intervention required is as follows:

   i. *Wound care* with antiseptic dressing, antibiotics.

   ii. *Urinary sepsis* due to indwelling catheter or CIC, should be investigated through urine analysis and culture. Suitable antibiotics with a maintenance long-term therapy may be required. USG of KUB, uroflowmetry are suggested to evaluate urodynamic status.

iii. *Respiratory infections* specially in quadriplegic having poor respiratory drive may need appropriate antibiotic bronchodilators, oxygen inhalation, nebulization or even ventilatory support.

iv. *Bedsore* to be cared with antiseptic dressing, frequent turning in the bed. For infected sores antibiotics are frequently suggested. Specialized bed mattress is also put to reduce the pressure effects.

v. *Antispastic medications* including baclofen, tizanidine, etc. are to be prescribed as and when required. Botulinum toxins, Baclofen pump are also in use sometimes.

All these approaches are elaborately discussed in the respective chapters of this book. However, there may be so many/complicating medical factors including deep venous thrombosis, heterotrophic ossification, reflex sympathetic dystrophy, etc. which are to be managed accordingly (discussed in other chapters).

5. *Therapeutic and orthotic intervention:* Plays a major role in SCI rehabilitation. The paralyzed limb and the part of trunk are gradually conditioned to regain functional capability. Different techniques, positioning and training are provided in a graded manner by the physiotherapist and occupational therapist with the aim of the highest level of functional regain and return to a productive and fruitful life. Different orthotic interventions are of immense importance for stability, protection and functional activation of the spine and the limbs as and when required. Various functional training and wheelchair selection and training for complete paraplegic or quadriplegic are integral part of the rehabilitation process.[13-15] A good nutritional support is mandatory for the growth of lost muscles and metabolic balances. All these are discussed in the subsequent chapters.

6. *Long-term rehabilitation in SCI:* It is aimed towards the maximum fitness and capability, that can be maintained at home, society and job place. As an acute rehabilitation phase should always be a center-based program, the specific measures and planning are to be accomplished before discharge.

The Predischarge Preparation

The medical stability, physical condition and psychological adaptability are tested and checked before discharge. A scientific occupational and vocational predischarge assessment is usually done based on which the long-term care and rehabilitation guidelines are provided. The paraplegics are to be properly trained for wheelchair mobility in different places and situations and the transfer techniques from wheelchair to bed or wheelchair to car, toilet or any other sitting place. Training for using lower limb orthosis like HKAFO, KFO, AFO, etc. is to be properly provided for functional purposes. Skin care in patients with poor sensations is to be taught before discharge.

The home modification such as using ramps and elevations, wheelchair—friendly, door and floor, appropriate height of the bed for easy transfer between wheelchair and bed, environmental control units like remote controls, power points, control lights, etc. are to be made and arranged when the patient is discharged. Various adaptive devices are also in use to achieve better functional capability. The patient is taught to self clean intermittent catheterization and to identify the signs of UTI. Proper bowel care includes laxatives, prokinetics, timed evacuation, etc. Specialized bed like alternating air pressure/inflatable mattress is to be arranged and the patient is instructed proper skills and habits to the ways to prevent formation of pressure sore. Proper nutritional care as per the direction of a qualified dietician is always recommended. A home rehabilitation program including necessary physiotherapy, occupational therapy is of immense help for further betterment of functional status. An adjustment in life style changes is to be reassured by proper psychological counseling and support. Friends, relatives and the professional colleagues are to be prepared to accept the patients disability in a careful manner. The prevocational and vocational planning and guidelines are to be formulated scientifically as discussed in a separate chapter. A paraplegic on wheelchair should scientifically remodulate the outdoor mobility with arrangement of proper vehicle for transportation from home to the job site. Job site modification is an important issue and is the responsibility of the employer. The rehabilitation personnel and the patient with his family members work together with the employer for such modification. The nature of job may be changed for patients who were engaged in outdoor and fieldworks before attack. The vocational counselor determines the suitable job profile considering the educational qualification, patient's interest and the disability.[16-18] The psychological stability, motivation and zeal also count a lot. All these are ways are discussed in detail in other chapters.

The long-term care and rehabilitation requires good teaching and training of the patient regarding his ailment, disability and the medical problems which may arise from time to time. Periodic checkup by a qualified physiatrist is an essential part of the long-term rehabilitation to ensure a safer future and survival.

Long-term Care for Quadriplegics

Quadriplegics are further challenged upon returning to the community. A careful predischarge assessment, planning and guidelines are formulated and discussed with the patient and the family members. Quadriplegics lacking the capability for propulsion of wheelchair are obviously dependent patients and trained attendants or family members are to be appointed for maintaining a smooth life. The feeding, handling, caring and transferring of the patient requires proper training of the attendant and the patient. The attendant must be aware of different medical problems like development of pressure sore, urinary and chest infections, autonomic dysreflexia, etc. Patient with high cervical lesion (C2 – C3) requires good respiratory support system with a home arrangement of O_2, nebulizer, mask and a suction machine, operation of which should be taught to the attendant. Routine and regular chest physiotherapy, breathing exercises, spirometric training is also mandatory to improve or maintain a good respiratory status. Proper balanced and high protein nutrition is to be supplied. And periodic checkup of blood biochemistry like lipids, liver function and renal function tests are essential. Intermittent clean catheterization with maintenance of intake-output chart and periodic ultrasound of kidneys, ureters and bladder (KUB) for proper evaluation and management of urinary problem is necessary. Transferring the patient from a bed to wheelchair or a wheelchair to bed requires scientific techniques to avoid injury or skin abrasions (increased risk secondary to poor sensation). A modified wheelchair with toileting attachments is usually used for such patient. Different adaptive devices are used for some of the hand activities including feeding, writing or controlling home units like powered switches of light, TV, etc. who has gained some power in the upper limbs. Such adaptation and modification are planned and designed scientifically after scrutinizing the spared muscular function thoroughly. Outdoor mobility of high cervical quadriplegic is more restricted than the lower segment injured persons **(Fig. 19.2)**.[19,20]

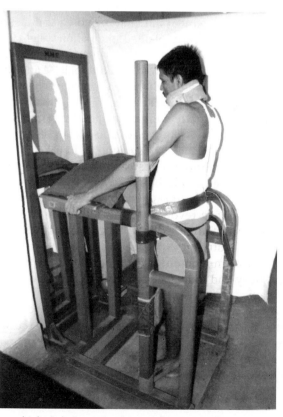

Fig. 19.2: A quadriplegic being trained to stand in a specially made "stand-in-frame"
(For color version, see Plate 6)

Modern Technologies in Spinal Cord Injury Rehabilitation

Numerous clinical and research studies have been conducted so long in various medical and rehabilitation institutes to conquer disabilities after spinal cord injury. Since, the early 70s, the electrical the nerves was being tried. In 80s and 90s, researchers were focused on kinetic and functional benefits of the paralyzed areas, ressulting in innovations like functional electrical stimulation (FES).[21]

Different studies on gait modification system have been practically implemented through the achievement of functional movement by different types of stimulation apparatuses. Intensive multichannel electrical stimulation, dual channel stimulators, bionic electrical garment, electrical acupuncture, dropped foot stimulator has been evolved as a measure to improve functional capacities of hands and lower limbs for specific task oriented jobs. Electrically powered orthosis are fitted in the limbs for neuromotor functional activities, such as, orthosis to improve hand grasps and to assist.[22-25]

Electrical stimulation with surface electrodes may not be sufficient to activate deep muscle groups. Some studies demonstrated that epimysial electrodes via surgically placed electrodes in the deep muscles and stimulation of these electrodes can augment function including ambulation. The safety and effectiveness of a practical implanted stimulation system for patients who do not regain hip instability after an upper motor neuron lesion has been demonstrated in these studies (Waters RL, Campbell JM and Nakai R 1988).[26]

Recent advances in modern rehabilitation technology recommends to reverse learned non-use through different forced-use training. Specialized biofeedback therapies, body weight supported treadmill ambulation training, robotic exercises, etc. contributes a modern result-oriented re-education system for people with spinal cord injuries.[27,28]

The conventional training of transfer, simple mat activities, manual exercise therapies are largely being supplemented by motor-driven, software-controlled, and therapeutic equipment and mobility aids. These technologies have revolutionized the active training procedures including muscle strengthening, spasticity reduction and rediscovering the residual muscle strength, promoting mobility and walking, etc. A continuous passive movement system recently has been modified to modulate spasticity and tone, using motorized software operated bicycles (**Fig. 19.3**).[29,30]

Patients confined to bed also may be trained with such bedside units to initiate remobilization and prevent contracture, pressure sore and thrombosis (**Figs 19.4 to 19.7**).

Management of Chronic Pain in SCI Patients

Chronic pain in spinal injury is frequently *neuropathic* rather than *nociceptive* in nature.

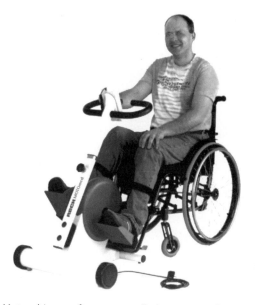

Fig. 19.3: MMT I—Motor-driven, software-controlled movement therapy system for passive, active and antispastic muscle training for paraplegics, quadriplegics and hemiplegics
(For color version, see Plate 7)

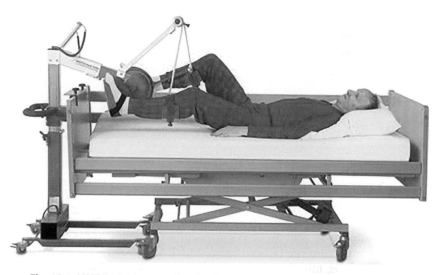

Fig. 19.4: MMT II—Patients confined to bed are trained with bed attached unit far remobilization and preventing contracture, pressure sore, thrombosis, etc.
(For color version, see Plate 7)
Courtesy: Hospimedica International

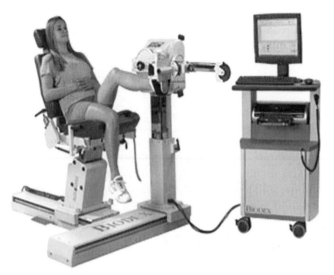

Fig. 19.5: Computerized strength and muscle function evaluation system (BIODEX)
(For color version, see Plate 8)
Courtesy: Hospimedica International

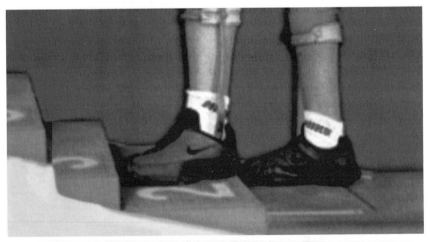

Fig. 19.6: Adjustable step height with push button control for SCI and stroke patients
(For color version, see Plate 8)

Pain immediately after injury is a direct effect of neural injury associated with other musculoskeletal damages, which is treated with medicines including NSAIDs, muscle relaxants, opioids, etc. The neuropathic chronic pain is managed with different rehabilitation measures and drugs. These include:

- *Exercise programs:* Different stretching maneuvers, flexibility and strength training including different physical and occupational therapies, massages and chiropractic therapies, etc. are primary recommendations.

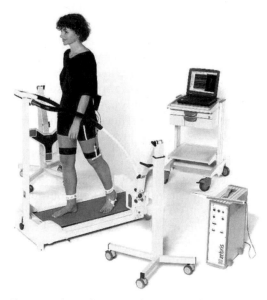

Fig. 19.7: Three-dimensional motion analysis system
(For color version, see Plate 8)

Heat and cold therapies (in cases of sensory impairment, these are to be avoided), hydrotherapy, different muscle relaxation techniques are also useful measures.

- *Transcutaneous electrical nerve stimulation (TENS):* With TENS, electrical impulses are applied through the electrodes attached to the skin (connected to a stimulator). It interrupts transmission of pain signals from small sensory nerves at the sight of pain.[31]
- *Other electrical modalities:* Various electrical modalities are used to minimize the localized pain syndromes like SWD, IFT, Faradic electrical stimulation, etc. as and when required.[32,33] Behavioral modification has got immense value to counteract the psychological inclination and dependency. A good number of patients need supportive psychotherapy to break the psychobehavioral component of chronic pain.[34]

Advanced Interventional Pain Management Systems

- *Therapeutic nerve blocks* include epidural block and neurolytic blocks. Local anesthetics, steroids are used for epidural blocks and alcohol, phenol or steroids are injected in the epidural space targeting neurolysis or specific nerve roots.[35]
- *Cryoanalgesia:* A probe is used to freeze neural tissues to damage nerves and interrupt sensory input.[36]
- *Radiofrequency* energy is applied through a probe inserted percutaneously, which coagulates nerves thermally which is an effective neuroablative procedure to relieve pain. It may be repeatedly used.[37]

- *Neuromodulation* therapies are implantable therapies with electrical impulses (spinal cord stimulation) or drug administration systems (DAS). Different implantable drug pumps deliver precise doses of medication on intrathecally directly in the spinal canal.[38]
- *Surgical neuroablation* deals with different types of surgical procedure like surgical division of a tract in the spinal cord (cordotomy), selective destruction of a nerve (rhizotomy), etc. These procedures are often considered as the last option for relieving the chronic spinal pain.[39]

Assistive Technology for People with Spinal Cord Injuries

Assistive technologies (ATs) can provide support for ADL, community participation, and vocational professional field, outdoor mobility, indoor mobility and recreation and control of home and office environment.

A thorough AT assessment should be performed by the rehabilitation team headed by a Physiatrist. Evaluation is focused on the individuals physical abilities (like strength, endurance, flexibility), cognitive abilities (like comprehension, decision making, etc.), living environment (like home work school), sensory function (like tactile sensation, hearing, vision), support system (like family assistance, professional assistance, organizational helps and the affect (like acceptance of disabilities) [Rose, Marie Cooper, et al. University Pitts Burgh].[40]

The AT consideration for a home environment must include ramps, stairs, lifts and wide doorways. The community activities like tasks such as shopping, using an automated tailor machine or eating in a restaurant, all need good AT fittings and training **(Figs 19.8A to H)**.

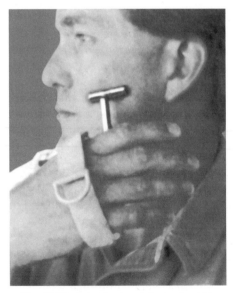

Fig. 19.8A: Adaptive hand device for ADL
(For color version, see Plate 9)

Electrically Powered Wheelchair

People with high-level tetraplegia because of functional motot limit, various customized control devices, electrically powered wheelchair (EPW) have been manufactured. Microswitching mechanisms that can be activated by mouth (sip and puff) or other parts of the body like feet, head, etc. Special sitting systems, transportability, technological controller programmability, suspension elements, shock and vibration decreasing elements, etc. are important adjunct of EPW in the modern period. More advanced systems and devices are being added day to day. However, proper training should be provided to use such EPW must be followed.[41,42]

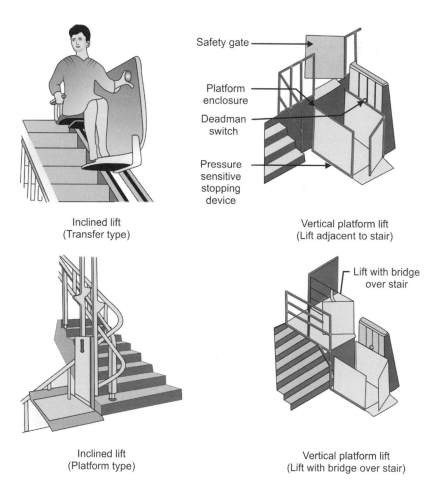

Inclined lift
(Transfer type)

Safety gate

Platform enclosure

Deadman switch

Pressure sensitive stopping device

Vertical platform lift
(Lift adjacent to stair)

Lift with bridge over stair

Inclined lift
(Platform type)

Vertical platform lift
(Lift with bridge over stair)

Fig. 19.8B: Door and staircases modified

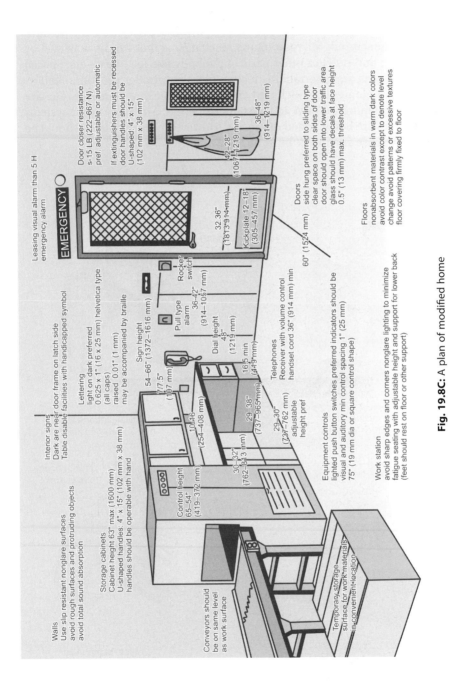

Fig. 19.8C: A plan of modified home

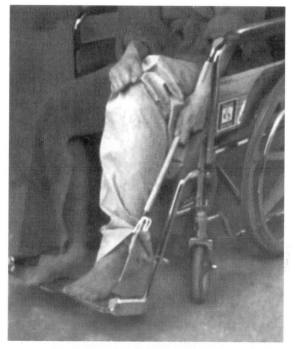

Fig. 19.8D: Assistive devices for self-care
(For color version, see Plate 9)

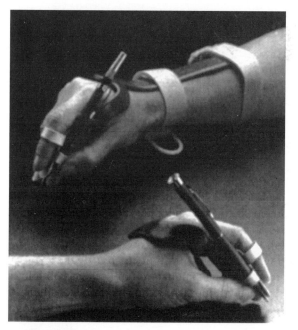

Fig. 19.8E: Adaptive hand devices for pen holding

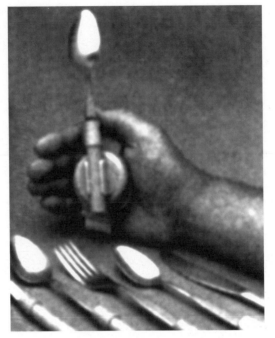

Fig. 19.8F: Adaptive hand device for spoon holding

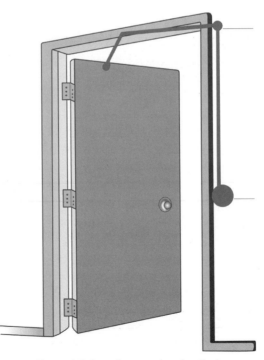

Fig. 19.8G: Door for a paralyzed patient

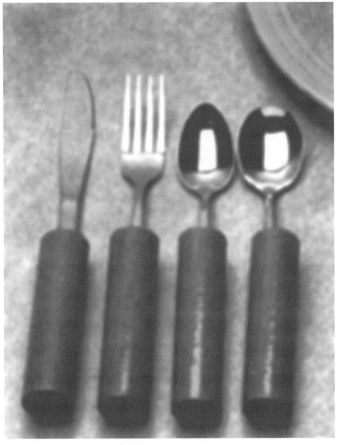

Fig. 19.8H: Specially made spoon handles
(For color version, see Plate 9)

Augmentation and Alternative Communication System

This modern and comprehensive system of augmentation and alternative communication system (AACS) has been popular with the goal to optimize the communication capability of the individuals with significant communication disorder. AACS refers to any communication approach that supplements or replaces natural speech or writing.[43,44]

Computer Access

The disability-friendly operating system and application are coevolved with specialized pointing devices or press button system. The mouse and the track pad are the familiar pointing devices while other devices include track ball and the track point. The pointing devices which are commonly prescribed in tetraplegics are touch screens, head mounted mouse emulators, mouse keys, etc.[45,46]

Rehabilitation of Spinal Cord Injury Patients

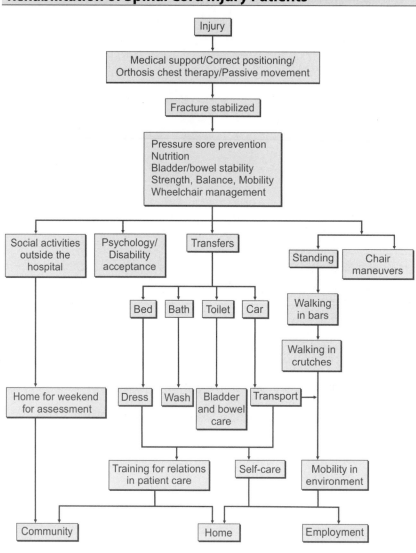

Reintegration of a Spinal Cord Injury: Person

SCI Rehabilitation: A Science with Care

A successful SCI rehabilitation requires the following factors—(Spinal cord).

S: *Specialized care:* Accept every patient as a special case with proper importance and care.

P: *Physical:* Rehabilitation should be multidisciplinary team program.

I: *Injury care* with surgery/immobilization.

N: *Nutritional* support with a high protein and balanced menu serving as per requirement.

A: *Assessing* the patient's disabling factors, the neuromuscular, skeletal, metabolic, urinary, cardiorespiratory and psychological parameters repeatedly.

L: *Listening* the patient with patience, following the emotions and expectations of the individual.

C: *Choosing* proper and scientific rehabilitation care and by rehabilitation specialists, technicians and required aids and equipment.

O: *Offering* an updated rehabilitation service along with best social, professional and family support and adaptation modules.

R: *Restricting* the risk factors and life-threatening medical conditions by enthusiastic treatment framing and preventive measures.

D: *Disability*, depression and dark life should be felt by all the service providers and to reassure the distressed with an enlightened rehabilitation process.

References

1. Huges JT. The Edwin smith surgical papyrus: An analysis of the first case report of spinal cord injuries. Paraplegia. 1988;26(2):71-82.
2. Munro D. The treatment of urinary bladder in case with injury of the spinal cord. American Journal of Surgery. 1937;38(1):120-36.
3. Fred H Geisler. Spinal cord injury. The Lancet. 2002;360(9348):1883-4.
4. Annual Report for the Model Spinal Cord Injury Care System. NSCISC; 2005.pp. 1-116.
5. Frankel, et al. Long-term survival in spinal cord injury: A fifty-year investigation. Spinal Cord. 1998;36:266-74.
6. McKinley, et al. Long term medical complications after traumatic spinal cord injury: A regional model system analysis. Archive of Physical Medicine and Rehabilitation. 1999;80(11):1402-10.
7. Middlton, et al. Patterns of morbidity and rehospitalisation following spinal cord injury. Spinal Cord. 2004;42:359-67.
8. Sumida, et al. Early rehabilitation effect for traumatic spinal cord injury. Archive of Physical Medicine and Rehabilitation. 2001;82:391-5.
9. Dobkin, et al. The evolution of walking related outcomes over the first 12 weeks of rehabilitation for incomplete traumatic spinal cord injury: The multicenter randomized spinal cord injury locomotor trial. Neurorehabilitation and Neural Repair. 2007;21:25-35.
10. Heinemann, et al. Relationship between disability measures and nursing effort during medical rehabilitation for patients with traumatic brain and spinal cord injury. Archive of Physical Medicine and Rehabilitation. 1997;78(2):143-9.
11. Adams, et al. Bedside monitoring of spinal cord injuries. American Journal of Critical Care. 2005;14:85-6.
12. Horton, et al. The value of nursing: A literature Review. Nursing Ethics. 2007;14:714-40.
13. Lobley, et al. Orthotic design from the new England regional spinal cord injury center-Suggestion from the field. Physical Therapy. 1985;65(4):492-3.
14. Jacobs, et al. Exerciser recommendation for the individuals with spinal cord injury: Review article. Sports Medicine. 2004;34(11):727-51.

15. Pamela F and Lind. The treatment of spinal paraplegia at stoke Mandeville. Australian Journal of Physiotherapy. 1955;1(3):112-7.
16. Cox, et al. The need for a multidisciplinary outreach service for people with spinal cord injury living in the community. Clinical rehabilitation. 2001;15:600-6.
17. Woolsey. Rehabilitation outcome following spinal cord injury. Archive of Neurology. 1985;42:116-9.
18. Curtiset, et al. Spinal cord injury community followup: Role of the Physical Therapist. Physical Therapy. 1986;66:1370-5.
19. Marino, et al. Neurogenic recovery after traumatic spinal cord injury: Data from the model spinal cord injury system. Archive of Physical Medicine and Rehabilitation. 1999;80(11):1391-6.
20. Carpenter C. The experience of spinal cord injury: The individuals perspective-Implication for rehabilitation practice. Physical Therapy. 1994;74(7):614-28.
21. Phillips CA. Functional electrical stimulation and lower extremity bracing for ambulation exercise of the spinal cord injured individual: A medically prescribed system. Physical Therapy. 1989;69(10).
22. Volker Dietz, et al. Locomotor activity in spinal man: Significance of afferent input from joint and load receptors. Brain. 2002;125:2626-34.
23. Rowley DI. Helping the paraplegic to walk. Journal of Bone and Joint Surgery. 1987;69B:173-4.
24. Mayr, et al. Prospective, blinded, randomized crossover study of gait rehabilitation in stroke patient using the locomat gait orthosis. Neurorehabilitation and Neural Repair. 2007;21:307-14.
25. Waters RL, et al. Therapeutic electrical stimulation of the lower limb by epimysial electrodes. Clinical Orthopaedics and Related Research. 1988;233:44-52.
26. Dietz and Muller. Degradation of neural function following a spinal cord injury: Mechanism and counter measures. Brain. 2004;127:2221-31.
27. Wolpaw JR. Control of two-dimensional movement signal by a noninvasive brain-computer interface in humans. Proceedings of the National Academy of Sciences. 2004;101(51):17849-54.
28. Edelle Carmen. Spinal cord control movement: Implication for locomotor rehabilitation following SCI. Physical Therapy. 2000;80:477-84.
29. Waters, et al. Energy cost of paraplegic locomotion. Journal of Bone and Joint Surgery, Am. 1985;67:1245-50.
30. Gersh and Wolf. Application of transcutaneous electrical nerve stimulation in the management of patients with pain, state of the art update. Physical Therapy. 1985;65:314-36.
31. Nora, et al. Short-wave diathermy: A review of existing clinical trials. Physical therapy reviews. 2001;6(2):101-18.
32. White, et al. Electroanalgesia: Its role in acute and chronic pain management. Anesthesia and Analgesia. 2001;92:505-13.
33. Swanson, et al. Result of behavior modification in the treatment of chronic pain, Psychosomatic Medicine. 1979;41(1).
34. Edwards. Management of pain in the critically ill. Journal of Intensive care Medicine. 1990;5(6):258-91.
35. Lloyd JW, et al. Cryoanalgesia: A new concept to pain relief. Lancet. 1976;30(2):7992.
36. Kaparal and Mekhail. Radiofrequency ablation for chronic pain control. Current Pain and Headache Report. 2001;5(6):517-25.

37. Katz PS. Intrinsic and extrinsic neuromodulation of motor circuits. Current Opinion in Neurobiology. 1995;5:799-808.
38. Jorge Roberto. Percuteneous radiofrequency spinal rhizotomy, Applied Neurophysiology. 1983;46(1-4):138-46.
39. Rose Marie Cooper, et al. Assessing the influence of wheelchair technology on perception of participation in spinal cord injury. Archive of Physical Medicine and Rehabilitation. 2004;85(11):1854-8.
40. Winyard, et al. The use and usefulness of electrically powered indoor wheelchair. Oxford Journals-Rheumatology. 1976;15(4):254-63.
41. Fass, et al. Durability, value and reliability of selected electric powered wheelchair. Archive of Physical Medicine and Rehabilitation. 2004;85(5):805-14.
42. Beukelman, et al. Augmentative and alternative communication for adults with acquired severe communication disorder. Augmentative and Alternative Communication. 1988;4(2):104-21.
43. Martin L Albart. Treatment of Aphasia. Archive of Neurology. 1988;55:1217-419.
44. Mcfarland, et al. Design and operation of an EEG based brain-computer interface with design signal processing technology. Behavior Research Methods-Instrument and Computers. 1997;29(3):337-45.
45. Raymond Quist W, Doreen Blischak M. Assistive communication devices: Call for specifications. Augmentative and Alternative Communication. 1992;8(4):312-7.
46. Floris, et al. The tetraplegic patient and the environment, Chapter-5, Surgical Rehabilitation of the Upper Limb In Tetraplegia by Vincent R. Hentz, Caroline Leclercq. 2002:45-55.

20

Therapeutic Rehabilitation and Medical Management of Spasticity

Rupam Sinha, S Ziauddin, Mouli Madhab Ghatak

Spasticity has been defined as a motor disorder characterized by a velocity-dependent increase in the tonic stretch reflexes (muscle tone) with exaggerated tendon jerks, resulting from hyperexcitability of the stretch reflex as one component of the upper motor syndrome (Lance 1980)[1], it is likely that it affects millions of people worldwide.[2]

Spasticity can lead to loss of coordination, loss of function, pain, and permanent muscle shortening, or contracture. Spasticity does not always require treatment, but when it does, a wide range of effective therapies—used alone or in combination—is now available.[3]

Pathophysiology

The production of spasticity is due to overactivity of the alpha motor neuron (α-MN) pool, which also causes some of the other 'positive' manifestations mentioned above. Lesions of the corticospinal tracts cause muscle weakness, loss of dexterity and a Babinski response, but no sign of spasticity. Loss of descending input from cerebral cortex and basal ganglia, through medial and dorsal reticulospinal and vestibulospinal fibers, is thought to be important in causing impaired modulation of monosynaptic input from primary afferent (la) fibers (segmental myotatic reflex), and polysynaptic afferent input from cutaneous receptors and Golgi tendon organs contributing to α-MN hyperexcitability. Spinal inter neurons play a critical part in this modulation, in particular through presynaptic and reciprocal (la) inhibition. Inappropriate muscle co-contraction may arise through reduced reciprocal (la) inhibition impeding voluntary limb movement. Moreover, nociceptive and motor pathways have considerable influence on each other, emphasising the clinical significance of pain management in treating spasticity.[4, 5]

Spasticity: Spinal Model

- Elimination of inhibition on segmental polysynaptic pathways
- Sluggish, progressive rise of excitatory state through cumulative excitation
- Afferent activity from one segment may lead to muscle response several segments away
- Agonist and antagonist may be overexcited.

Spasticity: Cerebral Model

- Enhanced excitability of monosynaptic pathways
- Speedy build-up of reflex activity
- Prejudice toward overactivity in the antigravity muscles and the development of hemiplegic posture.

Factors Related to Movement Dysfunction after Stroke[6, 7]

- Muscle tone increased
- Exaggerated tendon reflexes
- Clonus may be present
- Released flexor reflexes
- Babinski sign may be present
- Mass synergy patterns seen
- Loss of finger dexterity
- Weakness
- Inadequate force generation
- Slow movements
- Loss of selective control of muscles and limb segments.

Changes in Spastic Muscle

- Stiffness
- Contracture
- Fibrosis
- Atrophy.

Positive and Negative Roles of Spasticity

Individuals with spinal cord injury (SCI) may take advantages of their muscle spasms to help them perform common activities of daily living. For example, some people may learn to use their spasms to help empty their bladder, transfer, dress, and even stand or walk. However, initially, some patients with stroke experience motor impairments of the contralateral limb(s). Abnormal reflexes associated with spasticity were considered to be the major determinant of these motor impairments, a recent study, conducted in a clinical setting, has reported that 39% of patients with first-ever stroke are spastic after 12 months.[8]

Possible Advantages of Spasticity

- Maintains muscle tone and mass.
- Decreases bone loss and reduce the risk for osteoporosis.
- Increases metabolic requirements such as promoting blood circulation and improving breathing.
- Helps performing daily self-care routines such as assisting in pressure reliefs to prevent pressure sores and emptying reflex bladder and bowel.
- Helps performing daily functions such as picking up items, transferring or walking with braces.
- Warns when there is a problem in areas where the body has no feeling.

Possible Disadvantages of Spasticity

- Limits range of motion.
- Causes pain on joints and muscles due to over stress.
- Interferes with activities of daily living (ADL).
- Causes unwanted bladder or bowel release.
- Interferes with other activities such as sexual activity, sleeping, changing position, sitting or transferring.
- Affects posture and ability to sit comfortably, maintain balance or change positions.
- Causes scraping of the skin and increase the risk for pressure ulcers.
- Adds to cost of medications and attendant care.

Movement Problems Associated with Spasticity

When a muscle does not act through its full range of motion regularly, its tendons shorten. This makes stretching the muscle difficult; the muscle may develop fibrous scar tissue and further preventing full range of motion. The end result of untreated dynamic contracture is a permanently fixed contracture which is often painful. It may also give rise to a permanent abnormal posture.

Activities of daily living: The inability to control independent limb movements may represent increased difficulty in activities of daily living such as dressing, toileting, bathing, eating, and grooming.

Hygiene: Hypomobile, contractured joint limits the limb movements and prevent access to such areas as the buttocks, armpit, or pubic regions, thus interfering with hygiene. Odor and skin breakdown may occur. Bowel and bladder emptying may also become laborious.

Mobility: Spasticity in the leg muscles may interfere with mobility, seating, and transfers, such as from bed to wheelchair or from sitting to standing.

Comfort: Spasticity may interfere in the comfort levels of the life, such as frequent turning, lifting buttocks or changing positions to prevent joint pain and pressure sores is difficult, even spastic feet prevents comfortable fittings of shoes.

Assessment

Assessment of spasticity includes both identifying which muscles or muscle groups are hyperactive, and also determining the effect of spasticity on patient's activities of daily living (ADL). An upper motor neuron syndrome often leads to the development of stereotypical patterns of deformity secondary to agonist muscle weakness, antagonist muscle spasticity and changes in the rheologic (stiffness) properties of spastic muscles. Identification of the spastic muscles that contribute to deformity across a joint allows proper targeted therapeutic approach and success.

Upper extremity flexor patterns	Major involved muscles
• Adduction and internal rotation of the shoulder • Flexion of the elbow and wrist • Pronation of the forearm • Flexion of the fingers and adduction of the thumb	• Pectoralis major • Latissimus dorsi • Teres major • Biceps • Brachioradialis • Brachialis • Pronator teres and quadratus • Flexor carpi radialis or ulnaris • Flexor digitorum profundus and superficialis • Adductor pollicis

Lower extremity flexor patterns	Major involved muscles
• Hip adduction and flexion • Knee flexion • Ankle plantar flexion or equinovarus positioning	• Adductor magnus • Iliopsoas • Hamstrings (medial is more involved) • Tibialis posterior • Soleus • Gastrocnemius

Most common extensor patterns	Major involved muscles
• Knee extension • Equinus and/or valgus ankle • Great toe dorsiflexion or excessive toe flexion	• Quadriceps femoris • Medial hamstrings • Gastrocnemius • Tibialis posterior • Extensor hallucis longus • Toe flexors • Peroneus longus

Progress can be assessed using spasticity rating scales. The most popular system is the Asworth Scale. The scale grades the resistance of a relaxed limb to rapid passive stretch in five stages. Zero relates to normal or lowered muscle tone and 4 relates to a state in which passive movement of the affected limb is impossible.[9,10]

Spasticity Treatment Planning

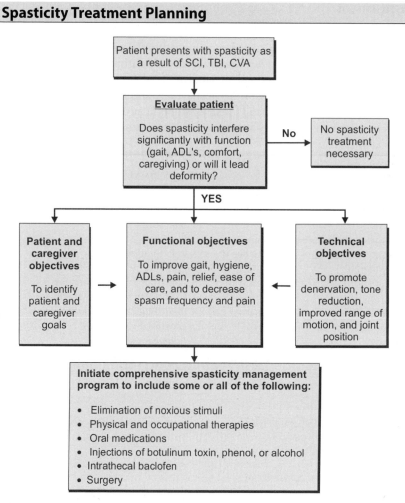

Abbreviations: SCI, spinal cord injury; TBI, traumatic brain injury; CVA, cerebrovascular accident; ADL, activities of daily living.

Therapeutic Approaches in the Treatment of Spasticity

Patient education: It is the most important part of spasticity rehabilitation, the patient and their caregivers should be fully educated about the cause and nature of spasticity. Simple factors some time give rise severe spasticity, such as poor sitting or lying postures, tight fitting garments or accessories, tight catheter leg bag straps, etc. even skin contact with a small noxious stimuli like- pin, medicine foil, ointment caps can elicit spasticity.[11,12]

Positioning: Proper and correct positioning is an important aspect of spasticity management. General principle of positioning is to place and keep the spastic part/limb in a fashion which allows a passive stretch in the spastic muscle or prevents the development of spasticity in a spasticity-prone muscle. As an example, supine lying in bed, which is commonly seen in the general medical ward may easily exacerbate extensor spasm. The primary principle of seating is that the body should stay in a balanced, symmetrical and stable posture which is comfortable and can maximize activities. Now a days various types of customized sitting arrangements are available. Additional fittings or accessories for a good seating arrangement, like-foot straps, knee block, adductor pommels, lumbar support, lateral trunk supports and a whole variety of head and neck support system.[13,14]

Relaxation techniques: Relaxation techniques are methods, processes, procedures, or activities those helps a person to relax; to attain a state of increased calmness; or otherwise reduce levels of anxiety, stress or tension. Spasticity may also be reduced by the use of relaxation techniques by a progressive tensing and relaxing an individual muscle (Jacobson), accompanied by deep breathing techniques and contrast methods. Relaxation techniques those effectively reduce spasticity may include-conscious breathing, progressive relaxation techniques and physiological relaxation techniques (Laura Mitchell, 1957).[15,16]

Passive movements: Lack of movement may result in permanent contracture of a joint, therefore it is essential to move a joint through its complete range of motion regularly. Passive movements are produced by an external force during muscular inactivity, frequent passive movement prevents contracture.[17,18]

Stretching: Stretching forms the basis of spasticity treatment. Stretching helps to maintain the full range of motion of a joint, and helps prevent contracture, or permanent muscle shortening. Passive stretching uses forced motion to restore the normal range of motion when this range is limited by loss of soft tissue elasticity. Its effect on muscles is to lengthen the elastic portion of the muscle passively, allowing greater length and hence greater range at the affected joints. However, "any increase in range obtained by forced motion will be lost unless maintained by active motion or by supportive devices".[19,20]

Weight bearing: Regular standing in a tilt board or standing frame relieves spasticity and prevent contractures.

Strengthening: Spasticity often leads to loss of strength in both the spastic muscles and adjacent muscles. Strengthening exercises are aimed at improving the strength to affected muscles so that, as tone is reduced through other treatments, at least the strong muscle can reactivate the affected limb. Special techniques like proprioceptive neuromuscular facilitation (PNF) can be effectively used to improve biomechanical balance in the muscle groups along with other specific exercises.

Orthoses and serial casting: An important goal of application of othoses and serial casting is to prevent and treat abnormal limb posture and prevent contracture due to spasticity, the appropriate use of orthoses and serial plaster casting have shown successful maintenance of muscle stretch. Orthotic prescription depends on the type of hypertonicity or contracture that needs to be corrected and the degree of voluntary limb movement. Improvements in walking pattern have been demonstrated with ankle foot orthosis in patients with equinovarus deformity. Thermoplastic splints are recommended for the arm while rigid or hinged polypropylene splints are needed to withstand heavy forces generated during walking. Inflatable pressure splintage is used when rigid splints are not tolerated, particularly for severe finger flexion. Lycra orthoses offers an alternative to thermoplastic and polypropylene splints for postural management of the upper limb.[21-23]

Electrical stimulation: Neuromuscular electrical stimulation over the agonist or antagonist spastic muscles is another method of reducing spasticity. There is some evidence that electrical stimulation of the antagonist muscles can reduce spasticity immediately following treatment. It has also been claimed that spasticity reduction by this method is achieved without any muscle weakness or paralysis. Bogataj et al found that neuromuscular electrical stimulation may amplify sensory inputs into the central nervous system and so accelerate nervous plasticity and lead to faster motor learning. It has been claimed that electrical stimulation may reduce muscle tonicity via the reduction of the stretching reflex, causing lower spasticity and allowing a larger range of motion, and preventing soft tissue stiffness and contracture.[24,25]

TENS: Transcutaneous electrical nerve stimulation (TENS), more commonly referred to as TENS, is an, application of electrical current through the skin for pain control (APTA, 1990). The unit is usually connected to the skin using two or more electrodes. A typical battery-operated TENS unit is able to modulate pulse width, frequency and intensity. Generally, TENS is applied at high frequency (>50 Hz) with an intensity below motor contraction (sensory intensity) or low frequency (<10 Hz) with an intensity that produces motor contraction (Robinson and Snyder-Mackler, 2008). Recent studies have shown TENS can be effectively reduce spasticity if used in a range of proper frequency regularly.[26-28]

EMG biofeedback: EMG-biofeedback is the use of an electrical monitor that creates a signal—usually a sound—as a spastic muscle relaxes. In this way, people with spasticity may be able to train themselves to reduce muscle tone consciously. There has been little research testing the effectiveness of biofeedback for reducing spasticity.[29]

Therapeutic massage: Massage is an ancient manipulative technique or art which is used to reduce pain, swelling and to promote relaxation through decades. Many researches have proved that therapeutic massage improves mobility of the tissue and prevents contractures, it has many local physiological effects as well as CNS effects, various studies have shown that proper therapeutic massage can inhibit á-motor neuron excitability and application of petrissage can significantly reduce H-reflex amplitude. Moreover, massage produces general body relaxation which also helps control spasticity. Few recent studies have also revealed that abdominal massage over ascending and descending colon helps in spastic bowel management.[30,31]

Cryotherapy: The application of cold results in a reduction of the amplitude of the compound motor action potential. Cold also slows nerve conduction and decreases muscle spindle activity. These factors can all lead to an overall inhibition of the monosynaptic stretch reflex. Spasticity may also be reduced by cold through an inhibition of sensory afferents. An important finding in a number of studies that have examined the effects of cooling on spasticity is that, often, there is an initial increase in spasticity, perhaps due to an increase in alpha motorneuron activity.[32,33]

Thermotherapy: Heat may also be used to reduce spasticity. The effects of heat are typically lesser than cold because an increase in blood flows in response to heat cools the target area very quickly. Superficial heat may be administered through hot packs, whirlpool, paraffin, fluidotherapy, and microwave diathermy. Deeper heat may be administrated by ultrasound, short-wave diathermy.[34]

Shockwave therapy: Shock waves are defined as a series of single sonic pulses characterized by high peak pressure (100 MPa), fast pressure rise (10 ns), and short duration (10 s). Different studies and clinical experiments have demonstrated the efficacy of shock waves in the treatment of bone and tendon diseases. The persistent clinical effects of shock wave treatment on muscular contractures has been reported to produce reduction in hypertonia in neurological patients after shock wave therapy. Possible use of shock wave treatment in patients experiencing muscular hypertonia may be advocated. However, more evidence-based research is indicated in this purpose.[35,36]

Constraint-induced movement therapy (CIMT): Constraint-induced movement therapy (CI) forces the use of the affected side by restraining the unaffected side. With CI therapy, the therapist constrains the survivor's unaffected arm in a sling. The survivor then uses his or her affected arm repetitively and intensively for few weeks. Dr Edward Taub, a professor of psychology at the University of Alabama in Birmingham, developed CI therapy. Various studies has been done on CIMT and proved its efficacy in stroke rehabilitation, few recent studies suggested that modified CIMT in combination of botulinum toxin type A can significantly reduce spasticity.[37,38]

Bobath approach: The Bobath approach advocates reduction of spasticity and primitive postural reflexes prior to facilitating voluntary activity in paretic muscles through attention to trunk posture and controlled muscle stretch of the limbs. Reduction in segmental reflex hyperexcitability through inhibition of distal segmental reflexes via Ib inhibitory interneurons is the basic mechanism.[39]

The Brunnstrom approach: The Brunnstrom approach suggests techniques to promote activity in weak agonists by facilitating contraction of either corresponding muscles in the unaffected limb or proximal muscles on the paretic side. This technique focuses on individual muscle groups with the underlying concept that stimulation of the weak agonist muscle will result in Ia mediated reciprocal inhibition in the spastic antagonist muscle.[40]

Watsu approach: Watsu is a new therapeutic technique that incorporates static passive stretches and a structured sequence and of passive limb, head and neck movements or patterns performed at warm water surface level. Warm water is beneficial to release muscle tone and to reach deep physical and mental relaxation (Vargas, 2004). Once the patient is relaxed, physical flexibility and mobility are more easily achieved in the submerged condition with weightlessness. The patient is cradled and supported by the practitioner while the various movement sequences are carried out at water surface level. In this way, Watsu may be beneficial for patients with spastic disorder.[41,42]

Hydrotherapy: Hydrotherapy is one of the oldest therapeutic methods for managing physical dysfunctions. Water has complex thermal, and inherent mechanical forces of buoyancy, pressure, cohesion, and viscosity that play a role in the effects produced on the body from hydrotherapy. The supportive, assistive, and resistive qualities of the water make it possible for patients to begin range of motion, strength, and endurance exercise. Various researches have shown that hydrotherapy may effectively reduce spasticity.[43]

Vibration of antagonistic muscles: Mechanical vibration (150–160 Hz) may be used to reduce muscle spasticity in the upper motor neuron diseases; researches found that vibration can produce reciprocal inhibition of motor neurons of antagonist muscles and may reduce the spasticity. However, more evidence is still needed to establish this theory.[44]

Medical Management of Spasticity

The medical and pharmacological treatment of spasticity after stroke or SCI is evolving rapidly in recent days. The abnormal muscle tone may be partially modified by oral administration of drugs acting on neurotransmitters or neuromodulators in central nervous system or on peripheral neuromuscular sites. Many newer drugs have been tried with variable results but none has been proved to be a consistently effective in reducing the spasticity.

Among the widely used antispastic drugs centrally acting diazepam, a long acting benzodiazepine is one of the old agent which increases the inhibitory effects of neurotransmitters,[45] gamma-amino butyric acid (GABA) at CNS synapses. Diazepam therapy is started with 5 mg at bed time which can be increased to 10–15 mg according to the patient's requirement. But patients using this drug, frequently complain of fatigue or weakness in day time and these adverse effects have restricted the use of diazepam as an antispastic agent.[46] Among the other widely used oral medications Baclofen has GABA inhibitory effect and capable of inhibiting both monosynaptic and polysynaptic reflexes at spinal level. The recommended dose of Baclofen starts from 5 mg/day and gradually may be increased up to 60–80 mg/day.[47]

Dantrolene sodium, another antispastic agent is typically a peripherally acting muscle relaxant and well accepted because of the lack of its CNS effects. It may be used 25 mg, 3–4 times per day or may be increased up to 400 mg/day.[48,49]

Tizanidine hydrochloride is a centrally acting α2-adrenergic agonist and is recently used by practitioners with more comfort and better efficacy. Dose varies from 4 mg/day to maximum 36 mg/day.[50]

Apart from these frequently used medications, drugs like clonidine (an antihypertensive), and gabapentin are also used as antispastic agents, but efficacy of those agents require more clarification through further researches.[51]

Focal Chemical Neurolytic Agents

Neurolysis of peripheral nerve can be achieved by local perineural or intramuscular injection of Phenol or Botulinum toxin type A, both these agents have proven efficacy in reduction of spasticity, but their action lasts for a limited period. In larger muscles the recommended dose of Phenol is 2–3 mL of 5% phenol and should be injected perineurally by a trained doctor. Intramuscular use of phenol is also effective but is more painful. Perineural injection is a better choice but may induce causalgia. The reduction of spasticity by injection phenol lasts from a few weeks to years.[52,53]

Chemodenervation by Botulinum Toxin (BOTOX) is another widely used modern pharmacological therapy for management of spasticity. It binds the presynaptic acetylecholine vesicles at neuromuscular junction, resulting in prevention of release of excitatory neurotransmitters. In stroke and SCI, spastic muscle often requires BOTOX for release of particular muscle for functional purpose as well as to prevent spasticity related complications like development of ulcers in finger webs in clinched fist. Larger group of muscles usually require 300–400 units of Botulinum Toxin to obtain antispastic effects and it is to be repeated every 4–6 months as judged by re appearance of spasticity.[54-57]

After any of these two injections a good physical rehabilitation programme including physiotherapy and occupational therapy is highly essential intervention to stretch the spastic muscles and also to regain functional capacity. 'BOTOX' is potentially a safe drug, very few complications are reported till now.

Intrathecal Baclofen Pump for Treatment of Spasticity[58-61]

Introduction

Intrathecal Baclofen (ITB) infusion using implantable and programmable intrathecal infusion pumps is an established therapeutic option used for last three decades. It is extremely effective in spasticity control in selected patients with spasticity of various origins. ITB Therapy (Intrathecal Baclofen Therapy) is a treatment for individuals with severe spasticity—tight, stiff muscles which can be a symptom of cerebral palsy, multiple sclerosis, brain injury, spinal cord injury, or stroke.

Indications of ITB Pump Placement

1. Spasticity secondary to multiple sclerosis.
2. Spasticity secondary to spinal cord injury.

3. Stroke related spasticity.
4. Cerebral palsy.
5. Spasticity secondary to brain injury.
6. Stiff man syndrome.
7. Spasticity of unusual origin like hemochromatosis, superficial hemosiderosis etc.

How does ITB Therapy Work?

The ITB therapy delivers a medication called Lioresal® Intrathecal (baclofen injection) directly to the intrathecal space where fluid flows around the spinal cord. The medication is administered in small doses using the Medtronic SynchroMed® programmable pump. The pump is surgically placed under the skin of the abdomen and connected to a thin tube called a catheter. Once in place, the pump and catheter deliver Lioresal Intrathecal directly to the spinal fluid where it is most effective. Delivery makes the difference with ITB Therapy. Because a small amount of medication is delivered directly to the spinal fluid, spasticity can be significantly decreased while possible side effects that often accompany oral medications may be reduced.

Patient Selection

An individual with severe spasticity who experienced intolerable side effects from oral medications and/or found other therapies ineffective may be a candidate for ITB Therapy. A screening test determines if ITB Therapy may work for an individual. During this test, a health care professional injects a test dose of Lioresal Intrathecal into the fluid around the spinal cord. If the spasticity is significantly reduced, the person may be considered a candidate for ITB Therapy. In clinical studies, ITB Therapy reduced spasticity in 97 percent of people with severe spasticity due to multiple sclerosis and spinal cord injury, and in 86% of people with severe spasticity due to cerebral palsy or brain injury.

Technique of Implantation

The most common used implantable, programmable drug delivery system used today is the Medtronic SynchroMed® Infusion System (Medtronics, Minniapolis, MN). This system has been commercially available since 1988 and consists of the following components:
- An implantable, programmable pump **(Fig. 20.1)**
- An intrathecal catheter **(Figs 20.2A and B)**
- An external programmer **(Fig. 20.2C)**

Implantation of a drug infusion system is generally done after the trial. After obtaining informed consent implantation procedure is scheduled. Implantation of the catheter and pump is usually done under general anesthesia. The patient is then placed in lateral position with the side the pump is to be placed facing up. Fluoroscopy is used to identify the appropriate

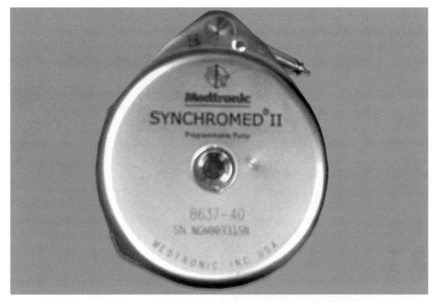

Fig. 20.1: Implantable, programmable Medtronic SynchroMed® Infusion System
(Medtronics, Minniapolis, MN) pump
(For color version, see Plate 10)

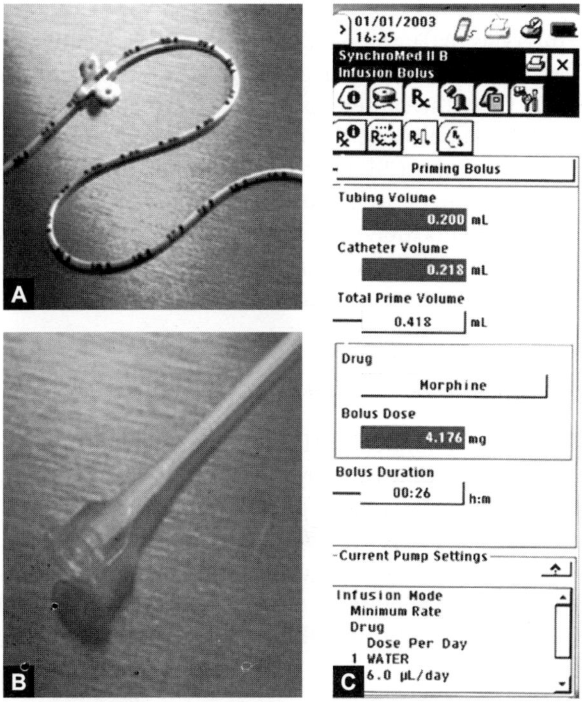

Figs 20.2A to C: Implantable, programmable Medtronic SynchroMed® Infusion System
(Medtronics, Minniapolis, MN) pump catheter (A), connection (B) and programmer screen (C)
(For color version of figures 20.2A and B, see Plate 10)

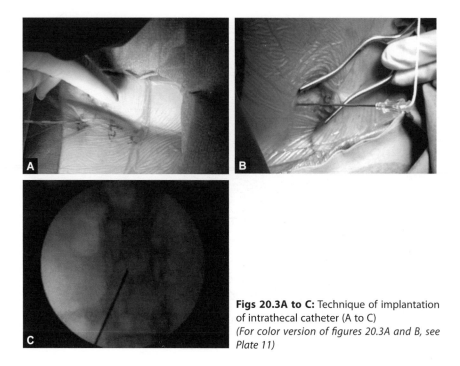

Figs 20.3A to C: Technique of implantation of intrathecal catheter (A to C)
(For color version of figures 20.3A and B, see Plate 11)

intraspinous intervals. A Tuohy needle is inserted and catheter is placed in the appropriate spinal location corresponding to the patient's pain pattern **(Figs 20.3A to C)**. Once the catheter is in place a skin incision is made around the entry site of the needle and the catheter is anchored to the underlying fascia after confirming the CSF flow and withdrawing the needle. Then an abdominal incision is made to create a subcutaneous pocket for the pump **(Fig. 20.4)**. The catheter is then tunneled to the pump pocket and connected to the pump. Pump is then placed in the pocket and secured. An external programmer is used to communicate with the pump to change parameters to optimize spasticity control.

How is the ITB Pump Controlled and Refilled?

SynchroMed is the only surgically placed drug infusion system that can be programmed from outside the body. When necessary, a clinician uses a computer-like external programmer to adjust the drug dose and/or infusion rate. This ensures that the most effective amount of Lioresal Intrathecal needed to reduce the spasticity is received. The programming is usually done every 2–3 months when the pump is refilled. To refill the pump, the clinician injects Lioresal Intrathecal through the skin into the pump's drug reservoir.

Benefits

The ITB therapy is a US Food and Drug Administration approved treatment for severe spasticity. Thousands of people receive ITB therapy to reduce their

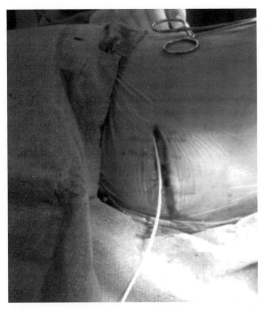

Fig. 20.4: Technique of making a subcutaneous pocket for the pump placement
(For color version, see Plate 11)

spasticity. In studies, people have reported that ITB Therapy helped them be more independent, allowing them to feed or dress themselves, sit more comfortably, or transfer more easily. Caregivers also reported that care is easier with ITB Therapy.

In our experience of over 200 pumps we have found 90% or more improvement in spasms and similar improvement in spasticity after ITB pump placement.

Side Effects or Complications

Possible side effects may include loose muscles, sleepiness, upset stomach, vomiting, headaches, and dizziness. The most common device-related complications reported involve catheter kinks, dislodgment, and breaks. Overdose, although rare, may lead to respiratory depression, loss of consciousness, reversible coma, and in extreme cases, may be life-threatening. However, almost all patients who experienced adverse events in the clinical studies continued with the therapy. Also, as with any surgical procedure, complications can occur after the pump is placed. Since the pump and catheter are placed beneath the skin, infections can develop and are generally related to the healing of the surgical incision, not long-term use of ITB therapy.

References

1. Lance JW. The control of muscle tone, reflexes, and movement: Robert Wartenberg lecture. Neurology. 1980;30:1303-13.

2. Feigin VL. Stroke epidemiology: a review of population-based studies of incidence, prevalence, and case-fatality in the late 20th century. Lancet Neurology. 2003;2(1):43-53.
3. Michael R Barnes. Management of spasticity. Age and Ageing. 1998;27:239-45.
4. Parziale JR. Spasticity: Pathophysiology and management. Orthopedics. 1993;16(11):1212.
5. Bipin B Bhakta. Management of spasticity in stroke. British Medical Bulletin. 2000;56(2):476-85.
6. O'Dwyer, et al. Spasticity and muscle contracture following stroke. Brain. 1996;119:1737-49.
7. Dimitrijević MR, Nathan PW. Studies of spasticity in man. I. Some features of spasticity. Brain. 1967;90(1):1-30.
8. Nathaniel, et al. Clinicophysiologic concepts of spasticity and motor dysfunction in adults with an upper motoneuron lesion. Muscle and Nerve. 1997;20(S6):1-14.
9. Richard W Bohannon, Melissa B Smith. Interrater reliability of a modified ashworth scale of muscle spasticity. Physical Therapy. 1987;67(2):206-7.
10. Ashby, et al. The evaluation of "spasticity". Canadian Journal of Neurological Science. 1987;14(3):497-500.
11. Rodgers H. Randomized controlled trial of a comprehensive stroke education program for patients and caregivers stroke. 1999;30:2585-91.
12. Evans RL. Family intervention after stroke: Does counseling or education help? Stroke. 1988;19:1243-9.
13. Michael Barnes P. Medical management of spasticity in stroke. Age and Ageing. 2001;30(s1):13-6.
14. Edward S. Neurological. Physiotherapy, problem solving approach. London: Churchill Livingstone, 1996.
15. Gardiner DM. The principles of exercise therapy, 4th edn. CBS; 2004. pp. 64-9.
16. Basmajian JV. New views on muscular Tone and relaxation. Canadian Medical Journal. 1957;77:203-5.
17. Godelieve, et al. Reduction of spastic hypertonia during repeated passive knee movements in stroke patients. Archives of Physical Medicine and Rehabilitation. 2002;83(7):930-5.
18. Paillard J, Brouchon M. Active and passive movements in the calibration of position sense; the neuropsychology of spatially oriented behavior. Dorsey Press. Homewood III. 1968;3:37-55.
19. Kisner C, Colby LA. Therapeutic exercise: Foundations and techniques, 3rd edn. F.A. Davis, 1996.pp.143-8.
20. Parziale, et al. Spasticity: Pathophysiology and management. Orthopaedics. 1993;16(7):801-11.
21. Shu, Mirka. A laboratory study of the effect of wrist splint orthosis on forearm muscle activity and upper extremity posture. Human Factors. 2006;48:499-510.
22. Mulcahey MJ. Upper limb orthoses for the person with spinal cord injury, Chapter-15, 203-212, AAOS atlas of orthoses and assistive devices, 4th edn. MOSBY, Elsevier.
23. Mark Gormley E, et al. A clinical overview of treatment decisions in the management of spasticity. Muscle and Nerve. 1998;20(s6):14-20.
24. Amir Bakhtiary H, et al. Does electrical stimulation reduce spasticity after stroke? A randomized controlled study. Clinical Rehabilitation. 2008;22:418-25.
25. Joodaki, et al. The effects of electrical nerve stimulation of the lower extremity on H-reflex and F-wave parameters. Clinical Neurophysiology. 2001;41:23-8.

26. Gulumser Aydýn, et al. Transcutaneous electrical nerve stimulation versus baclofen in spasticity: Clinical and electrophysiologic comparison. American Journal of Physical Medicine and Rehabilitation. 2005;84(8):584-94.

27. Levin, Chan. Relief of hemiparetic spasticity by TENS is associated with improvement in reflex and voluntary motor functions. Electroencephalogr Clinical Neurophysiology. 1992;85(2):131-42.

28. Potisk KP, et al. Effects of transcutaneous electrical nerve stimulation (TENS) on spasticity in patients with hemiplegia. Scandinavian Journal of Rehabilitation Medicine. 1995;27(3):169-74.

29. Steven L Wolf, Stuart A Binder Macleod. Electromyographic biofeedback applications to the hemiplegic patient: Changes in upper extremity neuromuscular and functional status. Physical Therapy. 1983;63(9):1393-403.

30. Margaret Hollis. Massage for therapist. Balckwell Science. 1998;2:34-5.

31. Harrington, Haskvitz. Managing a patient's constipation with physical therapy. Physical Therapy. 2006;86(11):1511-9.

32. Knutsson E. Topical cryotherapy in spasticity. Scandinavian Journal of Rehabilitation Medicine. 1970;2(4):159-63.

33. Price, et al. Influence of cryotherapy on spasticity at the human ankle. Archive of Physical Medicine and Rehabilitation. 1993;74(3):300-4.

34. Watanabe T. The Role of therapy in spasticity management. American Journal of Physical Medicine and Rehabilitation. 2004;83(Suppl):S45–S9.

35. Manganotti P, Amelio E. Long-term effect of shock wave therapy on upper limb hypertonia in patients. Affected by Stroke. Stroke. 2005;36:1967-71.

36. Ogden, et al. Shock wave therapy (Orthotripsy®) in musculoskeletal disorders, clinical orthopaedics and related research. Lippincott Williams and Wilkins. Inc. 2001;387:22-40.

37. Shu-Fen Sun, et al. Application of combined botulinum toxin type A and modified constraint-induced movement therapy for an individual with chronic upper-extremity spasticity after stroke. Physical Therapy. 2006;86(10):1387-97.

38. Page SJ, Levine P, Sisto S, et al. Stroke patients' and therapists' opinions of constraint-induced movement therapy. Clinical Rehabilitation. 2002;16:55-60.

39. Bobath B. Adult Hemiplegia: Evaluation and Treatment, 2nd edn. London, England, William Heinemann Medical Books Ltd, 1978.

40. Brunnstrom S. Motor behavior of adult patients with hemiplegia: Movement therapy in hemiplegia. New York, NY: Harper and Row; 1970.

41. Seung Chul Chon, et al. Watsu approach for improving spasticity and ambulatory function in hemiparetic patients with stroke. Physiotherapy Research International. 2009;14(2):128-36.

42. Dull H Watsu. Freeing the body in water. Middletown, CA: Harbin Springs Publishing; 1997. pp. 20-7.

43. Kesiktas, et al. The use of hydrotherapy for the management of spasticity, neurorehabilitation and neural repair. 2004;18(4):268-73.

44. Karl-Erik Hagbarth, Goran Eklund. The effects of muscle vibration in spasticity, rigidity, and cerebellar disorders. Journal of Neurology. Neurosurgery and Psychiatry. 1968;31:207-13.

45. Steen PA, Michenfelder JD. Cerebral protection with barbiturates: Relation to anesthetic effect. Stroke. 1978;9:140-2.

46. Lodde J, et al. Diazepam treatment to increase the cerebral GABAergic activity in acute stroke: A feasibility study in 104 patients. Cerebrovascular Disease. 2000;10:437-40.

47. Hulme, et al. Baclofen in the elderly stroke patient its side-effects and pharmacokinetics. European Journal of Clinical Pharmacology. 1985;29:467-9.
48. Pinder, et al. Dantrolene sodium: a review of its pharmacological properties and therapeutic efficacy in spasticity. Drugs. 1977;13(1):3-23.
49. Morgan KG, Bryant SH. The mechanism of action of dantrolene sodium. Pharmacology and Experimental Therapeutics. 1977;201(1):138-47.
50. David, et al. Open-label dose-titration safety and efficacy study of tizanidine hydrochloride in the treatment of spasticity associated with chronic stroke. Stroke. 2001;32:1841-6.
51. Durodami, et al. Should hypertension be treated after acute stroke? A randomized controlled trial using single photon emission computed tomography. Archive of Neurology. 1993;50(8):855-62.
52. Kuijk, et al. Treatment of upper extremity spasticity in stroke patients by focal neuronal or neuromuscular blockade: a systematic review of the literature. Journal of Rehabilitation Medicine. 2002;34(2):51-61.
53. Joann E Gallichio. Pharmacologic management of spasticity following stroke. Physical Therapy. 2004;84(10):973-81.
54. Bakheit, et al. A randomized, double-blind, placebo-controlled study of the efficacy and safety of botulinum toxin type A in upper limb spasticity in patients with stroke. European Journal of Neurology. 2001;86:559-65.
55. Lagalla, et al. Post-stroke spasticity management with repeated botulinum toxin injections in the upper limb. American Journal of Physical Medicine and Rehabilitation. 2000;79(4):377-84.
56. Cristina Sampaio, et al. Botulinum toxin type A for the treatment of arm and hand spasticity in stroke patients. Clinical Rehabilitation. 1997;11(1):3-7.
57. Das TK, Park DM, et al. Effect of treatment with botulinum toxin on spasticity. Postgraduate Medical Journal. 1989;65:208-10.
58. Albright AL, Barron WB, Fasick P, Polinko P, Janosky J. Continuous intrathecal baclofen infusion for spasticity of cerebral origin. JAMA. 1993;270(20):2475-7.
59. Rawlins P. Intrathecal baclofen for spasticity of cerebral palsy: Project coordination and nursing care. AJNN. 1995;27(3):157-63.
60. Loubser PG, Narayan RK, Sandin KJ, et al. Continuous infusion of intrathecal baclofen: Long-term effects on spasticity in spinal cord injury. Paraplegia. 1991;19:48-64.
61. Parke B, Penn RD, Savoy SM, Corcos DM. Functional outcome following delivery of intrathecal baclofen in patients with multiple sclerosis or spinal cord injury. Arch Phys Med Rehab. 1989;70:30-2.

21

Therapeutic Exercises for Spinal Cord Injuries

S Srinivas Rau

Introduction

An exercise program for spinal injured patients has to be realistic and achievable. A lot will depend upon the level of lesion and the individual patient's functional potential. Whenever a rehabilitation program is planned, a thorough assessment of the patient is necessary because a lot will depend upon the uninvolved muscles, which in turn have to be trained to compensate for the muscles which are totally paralyzed.

For convenience purposes, the physiotherapeutic management can be broadly categorized as acute care management and the subacute stage management.

General points regarding the conservative treatment of the acute spinal injured:
- The patient is turned on bed every 2–3 hours with proper care of fracture site till the patient is mobilized.
- The fractured site is treated with skull traction and or postural reduction by using pillows or rolls.
- Most cervical lesions have cones, skull traction, Halo traction or Halo traction with a vest. These may be maintained for a period of 6–8 weeks with regular checkup X-ray.
- Halo traction with vest is maintained for approximately 12 weeks until the fracture site is fully consolidated but the patient can be mobilized after 10 days of bed rest.
- New lesions admitted may usually have physiotherapy commenced immediately if medical stability is achieved.
- In the early days the patient should be treated twice daily during the week and once daily on weekends during the first 6 weeks when the risk of deep vein thrombosis is the greatest.
- Anticoagulant therapy may be started a couple of days after injury.

- After 6 weeks' treatment may be once a day. However, if there are chances of the patient developing contractures, loss of ROM treatment twice a day may continue.

Physiotherapy Assessment during the Acute Phase

Principles of Assessment

- To establish a functional level of the injury
- Establish short or long-term goals
- Design an effective treatment program.

Assessment is done for the following:

1. *Respiratory function:*
   - Test for respiratory capacity
   - Function of pulmonary muscles
   - Chest mobility.

The assessment should include the muscles the patient uses for quiet and deep breathing, the patients breathing pattern and chest excursion cough functions and vital capacity.

- *Breathing pattern*: It can be graded on a 4-point scale using the 4 components of respiration, i.e. diaphragm, chest, neck accessory, abdominals.
- A normal breathing pattern is equal use of diaphragm and chest, i.e. a 2D 2C pattern. The most common pattern of spinal injured is 4 diaphragm because of the lesions of the cervical and thoracic region have paralysis of intercostals and abdominals.
  The assessment is done in supine lying
- *Chest excursion*: Measured in supine at the levels of xiphoid or axillae.
- In spinal injured it may be reduced due to chest muscle paralysis or chest wall tightness.
- *Cough function*: This is assessed to evaluate the patient's ability to rid the lungs of secretions.
  It may be graded subjectively as:
  i. Functional cough.
  ii. Weak functional cough.
  iii. Nonfunctional cough.
- *Vital capacity*: This is measured in supine position with a spirometer.

2. *Motor control and ROM assessment:* These are done by the standard procedures. Usually the presence of trace (1+) is done. It is important to look for functional toe movements (sacral sparing), which is an important indication of an incomplete lesion.

- If there is spinal instability, use recumbent positions
- If there is cervical spine instability, then shoulder muscle strength should be tested without resistance to prevent the arm-neck-arm-chest muscles from moving the spine

- If there is low thoracic/lumbar instability, then hip muscles should not be resisted.

3. *Sensory assessment:* An assessment of the level of sensation loss, type of sensation lost should be recorded.

Physiotherapy Treatment during Acute Phase

Physiotherapy treatment in the acute phase can be broadly divided into:
1. Chest physiotherapy
2. Exercises for ROM.

Chest Physiotherapy

This will vary according to the individual patient's level of injury and respiratory status.

Diaphragmatic breathing should be encouraged. Manual contacts and facilitation can be given by placing hands below the sternum.

A manual compressive force can be applied to facilitate expiration, which can be followed by a deeper inspiration.

Air shift maneuver: This is a simple method of chest expansion. The patient takes in a deep inhalation, holds it by closing the glottis, relaxes the diaphragm, which allows the air to shift from the lower to upper thorax. This method allows a chest expansion of about half inch to two inches.

Glossopharyngeal breathing (GPB) or Frog breathing: In this method, the tongue, laryngeal and pharangeal muscles are used for respiration. This improves vital capacity, increases cough force, and chest expansion. About 8–12 deep sighs are taken on every one-hour.

Manual chest expansion: This is indicated when chest expansion of 2 inches is not achieved by the above methods. Stretchings are done segmentally by the therapist to the lower, middle and upper chest.

Method: Start in supine position. The therapist places one hand under the patient's ribs with the tips of fingers resting on the transverse process of the spine. The second hand is placed on the chest with the heel of the hand lateral to the sternum. By using a 'Wringing' type of movement, bring the hands together. Progress upwards to move the whole chest wall.

Contraindication: When there are fractures of ribs.

Manual coughing: This is indicated when there is a nonfunctional cough.

Method: In supine. The therapist places interlocked hands on the abdomen or epigastric area. The heel of the lower hand is placed above the umbilicus and 2 inches below the xiphoid, fingers are spread.

The patient is then asked to inhale maximum and attempt to cough. The therapist compresses the abdomen by quickly pushing down and inwards when the patient exhales.

Exercises for ROM

ROM must be monitored and recorded periodically:
- Remember that joints are paralyzed and can be damaged easily
- Remove bottles, pillows, etc. before commencing exercise program
- Be careful not to pull on the catheter
- Ensure that the bed is flat.

Passive or Active Movements

It is the choice of the therapist to start passive movements distally or proximally. There may be reasons for starting at either, e.g.
a. Normal movement principles advocate working from central or proximal points.
b. Can the hand, wrist and elbow be adequately mobilized prior to moving the shoulder?
c. Pain in a stiff shoulder may increase tone and anxiety and prevent movement at the distal joints.

OR

a. Starting treatment at hand may encourage a good rapport with the patient.
b. Distal treatment may enable patient to relax before progressing to more painful joints **(Fig. 21.1)**.

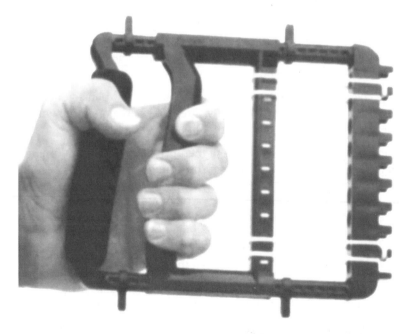

Fig. 21.1: Grip strength training
(For color version, see Plate 12)

Passive Movements for Upper Limbs

Hand and Wrist

Fingers: MCP flexion/extension with IP in extension. IP flexion/extension with MCP flexion/extension. This may be done with all fingers together or individually. It is important to maintain 90° of MCP flexion for a tenodesis grip. Ensure that MCP joints are not hyperextended while IP joint movements are done and the wrist is in extension during finger flexion.

Thumb: IP flexion/extension. CMC flexion/extension. CMC abduction/adduction. Opposition. Ensure that thumb movements are within normal ROM. Overstretching into abduction/adduction/extension may impair a potential tenodesis grip.

Wrist: Flexion/extension. 90° of wrist extension will be necessary to have a comfortable lifting position for the hand in a C5 - C6 lesion. The tenodesis grip for a C6 lesion offers a basic grip. This is by the action and shortening of the wrist extensors and flexors passing over the joints of the wrist and fingers. Therefore, movements should not jeopardize this function. Wrist extension should be accompanied by finger flexion and wrist flexion accompanied by finger extension. Radial and ulnar deviation should also be performed.

Elbow: Flexion—extension movements. Combining flexion with supination and extension with pronation. This ensures a full stretch on the biceps, which is essential for maintaining full elbow extension. Without this a C5 - C6 patient will not be able to achieve a lift. Wrist extension should be combined with elbow extension as this position is necessary for lifting.

Pronation: Supination—loss of passive pronation in a C5 lesion may lead to difficulties in hand-mouth functions.

Shoulder: Mobilization of scapula. This should precede shoulder movements to prevent unwanted pain and trauma and to facilitate full ROM.

Flexion: Extension—shoulder flexion with external rotation should be done with the elbow in extension and with adequate support to the elbow, wrist and hand. Encourage active depression of the shoulder where possible to minimize impingement of the head of humerus with the acromion.

Internal: External rotation—Reduction in ROM of external rotation is often the first development of limitation of ROM of the shoulder joint. Abduction-adduction, rhomboid stretches, trapezius stretch. All should be performed carefully **(Fig. 21.2)**.

Arm Position Regime with Arm Boards for Cervical Lesions

Supine: Both arms on boards. Shoulders abducted, laterally rotated elbows extended, i.e. crucifix position.

From the above, it can be seen that functional walking can be accomplished by patients with lesions below T10.

However, standing is important for the physiological gains that it provides.

Advantages of Standing

- Prevent contractures
- Decrease osteoporosis
- Stimulate circulation
- Decrease spasticity
- Aid renal function
- Additionally increases cardiovascular fitness
- Psychological.

Disadvantages of Standing

- Very hard work
- Risk of falling
- Long-term damage to shoulders if using crutches.

All paraplegics especially with lesions of T10 and below should be encouraged to stand and walk.

Bracing in Paraplegics

To be considered for bracing, the patients should fulfill the following criteria:
- No contractures of hip, knee and ankle
- No skin problems
- Wheelchair rehabilitated
- Motivated
- Realistic
- No signs of osteoporosis
- Able to take weight on arms
- Others like spasticity, blood pressure.

Points to Consider for Bracing

- Explain functional limitations to the patient
- Physiological effects of standing and walking related to calcium excretion is controversial
- Energy consumption
- Ambulation needs high physical endurance and high frustration levels
- Above average upper extremity strength is needed.

Gait Training

- Average duration 3–6 months
- Should begin in parallel bars
- Patient should develop a balance point, i.e. a 3-point base of support

- Must learn to keep CG posterior to hips
- Should learn more than one gait pattern in parallel bars
- 4-point gait is safest because it always has 3-points of contact, but it is slow and energy consuming
- Progress to elevation, start in small wide steps **(Figs 21.4A to D)**.

Gait Expectations of Complete Paras

Level of injury	Gait used
T1 - T8	Swing-to with KAFO may use crutches
T8 - T10	Swing-to and swing-through with KAFO and crutches. Walking likely to be an exercise than functional
T10 - L2	Swing-through and 4-point with KAFO and crutches. May need wheelchair for part of day. Walking can be fully functional
L2 - L4	AFO with crutches/stick. Wheelchair not required
L4 - L5	May/may not use orthosis Wheelchair not required. May need sticks/walking aids

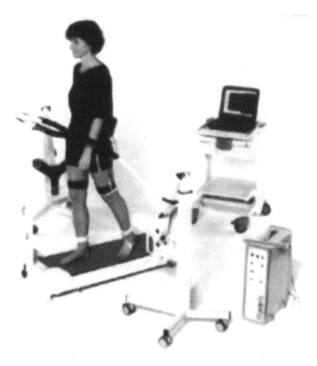

Fig. 21.4A: Three-dimensional motion analysis system

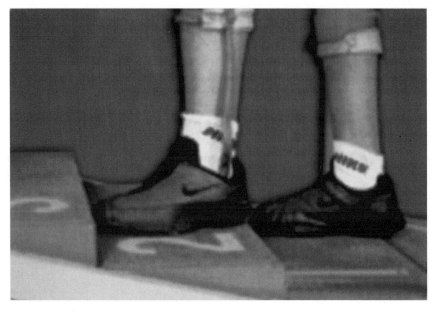

Fig. 21.4B: Calipers for gait

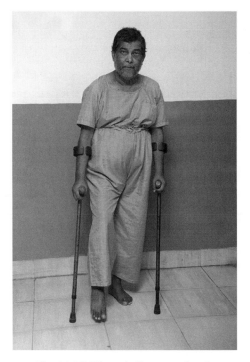

Fig. 21.4C: Bilateral elbow crutch gait
(For color version, see Plate 13)

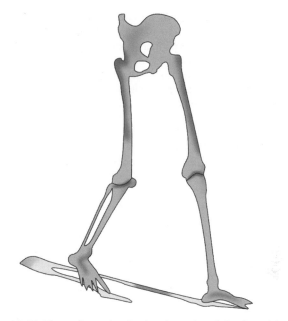

Fig. 21.4D: Three-dimensional animation using skeletal models

Bibliography

1. Behrman, Harkema. Locomotor training after human spinal cord injury: A series of case studies, Physical Therapy. 2000;80(7):688-700.
2. Bromley I. Paraplegia and tetraplegia.
3. Burke, et al. Response to passive movement of receptors in joint, skin and muscle of the human hand. Journal of Physiology. 1988;402:347-61.
4. Dejan, et al. Neurorehabilitation of upper extremity of humans with sensory motor impairment. Neuromodulation. 2002;5(1):54-67.
5. Dietz, et al. Locomotor activity in spinal cord injured person. Journal of Applied Physiology. 2004;96:1954-60.
6. Eng JJ, et al. Use of prolonged standing for individual with Spinal Cord Injury. Physical Therapy. 2001;81(8):1392-99.
7. Field Fote. Spinal cord control movement. Implication for locomotor rehabilitation following Spinal Cord Injury. Physical Therapy. 2001;80(8):477-84.
8. Grundy D, Russel J. ABC of spinal cord injury. Later management and complications-I Br Med J (Clin Res Ed). 1986;292:743-5.
9. Hicks, et al. Long-term exercise training in person with spinal cord injury: Effect on strength, arm ergometry performance and psychological well-being. Spinal Cord. 2003;41:34-43.
10. Iles JF, et al. Vestibular-evoked muscle response in patients with spinal cord injury. Brain. 2004;127:1584-92.
11. Jacobs, et al. Exercise recommendation for individuals with Spinal Cord Injury. Sports Medicine. 2004;34(11):727-51.
12. Kennedy RH. The new view point toward spinal cord injuries. Annals of Surgery. 1946;124(6):1057-62.

13. Marsolais EB. Orthosis and electrical stimulation for walking in complete paraplegia. Neurorehabilitation and Neural Repair. 1991;5(1-2):13-22.

14. Martin, Craig. Early care of patients with Injury of the Spinal Cord. American Journal of Nursing. 1955;55(8):936-39.

15. Michele Basso D. Neuroanatomical substrates of functional recovery after experimental Spinal Cord Injury: Implication of basic science research for human Spinal Cord Injury. Physical Therapy. 2000;80(8):808-17.

16. Noreau, Shephard. Spinal Cord Injury: exercise and quality of life. Sports Medicine. 1995;4:226-50.

17. O'Sullivan SB, Schmitz TJ. Physical Rehabilitation: Assessment and Treatment.

18. Pallard, Brouchon. Active and passive movement in the calibration of position sense, The Neuropsychology of spatiality oriented behavior, Dorsey Press, Homewood III, Chapter-3 1968;37-55.

19. Philps, et al. Effect of spinal cord injury on the heart and cardiovascular fitness. Current Problems in Cardiology. 1998;23(11):641-716.

20. Stauffer, et al. Ambulation in thoracic paraplegia. Journal of Bone and Joint Surgery (Am). 1978;60:823-24.

21. Zakotnik, et al. Co-contraction and passive forces facilitate load compensation of aimed limb movements. Journal of Neurosciences. 2006;26:4995-5007.

22

Surgical Management of Spasticity

Milind Deogaonkar

Introduction

Spasticity is a common end result of spinal cord injury (SCI). It is not only extremely unpleasant for the patient and difficult to manage but often makes nursing these patients impossible, resulting in pressure sores and other complication. There are various definitions of spasticity. The most accepted and useful definition given by Lance is 'velocity dependant increase in tonic stretch reflexes (muscle tone) with exaggerated tendon jerks, resulting from hyperexcitability of stretch reflex, as one component of upper motor neuron syndrome'.[1] This characteristic (velocity dependant) differentiates it from other forms of rigidities seen in contractures, dystonias and Parkinson's disease. In practice, spasticity develops over a period of time after the SCI and the release of supraspinal inhibition may be complimented by reorganization of the denervated spinal structures as a response to the degeneration of descending fibers.

Pathophysiology, assessment and medical management of spasticity have been nicely described in the preceding chapter. Surgical intervention for spasticity is necessary when it is uncontrolled by medicine and physiotherapy.

Surgical Strategies for Management of Spasticity

Multiple surgical strategies are available for management of spasticity. They include spinal cord stimulation, intrathecal baclofen pumps and selective neuroablative procedures **(Fig. 22.1)**.

Spinal Cord Stimulation in Spasticity

Spinal cord stimulation (SCS) has been widely used in treatment of neurogenic pain. This involves placing electrodes percutaneously in the spinal canal

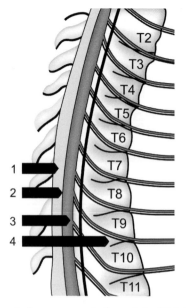

Fig. 22.1: Strategies for surgical management of spasticity. (1) Intrathecal baclofen pumps and spinal cord stimulation, (2) Myelotomies, (3) DREZotomies and posterior rhizotomies and (4) Peripheral neurotomies

in epidural space. They are attached to a pulse generator that sends out small electrical stimuli intermittently. The strength and frequency of these stimuli can be changed according to the clinical improvement. In spasticity management though, the effectiveness of SCS is equivocal. Especially in complete lesions, the SCS is not very effective. The underlying principle is, unless the dorsal columns have enough functional fibers, the SCS fails to work effectively. In spasticity due to non-traumatic myelopathies like multiple sclerosis or other such degenerative diseases, SCS is very effective.[2] In a study by Barolat,[3] 16 patients with severe spasms secondary to traumatic and nontraumatic myelopathy underwent epidural SCS. 4 patients had a complete motor and sensory spinal cord lesion. 6 of the subjects with an incomplete spinal cord lesion were ambulatory. All patients had previously undergone extensive trials with medications and physical therapy. All 14 subjects in whom a satisfactory placement of the electrode could be obtained had a reduction in the severity of the spasms. In 6 patients, the spasms were almost abolished. Extremity, trunkal and abdominal spasms were affected. Clonus in the upper extremities was consistently reduced. Marked improvement in bladder and bowel function was observed in each of 2 subjects. In over 1-year follow-up, 5 subjects showed persistence of the results, with less stimulation required to maintain the therapeutic effects. In Indian scenario where the cost of SCS is prohibitively high, this may not be a viable option.

Intrathecal Baclofen Pumps

Baclofen is a muscle relaxant medication commonly used to decrease spasticity. Spasticity is caused by an imbalance of excitatory and inhibitory input in the spinal cord. Baclofen [a gamma-aminobutyric acid (GABA) agonist] works by restoring the balance of excitatory and inhibitory input to reduce muscle hyperactivity. The transfer of baclofen through the blood-brain barrier is incomplete. So Penn and Kroin[4] directly administered baclofen in the intrathecal space. In this way, it allows more normal motor movements. This not only delivers the drug directly to the target tissue but also reduces the daily dose significantly and hence reduces the unwanted systemic side effects like dizziness, drowsiness, headaches, nausea and weakness. To avoid daily lumber punctures a programmable pump device was invented. It has a catheter (a small, flexible tube) and a pump. The pump–a round metal disk, about one inch thick and three inches in diameter—is surgically placed under the skin of the abdomen near the waistline. The pump stores and releases prescribed amounts of medication through the catheter. The pump is refilled by inserting a needle through the skin into a filling port in the center of the pump every 2–3 months. With a programmable pump, a tiny motor moves the medication from the pump reservoir through the catheter. Using an external programmer, adjustments can be made in the dose, rate and timing of the medication. This method is highly effective in controlling severe spasticity of spinal cord origin.[5] In a long-term (more than five years) study assessing 21 patients who received intrathecal baclofen given by programmable pump, clinical efficacy was established in reducing spasticity significantly.[6] All the patients had chronic disabling spasticity, which did not respond to oral antispasmolytic agents. Clinical efficacy was assessed by the Ashworth scale and spasm score. Compared with pretreatment values, there was a significant improvement in clinical efficacy (Ashworth scale and spasm score, $p < 0.05$). Baclofen pump still remains a very effective treatment option in treating disabling and intractable spasticity of spinal origin.

Selective Neuroablative Procedures

The goals of these procedures are to break local neural circuits that have escaped the supraspinal control without adding any more motor deficits. The segmental circuits consist of peripheral nerves, posterior roots, dorsal root entry zone (DREZ) and spinal cord. Ablative procedures thus consist of **(Fig. 22.1)**:
1. Longitudinal myelotomy.
2. DREZotomy.
3. Selective posterior rhizotomies.
4. Peripheral neurotomies.

Myelotomy

This involves splitting the spinal cord longitudinally between the anterior and the posterior horn cells of lumbosacral region. It is a major surgery and is only done in patients with complete spastic paraplegia with disabling spasms. The region of interest is generally approached after reaching the spinal canal through a midline posterior myelotomy **(Fig. 22.2)**. This in effect disconnects the anterior horn from the posterior horn cells and relieves spasticity. After the advent of baclofen pumps this surgery is rarely used.

DREZotomy

Selective destruction of DREZ has been commonly used for treating chronic intractable pain disorders for a long time. It has also been used for treatment of spasticity as it disconnects the local neural circuits that participate in development of spasticity.[7] It is useful for patients with severe and regional spasticity, possibly associated with chronic intractable pain, in one or both of the lower or upper limbs. This technique of DREZotomy consists of cutting only the ventral portion at the entry zone, including a large area up to the superficial layers of the posterior gray matter. The extent of the lesion is concerned not only with the junction between dorsal root and dorsal column (the entry zone), but also the more superficial layer of the dorsal horn, the gelatinosa area **(Fig. 22.2)**. Surgery is carried out at either the cervical or lumbar area depending on the spastic region. After a large laminectomy, the dorsal radicular spinal junction is carefully identified and a very delicate section is made by a blade (usually marked in millimeters) precisely at 45° in the ventromedial direction. The maximum depth of the lesion is 3 mm. In a paper by Sindou,[8] he published the results of 151 patients who underwent DREZotomy for lower limb hypertonicity. The patients were followed-up for a mean 5.6 years. He observed decreased hypertonia in 78% of cases (Ashworth scale, under 2), decreased painful spasm in 88% of the cases, and an increase in functional status. This procedure remains very useful in selected patients and when performed by surgeons familiar with it.

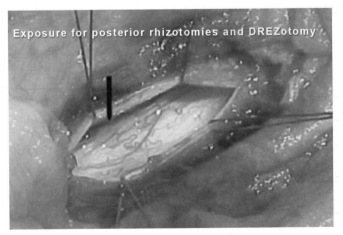

Fig. 22.2: Approach for the DREZotomy and posterior rhizotomy
(For color version, see Plate 13)

Selective Posterior Rhizotomy

Posterior rhizotomies can be done either surgically or by thermal or chemical lesioning. The procedure simply involves sectioning of posterior rootlets. In the preselected area, some rootlets in the posterior root are sectioned a few millimeters before they enter the posterolateral sulcus. Intraoperative stimulation of the rootlets is sometimes used as a guide for selection of the rootlets to be sectioned.

Peripheral Neurotomies

These are mainly used for focal spasticity, localized to a muscular group innervated by a single or few peripheral nerves. Preoperative selection consists of blocking these nerves by a long-acting anesthetic to see, if the focal spasticity improves. The main indication for the upper limb is in the spastic elbow, with section of the musculocutaneous nerve, and in spastic hand with section of the median and ulnar nerves. For the lower limb, the main indications concern the spastic hip and spastic foot where neurotomies of obturator and tibial nerves are used. The neurotomies must be done as distally as possible and limited to the fascicles innervating the hypertonic muscles.[9] The neurotomy must also be quantitatively selective.

Other Surgical Techniques

Other non-neurosurgical techniques such as tendon lengthening, tenotomy, muscular disinsertion, tendon transfers and osteotomies can also be used as an adjuvant to treatment of focal spasticity.

Conclusion

Surgical treatment in severe spasticity depends on the extent of the spasticity (local, regional or diffuse), residual motor activity and functional achievement due to the surgery. A variety of surgical procedures are available and their application varies according to the functional status of the patient. Intrathecal baclofen, SCS, ablative surgery and orthopedic procedures can give good functional results when used properly in a carefully selected group of patients.

References

1. Lane JW. Pathophysiology of spasticity and clinical experience with baclofen. In: Feldman RG, Young RR, Koella WP (Eds). Spasticity disordered motor control, Chicago. Year Book; 1980.pp.185-203.
2. Seigfried J. Treatment of spasticity by dorsal cord stimulation. Int Rehabil Med. 1980;2:31-4.
3. Barolat G, Myklebust JB, Wenninger W. Effects of spinal cord stimulation on spasticity and spasms secondary to myelopathy. Appl Neurophysiol. 1988;51(1):29-44.
4. Penn RD, Kroin JS. Continuous intrathecal baclofen for severe spasticity. Lancet. 1985;2:125-7.

5. Lazorthes Y, Sallerin-Caute B, Verdie JC, et al. Chronic intrathecal baclofen administration for control of severe spasticity. J Neurosurg. 1990;72:393-402.
6. Zahavi A, Geertzen JH, Middel B, Staal M, Rietman JS. Long-term effect (more than five years) of intrathecal baclofen on impairment, disability, and quality of life in patients with severe spasticity of spinal origin. J Neurol Neurosurg Psychiatry. 2004;75(11):1553-7.
7. Sindou M, Jeanmonod D, Mertens P. Surgery for dorsal root entry zone, microsurgical DREZotomy for the treatment of spasticity In: Sindau M, Abbot R, Keravel Y (Eds). Neurosurgery for spasticity, a multidisciplinary approach' Winn-New York, Springer-Verlag; 1991.pp.165-82.
8. Mertens P, Sindou M. La drézotomie microchiururgicale dans le traitement de la spasticité invalidante des membres inférieurs. Neurochirurgie. 1998;9:209-18.
9. Lazorthes Y, Sol JC, Sallerin B, Verdié JC. The surgical management of spasticity. European Journal of Neurology. 2002;9(Suppl 1):35-41.

23

Functional Restoration of Spinal Cord Injury Patients

Amit Pathak

Spinal cord injury (SCI) suddenly reduces an individual enjoying normal activity to a state of complete immobility and dependence upon others.

The rebuilding of lifestyle demands a creative, realistic and practical day-to-day adaptive approach to daily living skills, activities and tolerance.

Basic Principles

The following principles are basic to functional restoration:

1. Correlation of the therapy program with the medical condition of the patient, assessment information, motivation and goals of the patient, the family and home situation and medical and functional prognosis.
2. Use of therapeutic positioning of the body for rest and for therapy, using appropriate equipment and principles of body mechanics.
3. Development of therapeutic relationship between patient and therapist, patient and patient, and patient and group.
4. Use of purposeful activity and hand function (**Fig. 23.1**).
5. Use of activity analysis in:
   a. Choice of activity for evaluation and treatment
   b. Choice of treatment method related to the therapeutic value of the selected activity.
6. Use of the environment to aid in adjustment and adaptation by the patient for functional living:
   a. Adjusting the setting for appropriate and effective evaluation of the patient's functional level
   b. Adapting the level of stimuli for tolerance and interaction
   c. Adjusting for successful and satisfying daily living activity
   d. Insuring self-worth through productive and social activity.

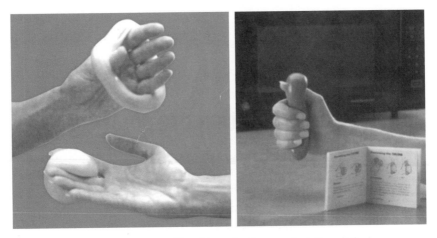

Fig. 23.1: Training of hand (coordination, manipulation, etc.)
(For color version, see Plate 14)

7. Use of adaptive devices and equipment to:
   a. Obtain maximum involvement in functional physical activity
   b. Provide independence in daily self-care activities
   c. Provide self-esteem and self-worth in task completion.
8. Use of community resources for:
   a. Successful community re-entry
   b. Social stimulation and benefit
   c. Independence in continuing rehabilitation goals.

Preliminary Training for Functional Activities

Lifting the buttocks by pushing on the arms is the basis of most of the activities of daily living (ADL). An effective lift depends upon balance and strength and upon knowing exactly where to place the hands and how to hold the shoulders, head and trunk.

In order to maintain balance while moving the first principle of body mechanics must be observed, i.e. the line of gravity must remain inside the base of support. To achieve this in sitting position with no muscle power around the hip joint, the head and shoulder must be kept forward of the hip joint. This position gives a mechanical advantage so that same strength achieves a higher lift.

Maneuvers Necessary for Functional Activities

- Lifting and moving
- Moving the paralyzed limbs
- Sitting up and lying down
- Rolling prone and turning on to the side.

Functional Independence

Following survival of spinal cord injury, the primary goal of rehabilitation should be in terms of independence.

ADL for the Paraplegic Patient

(A) Dressing
i. *Trousers*
- Position—sitting with knee flexed.
- Process—hold the top of trousers and flip the pants down to the hip.

  ↓

  Work pant legs over the feet and pull up to the hips

  ↓

  In semireclining position, roll from hip to hip and pull up the garment.
ii. *Shirts*
- Method of putting clothing on does not usually create a problem.
- Balance body by putting palms of hand on mattress on either side of the body.
iii. *Socks or stockings*
- Position—sitting on bed.
- Process—pull one leg into flexion with one hand and cross over the other leg.

  ↓

  Use other hand to slip sock or stocking over foot and pull it on.

(B) Eating
Eating activities should present no special problem for paraplegic patient.

(C) Hygiene and grooming
i. Spray hose is useful in bathing. Patient should keep finger over the spray to determine sudden temperature change.
ii. Long-handled bath brushes with soap insert are helpful for ease in reaching all parts of the body.
iii. Soap bars attached to a cord around neck may be helpful.

ADL for Quadriplegic Patient

(A) Dressing
i. *Minimal criteria for upper extremity dressing*
- ROM of shoulder flexion and abduction—0°–90°
  Shoulder internal rotation—0°–80°
  Shoulder external rotation—0°–30°
- Sitting balance may be achieved with bed rails or wheelchair safety belt.
- Fair to good muscle strength in deltoids, upper and middle trapezi, shoulder rotators, rhomboids, biceps, supinator and radial wrist extensor.

ii. *Additional criteria of lower extremity dressing*
- Fair to good muscle strength in pectoralis major and minor, serratus anterior.
- ROM of 0°–120° in knee flexion, 0°–110° in hip flexion and 0°–80° in hip external rotation.
- Ability to roll.

Suggestions for dressing
1. Zippers and Velcro fastening facilitate dressing.
2. Garments should be loose fitting.
3. Shoes can be one size larger than normally worn to accommodate edema and spasticity and to avoid pressure sore.

(B) Feeding
i. Level C5 and above require mobile arm supports or externally powered splints and braces. A wrist splint and universal cuff may be used to hold the eating utensils.
ii. A nonskid mat and plate with plate guard provide extra stability.
iii. A regular or swivel spoon/fork combination can be used when there is minimal muscle function (C4 – C5).
iv. Built up utensils may be useful for those with functional grasp or tenodesis grasp.

(C) Hygiene and grooming
Suggestions to facilitate hygiene and grooming:
i. Extend reach by using long-handled bath sponges with loop handle.
ii. Eliminate need to grasp wash cloths by using bath mitts.
iii. Hold comb and toothbrush with universal cuff.
iv. Use a clip type holder for electric razor.
v. Use skin inspection mirror with long stem and loop handle for independent skin inspection.

Functional outcome on the basis of level of injury is tabulated in **Table 23.1**.

Table 23.1: Functional outcome on the basis of level of injury			
Level	*Possible active mobility*	*Pattern of weakness*	*Functional capabilities and limitation*
C1-3	Neck control	1. Total paralysis of trunk, U/E and L/E 2. Dependence on respirator	1. Total ADL dependence 2. Can propel power wheel chair 3. Needs full time attendant care
C3-4	Neck movements, Scapular elevation	1. Paralysis of trunk, U/E and L/E 2. Difficulty in Breathing	1. Full time wheelchair user 2. Activities can be accomplished through use of mouthstick, e.g. typing, page turning, etc.

Contd…

Contd...

Level	Possible active mobility	Pattern of weakness	Functional capabilities and limitation
C5	Shoulder flexion, shoulder abduction up to 90°, elbow flexion, supination, scapular adduction, abduction, upward and downward rotation (weak)	1. Absence of elbow extension, pronation, and all wrist and hand movements 2. Total paralysis of trunk and U/E	1. Unable to roll over 2. Needs assistance in transfers 3. With good muscle power may be able to do U/E dressing with minimum assistance 4. With adaptive equipment can do feeding, light hygiene, telephoning, etc. 5. Can direct bowel and bladder management
C6	1. All movement of C4 and C5 scapular abduction and upward rotation 2. Shoulder extension and internal rotation, shoulder flexion, forearm pronation, radial wrist extension	1. Absence of wrist flexion, total paralysis of trunk and L/E 2. Low endurance	1. Able to perform many activities with tenodesis grasp 2. Roll from side to side in bed with aid of bedrails 3. Independent in wheelchair propelling with help of rim adaptations 4. Independent in managing communication devices with adaptive equipment
C7-8	1. All movements of C4, L5 and C6 2. Elbow extension 3. Ulnar wrist extension 4. Radial wrist flexion 5. PIP and DIP flexion	1. Weakness in trunk control affecting balance 2. Limited grasp, release and dexterity balance of incomplete innervation of hand intrinsics	1. Can transfer to and from bed and wheelchair independently 2. Can roll over, sit up in a standard bed 3. Can dress independently 4. Independent with eating 5. Tenodesis may helpful because of weakness of grasp 6. Can propel manual wheelchair (may need rim adaptations)
C8-T1	Forearm pronation, ulnar wrist flexion, MP flexion, thumb flexion and opposition	Paralysis of L/E trunk control weakness	1. Independent in bed activities, wheel chair transfer, self-care 2. Can manage manual wheel chair 3. Independent bladder and bowel care 4. Independent in management of communication devices
T4-T9	All arm functions partial trauma stability	Partial trunk paralysis and paralysis of L/E	1. Independent in self-care 2. Independent manual wheel chair and transfer 3. May use standing frame independently

Contd...

Contd...

Level	Possible active mobility	Pattern of weakness	Functional capabilities and limitation
T10-L2	Partial to good trunk stability	1. L/E paralysis 2. May have flaccid bowel and bladder	1. Independent in self-care, personal hygiene and housekeeping 2. Ambulates with difficulty using braces and crutches, but wheelchair is preferable for speed and energy conservation
L3-L4	1. Trunk control 2. Hip flexion and adduction 3. Knee extension	Partial paralysis of L/E, hip extension, knee flexion and foot and ankle movement	1. Independent in all activities as in above level 2. Can ambulate independently with short leg brace and crutches
L5-S3	Partial to full control of L/Es	Partial paralysis of L/Es Mostly in distal segment	1. Independent in all activities 2. May require limited bracing for ambulation 3. May have volitional bladder and bowel function

Bibliography

1. Anderson, et al. Performance of health-related quality of life instruments in a spinal cord injured population. Archive of Physical Medicine and Rehabilitation. 1999;80(8):877-84.
2. Barbeau, et al. Physical determinants, emerging concepts and training approaches in gait of individuals with spinal cord injury. Journal of Neurotrauma. 2006;23(3):571-85.
3. Barelay, Linda. Exploring the factors that influence the goal setting process for occupational therapy intervention with an individual with spinal cord injury. Australian Occupational Therapy Journal. 2002;49(1):3-13.
4. Bizzarine, et al. Exercise prescription in subjects with spinal cord injuries. Archive of Physical Medicine and Rehabilitation. 2005;86(6):1170-5.
5. Clayton KS, Chubon RA. Factors associated with the quality of life of long term spinal cord injured persons. Archive of Physical Medicine and Rehabilitation. 1994;75(6):633-8.
6. Gerhart, et al. Long-term spinal cord injury: Functional changes over time. Archive of Physical Medicine and Rehabilitation. 1999;80(8):877-84.
7. James Oat Judge. Balance training to maintain mobility and prevent disability. American Journal of Preventive Medicine. 2003;25(3) Supplement-2:150-6.
8. Kennedy. The new viewpoints toward spinal cord injuries. Annals of Surgery. 1946;124(6):1507-1062.
9. Michal S Atkins. Spinal Cord Injury, Section VI, Chapter-43, Occupational Therapy for Physical Dysfunction, 6th edn. Lippincott Williams and Wilkins; 2007. pp. 1131-69.
10. Sue Cox, et al. Spinal cord lesions, Chapter-16, Occupational Therapy and Physical Dysfunction, Principles, Skills and Practice, 5th edn. Churchill Livingstone, 2002.
11. Valent, et al. The effects of upper body exercise on the physical activity of people with spinal cord injury: a systemic review. Clinical Rehabilitation. 2007;21:315-30.

24

Management of Neurogenic Bladder, Sexual and Bowel Dysfunction in Spinal Cord Injuries

Mahima Agarwal, Mrinal Joshi

Neurogenic Bladder Dysfunction in Spinal Cord Injuries

Neurogenic bladder is a general term applied to a malfunctioning urinary bladder due to neurologic dysfunction, or insult, resulting from internal or external trauma, disease or injury. Bladder dysfunction is the most important cause of morbidity and mortality amongst long-term spinal cord injury individuals.

It has been recommended that any patients with known neurologic disease should be evaluated for neurogenic bladder dysfunction as a standard diagnostic approach.

Classification of Neurogenic Bladder

The aim of classifying neurogenic bladder is to facilitate better understanding of the pathophysiology behind the clinical findings, and to help in better management. Based on the data obtained from the neurourologic evaluation, a given voiding dysfunction can be categorized in a number of descriptive systems.

The functional classification system divides the voiding dysfunction into two categories: failure to store and failure to void. The flexibility and simplicity of this system makes it a widely used system. It can be easily expanded to include the etiologic basis of each category and thus form the expanded functional classification system, the storage and voiding phases of micturition are described separately and within each, various designations are applied to describe bladder and urethral function.

The classification system proposed by International Continence Society (ICS) is an extension of urodynamic classification system as depicted in **Table 24.1**. Lapides classification system divides bladder dysfunction into

Table 24.1: Classification of neurogenic bladder as given by International Continence Society	
Storage phase	*Voiding phase*
I. Bladder function	**I. Bladder function**
1. Detrusor activity • Normal or stable • Overactive – Neurogenic – Idiopathic	1. Detrusor activity • Normal • Underactive • Acontractile • Areflexic
2. Bladder sensation • Normal • Increased or hypersensitive • Reduced or hyposensitive • Absent	
3. Bladder capacity • Normal • High • Low	
II. Urethral function	**II. Urethral function**
• Normal closure mechanism • Incomplete closure mechanism	• Normal • Abnormal – Mechanical obstruction – Over activity – Dysfunctional voiding – Detrusor sphincter dyssynergia – Nonrelaxing urethral sphincter dysfunction

sensory neurogenic bladder, motor paralytic bladder, uninhibited neurogenic bladder, reflex neurogenic bladder and autonomous neurogenic bladder. This system remains one of the most familiar systems to urologists. Bors–Comarr proposed the terms balanced and unbalanced bladder which later helped in deducing the effectiveness of bladder management technique. Hald-Bradley classified bladder dysfunction according to the level of the lesion. Urodynamic classification system gave specific terms like detrusor overactivity (DO), detrusor areflexia (DA) and detrusor sphincter dyssynergia (DSD).

Important Terms

- Detrusor overactivity (DO)
    - It is a urodynamic observation characterized by involuntary detrusor contractions during the filling phase which may be spontaneous or provoked.
    - Phasic detrusor overactivity is defined by a characteristic wave form and may or may not lead to urinary incontinence. May be a sign of first sensation.

- Terminal detrusor overactivity is defined as a single, involuntary detrusor contraction, occurring at cystometric capacity, which cannot be suppressed and results in incontinence usually resulting in bladder emptying (voiding).
  - Neurogenic detrusor overactivity when there is a relevant neurological condition. This term has replaced the term "detrusor hyperreflexia".
  - Idiopathic detrusor overactivity when there is no defined cause. This term replaces "detrusor instability".
- Detrusor sphincter dyssynergia (DSD) is defined as a detrusor contraction concurrent with an involuntary contraction of the urethral and/or periurethral striated muscle.
- Detrusor areflexia is defined as an absence of any measurable detrusor contraction during filling or voiding phase.

Evaluation of Voiding Dysfunction

All spinal cord injury individuals, even those who are ambulatory and who do not complaint of any difficulty in bladder routine, should be, thoroughly evaluated for voiding dysfunction. Detailed clinical assessment should include urologic history (present bladder management technique, its acceptance, and problems, daily bladder diary, dysuria, and episodes of autonomic dysreflexia, if any). Physical examination should include complete sensory, motor neurologic examination along with anal tone, deep anal reflexes, deep anal pressure, bulbocavernosus reflex/clitoroanal reflex, and anal wink along with inspection of the abdomen, perineal skin and external genitalia.

Detailed evaluation of the upper and lower urinary tracts must be done whenever indicated. Twenty-four hours creatinine clearance is very useful to assess the damage that has occurred to kidneys as against the use of serum creatinine clearance alone. Objective evaluation in the form of urodynamic study with electrophysiological analysis of the pelvic floor muscles and sphincters is a must for proper management of bladder dysfunction. Cystoscopy can reveal pubic hairs or eggshell calculi that may be missed on radiography and serve as a nidus for bladder stones. Once a year, detailed bladder evaluation, is the recommended standard in spinal cord injury for first ten years, then evaluation should occur every other year.

Management of Voiding Dysfunctions

Management depends on the type of spinal injury, bladder behavior and practicality along with proper consideration for cognitive function of the individual. Achieving a successful bladder management program enables people with spinal cord injuries puts them back in control of their bodies again and helps them improve their self-confidence along with ensuring a good health. The main goals of bladder management include:

- Protecting upper urinary tracts from sustained high filling and voiding pressures (>40 cm water)

- Maintaining a balanced (< 20% of total bladder capacity as residual) and, continent bladder.
- Preventing recurrent complications like urinary tract infections, autonomic dysreflexia and incontinence.

Bladder Management Techniques

Nonpharmacological

Catheterization

Also referred to as cathing is a bladder emptying technique in which a flexible tube (catheter) is inserted into the urethra to drain urine.

Intermittent catheterization (IC): Sterile IC was first proposed by Guttman and Frenkel for patients with spinal cord injury (SCI) in the 1960s with a low rate of complications. In mid 1970s, Lapides et al reported the effectiveness of clean IC and it has been reported to be the safest method of management. Factors important for self-catheterization, apart from well controlled detrusor activity, include good bladder capacity, adequate bladder outlet resistance, absence of urethral sensitivity to pain with catheterization and patient motivation. IC whether performed acutely or chronically, has the lowest complication rate although urethral complications and epididymo-orchitis occur more frequently in those using IC than other methods. Important principals are to restrict fluids to 2L a day, and to catheterize frequently enough to keep the bladder volumes < 400 mL, i.e. every 4–6 hours. Prelubricated non-hydrophilic catheters and hydrophilic catheters have been suggested to be better than conventional PVC catheters.

External catheters: A viable option for bladder management in males is condom catheterization. It is associated with relatively fewer complications than indwelling methods but more complications than intermittent catheterization. It leads to incomplete drainage, which may lead to persistently high bladder pressures, recurrent urinary tract infection (UTI) and the likelihood of renal complications including glomerular filtration rate deterioration are common.

Indwelling catheterization (urethral and suprapubic): Though these methods are losing their popularity these days, but in cases where clean intermittent catheterization (CIC) is not a feasible option suprapubic catheter is generally preferred to avoid creation of a penoscrotal fistula, damage to the sphincter muscles, dilation of the urethra with leakage around the catheter, penile tip erosion and traumatic hypospadias.

Reflex Voiding and Bladder Expression Techniques

In males with tetraplegia and insufficient hand dexterity to perform CIC, drainage by reflex voiding with triggering maneuvers such as suprapubic tapping, scissoring actions of the fingers in the rectum or stroking inner thigh are sometimes used. Valsalva or Crede (pressing over the bladder) are discouraged because of high voiding pressures causing damage to the upper urinary tract.

Pharmacological Management

Anticholinergic Therapy for SCI-related Detrusor Overactivity

The body of the detrusor is comprised of smooth muscle that contains muscarinic receptors triggered by acetylcholine to cause muscle contraction. Therefore, to relax the detrusor and allow it to fill with higher volumes under lower pressure, anticholinergics may be used. Common marketed medications in this class used for overactive bladder include oxybutynin, tolterodine, fesoterodine, and more recently, trospium chloride, propiverine hydrochloride and M3-receptor specific medications darifenacin and solifenacin.

Toxin Therapy for SCI-related Detrusor Overactivity

Botulinum Toxin, Capsaicin and Resiniferatoxin

Anticholinergic medications remain first line therapy for detrusor overactivity, but the advantage of botulinum toxin over systemic administration of medications is that botulinum toxin is used focally in the bladder; thus, it avoids systemic side effects, for the most part. There is level 1a evidence (from several RCTs) that supports the use of onabotulinum toxin A injections into the detrusor muscle to provide targeted treatment for neurogenic detrusor overactivity and urge incontinence resistant to high-dose oral anticholinergic treatments with intermittent self-catheterization in SCI.

Capsaicin induces localized and reversible antinociception results from C-fiber conduction and subsequent neuropeptide release inactivation. Resiniferatoxin (RTX) is another vanilloid which has been studied for its similar beneficial effects; however, it has less irritation to the bladder and is therefore better tolerated. Both of these are still under experimental phase.

Intravesical instillation of oxybutynin and propantheline has also been studied for treatment of detrusor overactivity.

Nociception/Orphanin Phenylalanine Glutamine

Nociceptin/orphanin phenylalanine glutamine (N/OFG) is a pentadecapeptide that acts on sensory innervation of the lower urinary tract. It activates the G protein coupled receptor nociceptin orphan peptide and thus has an inhibitory effect on the micturition reflex. It supports N/OFG receptor agonists as a possible new treatment for neurogenic bladders of SCI patients.

Electrical Stimulation

Electrical stimulation, mostly anterior sacral root stimulation, has been used to enhance bladder volume and induce voiding. This approach has involved concomitant dorsal sacral rhizotomy and implantation of a sacral nerve stimulator. The combined effect of this is a more compliant bladder with more storage capacity under lower pressure and triggered voiding resulting in reduced incontinence, without the need to catheterize.

Intrathecal Baclofen and Clonidine

Though, it has been proposed that the use of intrathecal baclofen and clonidine may help in detrusor overactivity but evidences are weak and are not used until indicated for other issues like spasticity. With respect to bladder management, phosphodiesterase-5 inhibitors (PDE5) are postulated to promote relaxation of the detrusor muscle, thereby decreasing overactivity and increase capacity and compliance.

Enhancing Bladder Emptying Pharmacologically

Alpha-adrenergic Blockers for Bladder Emptying

These drugs target alpha adrenoreceptor blocker subtypes which may be implicated in a variety of mechanisms including bladder neck dysfunction, increased bladder outlet resistance, detrusor-sphincter dyssynergia, autonomic hyperreflexia or upper tract stasis.

Tamsulosin, moxisylyte, terazosin, phenoxybenzamine are some of the examples of the same.

Botulinum Toxin for Bladder Emptying

Injections of botulinum toxin A into the sphincter may improve emptying by reducing outlet resistance and thus may also reduce the episodes of autonomic dysreflexia.

Other Pharmaceutical Treatments for Bladder Emptying

4-aminopyridine is a potassium channel blocker, prolonging action potentials and increasing neurotransmitter release at the neuromuscular junction. Isosorbide dinitrate reduced external urethral sphincter pressure along with dyssynergic contraction; however, bladder pressures remained unchanged.

Surgical Treatment Options

Bladder augmentation and urinary diversion are two surgical options for incontinence due to bladder. Transurethral sphincterotomy and mesh stents are also used for retention of urine.

Neurogenic Bowel Dysfunction in Spinal Cord Injuries

'Neurogenic bowel' is the term used to describe dysfunction of the colon (constipation, fecal incontinence and disordered defecation) due to loss of normal sensory and/or motor control or both, as a result of central neurological disease or damage. There are two distinct patterns of clinical presentation of bowel dysfunction. Injury above the conus medullaris results in upper motor neuron bowel syndrome (reflexic/hyperreflexic) and injury at or below it will result in lower motor neuron bowel syndrome (areflexic) or a mixed picture can be seen.

Pathophysiology and Clinical Features

Hyperreflexic Bowel

- Loss or impairment of sensory perception of the need for defecation.
- Loss or impairment of voluntary control of the external anal sphincter.
- Intact reflex arcs through the conus medullaris maintain tone (reflex activity) in the anorectum.
- Tone in the external anal sphincter, colonic wall and pelvic floor, is increased resulting in reduced colonic compliance, overactive segmental peristalsis, underactive propulsive peristalsis, spastic external anal sphincter constriction. Modulation of colonic motor activity from the brain is lost and peristalsis and haustral movements continue though less effectively.
- Colonic transit time may be slowed throughout the colon.
- Discoordination between relaxation of the anal canal and rectal contraction (rectoanal dyssynergia).
- Constipation usually with fecal retention but reflex, uncontrolled evacuation of the rectum.
- Damage in the thoracic and cervical spinal cord also reduces or eradicates the patient's ability to use the diaphragm and abdominal muscles to voluntarily increase abdominal and therefore rectal pressure.

Areflexic Bowel

- Loss or impairment of sensory perception of the need for defecation.
- Loss or impairment of voluntary control of the external anal sphincter.
- Autonomic motor nerves are disrupted due to damage to parasympathetic cell bodies in the conus medullaris or their axons in the cauda equina.
- No spinal cord mediated peristalsis occurs and modulation of colonic motility by the brain is lost, resulting in a loss of effective stool transport in the descending and sigmoid colon and rectum.
- External anal sphincter is denervated and flaccid.
- Pressure in the internal sphincter is reduced, pelvic floor muscles are areflexic allowing the sigmoid colon and rectum to descend into the pelvis, reducing the anorectal angle and opening the rectal lumen. This leads to a risk of fecal incontinence through the lax sphincter, as well as constipation.
- Colonic transit time is considerably increased.

Complications

- Reduced quality of life
- Constipation

- Fecal impaction
- Megacolon
- Fecal incontinence
- Rectal prolapsed
- Hemorrhoids/anal fissure/tear/perianal abscess
- Stercoral perforation
- Autonomic dysreflexia
- Sigmoid volvulus, intestinal obstruction
- Superior mesenteric artery syndrome.

Aims of Neurogenic Bowel Management

- Avoid fecal incontinence
- Minimize or avoid constipation
- Manage evacuation within a reasonable time, generally suggested to be up to one hour
- Optimize comfort, safety and privacy
- Acceptable to individual
- Avoid autonomic dysreflexia and minimize other secondary complications
- Maintain short and long-term gastrointestinal health.

Neurogenic Bowel Management

Nonpharmacological (Conservative and Nonsurgical)

All interventions that form a part of multifaceted bowel management routine, target reduction of bowel transit time and decreasing the episodes of incontinence.

Dietary Fiber

Soluble fiber mixes with water in the intestine to form a gel-like substance, which acts as a trap to collect certain body wastes and then move them out of the body. Insoluble fiber absorbs and holds water, producing uniform stool and helping to push gut contents through the digestive system quickly. Insoluble fiber in appropriate amounts and with additional fluid intake can promote bowel regularity and improve constipation. Recommended intake in spinal cord injury (SCI) individuals is 15 g per day which can vary with requirement. Level of evidence in support of the same is weak and has to be substituted with other more appropriate interventions.

Stimulation of Reflexes in the Gastrointestinal Tract

Utilization of the preserved gastrointestinal reflexes can be beneficial in bowel management following SCI. The gastrocolic reflex is stimulated by gastric distention due to eating and can activate bowel motility and promote defecation. Digital stimulation of anorectal reflexes has been shown to result in increased rectal contractions and could be useful in bowel evacuation following SCI.

Manual Evacuation of Bowel

Manual evacuation of feces involves the use of a single gloved and lubricated finger to remove feces from the rectum. It is used by individuals with both hyperreflexic and areflexic bowel dysfunction. Manual evacuation is a key method in conservative bowel management practice. It reduces number of unplanned bowel evacuations. There is conflicting evidence on the effect of manual evacuation on duration of bowel evacuation.

Use of Suppositories

Rectal placement of chemical rectal agents (suppositories) is a very commonly used method of bowel management by SCI individuals. Bisacodyl and glycerine is the main ingredient in these suppositories. Their use reduces the total nursing time required and polyethylene glycol based suppository is significantly better than vegetable oil based bisacodyl suppositories as per total bowel care time is concerned.

Abdominal Massage

This maneuver beginning at the cecum and extending up to the rectum and anus has a low level of evidence and needs further research to support its use.

Functional Electrical and Magnetic Stimulation of Skeletal Muscles

There is strong evidence suggesting that functional electrical stimulation of abdominal muscles decreases the colonic transit time and a lower evidence for magnetic stimulation; also poor evidence for the efficacy of posterior tibial nerve stimulation. Some also support the use of functional magnetic stimulation on thorax and lumbosacral nerves to reduce transit time and symptoms of constipation.

Bowel Irrigation Techniques

Transanal irrigation is a process of facilitating evacuation of stool from the bowel by passing water (or other liquids) via the anus in a quantity sufficient to reach beyond the rectum into the colon. Pulsed water irrigation uses a pump to deliver intermittent, rapid pulses of warm water into the rectum/colon to break up stool and to stimulate peristalsis.

Assistive Devices

Standing table and washing toilet seat with biofeedback are some examples of devices that may assist in bowel care program.

Pharmacological Agents

Cisapride was initially used for bowel management. Prucalopride increases stool frequency, improves stool consistency and decreases gastrointestinal transit time. Metoclopramide may decrease time of gastric emptying. Neostigmine administered with or without glycopyrrolate, leads to a greater expulsion of stool.

Fampridine (potassium channel blocker) can increase the number of days with bowel movements.

Surgical Management

When individual with SCI have failed all conservative management options than a colostomy can be done, where the bowel loops are made to open on the abdominal wall. Alternatively antegrade irrigation can be done where irrigation is delivered via a surgically formed non-reflux stoma. Irrigation may be delivered via the stoma using a manual or powered pump, or by gravity. The Malone antegrade continence enema (MACE or ACE) is a continent catheterisable stoma, connecting from the external abdominal wall to the cecum, through which a catheter is inserted. An enema can then be given via the catheter.

Some authors also recommend surgical implantation of electrodes to stimulate anterior sacral roots. The sacral anterior root stimulator (SARS) employs electrodes implanted on to the second, third and fourth sacral anterior nerve roots to deliver short bursts of high voltage stimulation several times daily resulting in increased colonic activity, reduced constipation and sometimes defecation during the stimulation.

Bibliography

1. ACI management of neurogenic bladder for adults with spinal cord injuries, 3rd edition, 2014.
2. Awad RA. Neurogenic bowel dysfunction in patients with spinal cord injury, myelomeningocele, multiple sclerosis and Parkinson's disease. World J Gastroenterol. 2011;17(46):5035-48.
3. Bladder management following spinal cord injury: What you should know, consortium for spinal cord medicine and paralyzed veterans of America, 2010.
4. Krassioukov Al, Eng JJ, Claxton G, Sakakibara BM, Shum S. Neurogenic bowel management after spinal cord injury: a systematic review of the evidence. Spinal Cord. 2010;48(10):718-33.
5. Lance L Goetz, Adam P Klausner. Strategies for prevention of Urinary Tract Infections in Neurogenic Bladder Dysfunction. Physical Medicine and Rehabilitation Clinics of North America. 2014. pp. 605-18.
6. Samson G, DC Diana. Neurogenic bladder in spinal cord injury. Physical Medicine and Rehabilitation Clinics of North America. 2007;18:255-74.

25

Respiratory Care in Spinal Cord Injury

Parthasarathi Bhattacharya

Introduction

Respiratory complications accounts for significant morbidity, mortality and economic burden in the patients of spinal cord injury.[1-4] Atelectasis, pneumonia, ventilatory failure, pleural effusion, and pneumothorax/hemothorax were found to be frequent complications of SCI.[5,6] The leading causes of death in SCI are pneumonia, pulmonary embolism, sepsis, and coronary artery disease.[1,7,8] Hence, respiratory care is a very important and integral part of the care of the patients of spinal cord injury.

The issue has been discussed in the following fashion:
1. Understanding the physiology of breathing and the impact on the respiratory system in SCI
2. Respiratory problem in SCI
3. Assessment of respiratory problems in SCI
4. Prevention and treatment of the respiratory problems in SCI.

Understanding the Physiology of Breathing and Impact on Respiratory System in Spinal Cord Injury

Normal respiration has two components: (a) Inspiration and (b) Expiration. The inspiration is an active process of indrawing air from atmosphere and this is achieved by the synchronous activity of different types of inspiratory muscles that creates a negative intrathoracic pressure so that the air in the ambient atmospheric pressure is basically sucked into the lungs. On the contrary, the expiration is a passive process where the elastic recoil of the lungs and the thoracic cage slowly expels the air out of the lungs. The expiratory muscles come into play only when there are some obstructions or resistance in the airflow as in asthma or COPD or during production of cough.

The diaphragm, scalenes, and the intercostal muscles are the main muscles of inspiration. The diaphragm being the most important is innervated by the phrenic nerves with origin from cervical C3, 4, 5 spinal segments. Several other muscles play an accessory role in inspiration, especially in situations of high demand for ventilation. They include the trapezius, levator scapulae, pectoralis, serratus anterior, costal levators. In expiration, the intercostals and oblique abdominals play an active role.

The effect on spinal cord injury on ventilation (largely inspiration) is thus largely dependent on the level of spinal cord injury, the degree of damage (complete or incomplete), the duration of spinal shock and associated complications or effect of injury to the lungs, airway and the related structures. There could be complete or incomplete denervation of the respiratory muscles depending on the degree and site of the SCI. Complete denervation is said to occur when the motor denervation and the sensory feedbacks are absent while in case of incomplete or partial denervation some neurological activities persist below the site of injury leading to a variable functional compromise of the ventilatory muscles. However, even with preservation of the anterior horn cells of the phrenic nerve, spontaneous respiration may be depressed or absent soon after injury because of spinal shock. With this spinal shock, phrenic nerve function may take weeks or months to return resulting in prolonged ventilatory dependence.[9] This can lead to disuse atrophy of the diaphragm.

High cervical cord injuries affect the diaphragm as well as other muscles as mentioned. Patients with complete lesion above C4 develop acute hypoventilation from severe inspiratory muscle weakness and require mechanical ventilatory support especially in acute phase. Though respiratory failure is present virtually in cervical and thoracic spinal cord injury,[10] most of the patients with SCI above C3 die before reaching hospital. Those with complete lesion below C4 can breath independently after the acute phase provided that they have no associated pulmonary impairment. The patients with complete injury at C4 level pose a peculiar challenge since they have the potential to breath on their own but have very little reserve. In the patients below C3 lesion, any pulmonary compromise due to secretion, atelectasis or infection can result in ventilatory insufficiency and demand mechanical ventilation.

Lower-cervical injuries will affect the scalenes (innervated by cord levels C4 to C7), the intercostals (T1 to T11), the oblique abdominals (T6 to L1), and the rectus abdominus. Thus, injuries at C6 level or below do not usually require ventilatory support unless other pulmonary complications or injuries coexists. Among patients with incomplete lesions, the level of injury is not very clearly associated with the need for mechanical ventilatory support and even patients with C2 or C3 level injury sometimes do not require mechanical ventilation.

Paralysis of the abdominal muscles (T6 to T12) results in the inability to cough effectively. Poor ventilation and poor cough can lead to retained secretions, mucus plugging, and atelectasis. Atelectasis allows bacterial overgrowth and ultimately pneumonia. Furthermore, cervical lesions lead to a loss of sympathetic nervous system innervation. This, in turn, resulting a parasympathetic overactivity, leads to bronchoconstriction and increased mucus secretion in the lungs. This increased mucus compounded to the impaired clearance from poor cough invites infection.

Respiratory Problems in Spinal Cord Injury

Essentially the respiratory problems in SCI are of two types. It may be from the direct effect of the injury or may be from an aftermath of the injury **(Table 25.1)**.

The direct acute effect of injury is either motor or sensorimotor impairment leading to hypoventilation and respiratory failure. But the aftermath of SCI develop from a variety of interrelated factors present in varying proportion from a victim to other. It is important to understand the predisposing factors for the respiratory complications. They are:

a. Restriction of lungs
b. Ineffective or absent cough reflex
c. Atelectasis from restrictive effects and retained secretions
d. Chronic aspirations from dysphagia exacerbated by chronic ineffective cough function
e. Immobility leading to complications.

The restrictive defect: The restrictive defect derives from the impairment of the elastic properties of the lungs and the chest wall with paralysis of the diaphragm and the muscles. These lead to reduced static lung volumes and capacities.[11] Infact, the reduced vital capacity and the paradoxical motion of the abdominal muscles impart severe restrictions upon the lung function.

Table 25.1: Respiratory problems in spinal cord injuries

Direct
• High cervical spinal cord injury involving phrenic motor neurons/roots: diaphragmatic palsy and acute ventilatory failure. Associated loss of coughing ability with tracheobronchial secretions
• Lower SCI sparing the diaphragmatic innervation: partial ventilatory weakness with inability for effectual cough and retention of tracheobronchial secretions and pneumonia. They may result decompensation with development of ventilatory failure
• Problems for associated injuries associated to airway chest wall, etc.
Indirect
• Pulmonary thromboembolism from immobilization
• Atelectasis
• Aspiration leading to infection
• Bronchospasm
• Nosocomial infection
• Perioperative problems following surgical interventions of spinal cord injury

The impairment of cough reflex: Cough is a complicated and integrated function of the respiratory and glottic muscles. There is an inspiratory gasp followed by expiratory compression of the lungs against the closed glottis. Subsequent sudden opening up of the glottis leads to a sudden burst of airflow and expulsion of the trapped air in high velocity with shearing and clearing of the respiratory mucus. In SCI, the inspiratory capacity is decreased with diminished expiratory capacity for weakness of the muscles concerned. Depending on the level of injury, the effectiveness of cough is affected. This leads to a great rise of complications as pneumonia, atelectasis, respiratory insufficiency and respiratory failure.[12]

Predisposition to atelectasis: Atelectasis is a state of airlessness of lungs. Even in normal health with continuous tidal breathing the basal alveoli tend to collapse and this is prevented by exercise, yawning, and cough that forces open these closing alveoli intermittently. Atelectasis may be a cause or effect of lung restriction in SCI.[13] In SCI, redundant secretions from impairment of cough gets infected on top of the lack of the aforesaid natural process of opening up of the alveoli. Immediate post-traumatic atelectasis is seen in 36.4% of the victims; of them, about 30% (31.4%) develop pneumonia and another 22.6% develop respiratory failure.[14] Impaired secretion clearance is found to be the cause of atelectasis in post-traumatic patients in several studies.[5]

Risk of aspiration: In SCI, the risk of aspiration is increased. Severe features that lead to aspiration, are:
  a. Dysphagia
  b. Glottic and tracheal stenosis
  c. Ineffective cough
  d. Gastroesophageal reflux.

Esophageal dysmotility and impaired swallowing: This may occur in 30% of the patients.[15] An important cause is tracheal and glottic stenosis is prolonged intubation.[16] This can lead to dysphagia, odynophagia, dyspnea and dysphonia in these patients with occasional hypersecretion of mucus.[17] Consequently, these patients are more likely to aspirate.

Gastroesophageal reflux: Added to impaired airway clearance, GE reflux leads to aspiration of gastric contents. Such patients experience recurrent symptoms of asthma, bronchitis, bronchiectasis and laryngitis.[8] Aspiration can also lead to an ARDS like state leading to infection.[18]

Immobility: Physical exercise is an important component of normal airway clearance.[19] Exercise improve airflow, reduce the viscosity of the airway secretion by increased parasympathetic drive, promote release of certain endocrine hormones that affect the volume and viscosity of secretion.[20] These along with effective cough clears the airway. With ineffective cough, immobility leads to retention of secretion and subsequent infection. Another result of immobility is predisposition to formation of DVT which can lead to pulmonary embolism with lethal consequences.[21]

Other Problems

Obstructive sleep apnea (OSA): Elderly SCI patients appear to have more frequent OSA than general population; the possible relevant factors include patient selection, reduced ventilatory function for spinal cord damage, sleep posture and medication.[22]

Even late by months or years, the victims of SCI have continued risks for respiratory complications of atelectasis or pneumonia.[23] This could be because of a late neurological deterioration or lung disease or restrictive ventilatory impairment. The respiratory complications follow the victims for years as they survive and are found to be more with complete injuries.[24] This could lead to ventilatory failure that may occur weeks or month of SCI and is usually secondary to increased respiratory demand from pathologies like pneumonia or with gradual but progressive deterioration of pulmonary or neuromuscular function. This is called late ventilatory failure in SCI. The patient shows tachypnea, dyspnea, daytime drowsiness, unexplained erythrocytosis. This situation also merits ventilatory support.

Assessment of Pulmonary Function in Spinal Cord Injury

1. The assessment of pulmonary function with spirometry is difficult to achieve in SCI patient hence a modification of ATS guidelines has been proposed.[25] It requires two acceptable and reproducible efforts instead of there in the original ATS guidelines and acceptable expiratory time as 0.5 sec instead of 6 sec in the guideline. These modifications increased the reproducibility from 58–83% for FVC and 50–75% for FEV.[1]

2. *Limb muscle strength assessment:* There is a positive correlation between muscle strength and tone with PFT.[26]

3. *Chest X-ray*: Regular chest X-ray is important in order to detect missed out chest injury,[27] to detect pulmonary opacities as pneumonia, atelectasis, etc. However, supine chest X-ray can miss or underestimate a lot of pathology detected in CT chest and can overestimate the changes demonstrated in CT.[16,28] Pleural effusions are common despite normal supine X-ray in patients of SCI. Radiological evaluation are also important to diagnose subglottic stenosis.[16]

4. *Pulse oximetry*: Some patients of SCI can have nocturnal desaturation. In some patients with tetraplegic SCI, it is suggested that clinical history may not be a reliable indication of the risk for sleep disorder breathing in patients of cervical SCI.[29]

5. *Study of swallowing*: Effective swallowing is important to appreciate the risk of aspiration in patients of SCI having swallowing problems. Dysphagia is found to be present clinically in 22.5% of cases.[30] Patient with tracheostomy and anterior surgical approach one likely to develop dysphagia up to 48% of cases.

6. *Bronchospasm*: Bronchospasm is under recognized under the over shadowing restrictive defect in tetraplegic form of SCI[31] sympathomimetic metaproterenol is found to reduce this airway hyper-responsiveness[32] while ipratropium cannot.[33]

Respiratory Care in SCI

The respiratory care in SCI can be denoted in the following list:

Ventilatory Assistance

- Airway management
- Mechanical ventilation
- *Chronic ventilatory support:*
  - Nasal intermittent positive pressure ventilation (NIPPV)
  - Pneumobelt
  - Electrophrenic pacing
  - Glossopharyngeal breathing
  - Respiratory muscle conditioning
  - Posture.

Prevention

- *Neuromuscular weakness:*
  - Conditioning of respiratory muscle
  - Cough stimulation
  - Diaphragmatic breathing
  - Diaphragmatic pacing
- *Clearance of secretions:*
  - Postural drainage and tracheobronchial clearing
  - Insufflation-exsufflation
  - Cough induction
- Prevention of aspiration
- *Prevention of infections:*
  - Clearance of secretions
  - Care of swallowing and aspiration
  - Measures for prevention of nosocomial infection
  - Vaccination
- Prevention and treatment of factors that lead to complications from immobility (PTE, infections, etc.).

Associated Issues

- Nutrition and metabolic factors
- Treatment of OSA, traumatic fat embolism, etc.
- Care of skin, mouth, eye, and other organs
- Mental well-being
- Care of wound in other areas
- Care of the comorbidities.

Patient Education

Airway management: Patients of SCI with acute ventilatory failure needs immediate intubation. These patients need meticulous airway care with maintenance of alignment and provision of continuous cervical immobilization are an integral component of care in these patients. However, intubation in a case of cervical cord injury needs caution and appropriate modification not to disturb the destabilized spine. Nasotracheal or orotracheal incubate with help of FOB or laryngoscope has been practiced.[34] Tracheotomy is performed if the prospect of ventilation appears to continue over weeks or months. There could be several short or long-term complications of tracheotomy including infection, hemorrhage or pneumothorax, hemostasis to granuloma formation TOF and even erosion of artery and tracheal stenosis.[35] Cuffless tracheotomy tubes appear better for reducing the chance of stenosis and for allowing speech to the patients.

Ventilatory support: Ventilatory deficiency is manifested by tachycardia, diaphoresis and altered sensorium and ventilatory support is essential whenever there is evidence of ventilatory deficiency in victim of SCI. This may be in acute setting with requirement of complete of near complete ventilatory support and it is usually accomplished by intubation and subsequent use of ventilators. However, there are situations when such intensive management is not required, CPAP, BiPAP or GSB (Glossopharyngeal Breathing) may suffice in such cases. The predictors of need for ventilation are injury level above C5 segment complete lesion, copious sputum in the 1st week (postinjury) and pneumonia in lung collapse.[36] Patients with higher level of injuries and complete injuries are more likely to need mechanical ventilation.[36,37]

Ventilatory support has got several facts and facets to discuss. The nature and degree of support depends on the demand, the status of the underlying lung parenchyma and the airways. Thus, the mode and settings are adjusted accordingly. There has to be some mechanism to prevent atelectasis while ventilating a victim of SCI by use of 'sigh' or 'peep'. Proper tracheobronchial toileting is required to be ensured with all possible support to prevent or lessen the disuse atrophy of the ventilatory muscles especially when the injury is incomplete with very little chance of recovery. Expert hands are required to accomplish all these.

In chronic ventilatory support, tracheotomy is required though it interferes with speech. The noninvasive chronic ventilation can be accomplished by NIPPV, intermittent abdominal pressure respiration, electrophrenic pacing (EPR) and respiratory muscle conditioning. Noninvasive ventilation is either positive (NIPPV) or negative pressure ventilation (NNPV). Negative pressure ventilation can be done by total body chamber (iron lungs) or chest wraps that enables expansion of chest bellow creating negative pressure surrounding it.

The NIPPV has really replaced NNPV. The machine delivers airway pressure which is transmitted through an interface (facemask, mouth piece, nasal or oral device, etc.) to the patient's airway. The modern BiPAP ventilators are capable of compensating leak around the interface, providing PEEP, assuring volume delivery or attending a preset pressure with each breath (pressure control). They can have provision for back-up ventilation for situations when the breath is not initiated by the patient and simultaneous oxygen supplementation. They are lighter and can be transported easily. For an effective NIPPV, the patient must be able to cooperate and coordinate his or her breathing with the ventilator.

However, expert personnel is required for monitoring the patients on NIPPV. Noncooperative and drowsy patients are not fit for NIPPV. The management of tracheobronchial secretions is often a problem for such ventilation. In any situation of difficulty with NIPPV, the patient may need to be shifted to the conventional ventilators.

The motto of ventilatory support is to buy time to let the patient become capable of independently ventilating adequately. This means preparing the patient to take up its own breathing with the natural course of recovery. Expert respiratory therapist is essential to accomplish this job.

Weaning: This can be achieved by: (1) keeping the patient on partial support and by manipulating the ventilator to reduce the assistance; (2) removing the patient altogether from support for limited period of time intermittently and progressively increasing the support free duration; and (3) providing and alternate means of ventilatory support as (a) intermittent abdominal pressure ventilation, (b) glossopharyngeal breathing (GSB), and (c) electrophonic respiration (EPR). Finally, (4) use of noninvasive ventilation with manipulation (gradual reduction).[38-40] Patient with lower cervical cord injury are easier to wean than patient with high cervical SCI. Infact, the C2 level complete injury are not candidature for weaning because of expected inadequate diaphragm function.

Weaning should be attempted only in absence of cardiopulmonary problems and acute infections and the patient having a reasonable vital capacity.

Chronic Ventilatory Management

A segment of patients fails to get weaned from ventilator being dependent on ventilator at the time of death or discharge;[41] pneumonia being the common cause of death in them. The following may be helpful adjunct to them:

Chronic NPPV: This has been attempted in acute ventilatory insufficiency,[40,42] to facilitate weaning from invasive ventilator[43] and as a means of long term ventilatory support.[44] The risk of pneumonia is found lower in NPPV than in tracheotomised patients is both acute care with short term ventilation and also in home ventilation with part time or full time support.[44]

Pneumobelt: It may be an adjunct in noninvasive ventilatory support in a large series of neuromuscular diseases[45] and variable success from high level of satisfaction to intorability has been experienced in patients with high level cervical SCI.[45]

Nonmechanical ventilatory assistance: Varity of physical interventions have been attempted in case of ventilatory failure in SCI.

Respiratory muscle conditioning: Several techniques especially exercise schedules have been tried to improve the strength and in durance of diaphragm and accessory muscles.[46] They are namely stretching, incentive spirometry, inspiratory muscle training, abdominal weight training, Glossopharyngeal breathing, and other maneuvers. Abdominal weight training[47] inspiratory resistive muscle training[48] induced insufflation and resistance,[49] incentive spirometry,[50] multidisciplinary intervention of respiratory muscle exercise[51] have all shown significant improvement in lung function.

Electrophrenic respiration/diaphragmatic pacing: Pacing of phrenic nerves or diaphragm may help ventilation in tetraplegic patients by implanting a pulse generator.[52,53] This technique has some limitations; it is best effective with a viable phrenic nerve having its neurons at cervical segments intact and is limited by diaphragm fatigue and deconditioning that occur during the gap of paralysis and the implant of the device.[54] ERP cannot induce cough and can contribute to obstructive sleep apnea often demanding keeping of a tracheotomy tube.

Intermittent abdominal pressure respirator (pneumobelt): It is an exsufflation belt placed on the abdomen that helps expiration and used only in alert and upright positioned patients.[43] The belt swells up with air to pressure on abdomen helping the diaphragm to rise. When quickly deflated, there is passive inspiration.[43,45]

Glossopharyngeal breathing (GSB): This is a technique in which the patient gulps air bolus beyond the glottis with the help of the muscles of mouth, pharynx and larynx. It has been found to significantly increase the vital capacity (VC) in supervised training.[55] Apart, this also improves the audibility of the patient's voice.

Posture: In SCI, the effects of posture on VC of the patients are marked.[56] There is a reduction in VC from supine to sitting. This reduction is suggested to be from reduction in expiratory reserve volume rather than the mechanical advantage of the diaphragm.[57]

Drugs: Improvement of ventilatory muscle function has been attempted with regular short-term hyperbaric oxygen in chronic phage of injury with tetraplegia. It has shown some improvement in ventilatory muscle function in some patients.[58] Statistically, significant change is observed with oral anabolic steroid oxandrolone; there is also associated improvement in subjective symptoms.[59] A study with 4-aminopyridine, a potassium-channel blocker with potentials to enhance nerve conduction in demyelinated neurons has shown significant improvement in pulmonary function.[60] Researchers are trying to understand the mechanisms that unmask the inactive motor pathways that can potentially restore the function of the muscles paralyzed by a spinal cord injury. Theophylline, a drug used to improve the function of nerves or muscles that control breathing has been under trial. This is a kind of pharmacological management of the respiratory system to enhance the body's respiratory centers and restore function to respiratory muscles.[61]

Others Issues: Prevention and Treatment of Complications

Management of Secretion and Atelectasis

Secretion clearance: The amount of secretion and pulmonary infections are strongly associated with pneumonia.[30,37] Retained secretion may plug bronchi, lead to atelectasis and eventually pneumonia. A very high degree of efficient monitoring and aggressive efforts to clear the secretions are essential to prevent it. There are several methods to tackle secretion and atelectasis that includes postural drainage, chest percussion, active suctioning, assisted cough and rotating beds.

Intermittent positive pressure ventilation (IPPV) with breath stacking or mechanical insufflation-exsufflation with concomitant abdominal thrust and intrapulmonary percussive ventilation may be used to help clearing the secretion. Mechanical insufflation (Positive pressure ventilation with air stalking) is a common practice[38,39] and incidentally the tracheostomized patients prefer it than suctioning.[40] Rotating beds, assisted cough and multimodal respiratory therapy are used to clear secretions. Rotating beds were found to reduce the risk of pneumonia and length of ICU stays.[62-64]

No study is available regarding the role of mucolytics.

Assisted cough, imparting pressure on abdomen simultaneous to the cough, positive pressure insufflation and electrical stimulation of abdominal muscles have also been tried.[65-67]

Multimodal pulmonary therapy incorporate increasing the frequency (doubling) the routine suctioning and assisted coughing in addition to deep breathing and spirometry and even bronchoscopic clearing of bronchial section.[68] This has been found effective.

Prevention and Treatment of Infection

Nosocomial pneumonia is one of the leading cause of death due to hospital-acquired infections. It contributes to mortality ranging from 20% to 50%.[69,70] The highest risk is in the patients on mechanical ventilation (ventilator-associated pneumonia), in whom the entity has been best studied. As many as one-quarter of intensive care unit patients develop pneumonia.[71]

Incidentally, because of ventilatory failure the SCI patients are mostly kept in the intensive care areas where the chance of infection and also the chance of resistant infection is high. Approximately, 45% of healthy subjects aspirate during sleep, and an even higher proportion of severely ill patients aspirate routinely.[70] Although frequently regarded as partially protective, the presence of an endotracheal tube permits the aspiration of oropharyngeal material or bacteria of colonic origin. Depending upon the number and virulence of the organisms reaching the lung, pneumonia may ensue.

Nosocomial pneumonia and especially ventilator-associated pneumonia (VAP) is a common problem in the patients of SCI. They lead to significant morbidity and mortality in the intensive care unit (ICU). Overall, VAP is associated with an attributable mortality of up to 30%.

VAP is typically categorized as either early-onset VAP (occurring in the first 3–4 days of mechanical ventilation) or late-onset VAP. The common organisms responsible for the early-onset VAP is antibiotic-sensitive community-acquired organisms (e.g. *Streptococcus pneumoniae, Haemophilus influenzae,* and *Staphylococcus aureus*). Late-onset VAP is usually caused by antibiotic-resistant nosocomial organisms (e.g. *Pseudomonas aeruginosa,* methicillin-resistant *Staphylococcus aureus, Acinetobacter,* and *Enterobacter* species).

The pathophysiology of VAP is mostly through aspiration of oropharyngeal secretions containing potentially pathogenic organisms. Aspiration of gastric secretions may also contribute, though likely to a lesser degree. Tracheal intubation interrupts the body's anatomic and physiologic defenses against aspiration, making mechanical ventilation a major risk factor for VAP.

The prevention of nosocomial pneumonia especially VAP has got several things to do. They are available in the guideline of different critical care and infectious disease societies to which I wish to refer an interested reader. However, the important points are:

1. Hand washing and barrier precautions
2. Proper use of the nebulizers, humidifiers and other respiratory apparatus, humidifier, spirometers, anesthetic apparatus, etc.
3. Prevention of aspiration by semirecumbent position, bed rotation
4. Prevention of oropharyngeal colonization
5. Prevention of gastric hypochlorhydria
6. Observation of stringent ICU protocols
7. Others as vaccination, preventive antibiotics, etc.

It is to keep in mind that SCI is a special situation and many a times interventions related to movement of the patient is extremely difficult and often restricted.

Here, we wish to refer the reader to the CDC guideline for prevention of nosocomial pneumonia.[72]

Pneumococcal vaccination: It has been observed that irrespective of the post-injury, pneumococcal vaccination can raise immunity in the victims of spinal cord injury against respective types of *Streptococcus pneumoniae*.[73] Hence, ideally, patients of SCI should receive pneumococcal vaccination.

Prevention and Treatment of Complication of Immobilization

Pulmonary embolism: Fatal pulmonary embolism is a major cause of mortality in spinal cord injury.[74] This is because of stasis, hyperviscosity and associated compounding factors in the patient of SCI. Higher age, higher level of injury, higher BMI and more frequent serious infections had statistically higher prevalence of lethal PTE. LMWH appeared more effective in presenting the complication. Prevention of TE in spinal cord injury may be achieved by use one or more of the following:

1. Compression hose or pneumatic device alone or in combination with antithrombotic agents such as aspiration, dipyridamole or heparin. This

should be done in all patients for the initial two weeks of injury. It should be thoroughly inspected for proper placement and the condition of the underlying skin.

2. *Vena cava filter placement:* It is indicated in patients of SCI who have failed anticoagulant prophylaxis or who have a contraindication for anticoagulation. It is also indicated in complete motor paralysis due to lesion in the high cervical cord (above C2, C3), with poor cardiopulmonary reserve or with thrombus in the IVC despite anticoagulant prophylaxis.

3. *Anticoagulant therapy with LMWH (enoxaparin, tinzaparin) or adjusted dose of unfractionated heparin:* It should be initiated within 72 hours of spinal cord injury provided there is no active bleeding or coagulopathy. They should be continued for a long time (8 weeks for uncomplicated complete motor injury, 12 weeks or until discharge from rehabilitation for those with complete motor injury and other risk factors predisposing to increased risk for DVT and PTE. The duration of prophylaxis should be individualized depending on the need, medical condition and the functional status, support services and the risk of the patient.

4. USG of lower extremities or V/Q lung scanney in prophylaxis failure.

5. Mobilization or passive exercise once the patient is medically or surgically stable. With documented DVT, mobilization and exercise of the lower extremities should be withheld for 48–72 hours until appropriate medical therapy is implemented.

6. Training of health-care professionals to recognize signs and symptoms of DVT and apply prophylactic measures with appropriate monitoring the side effects of the agents used.

7. Patient and family education on recognition and prevention of DVT should be done. Here we wish to refer the reader to the relevant literature and guideline by the Paralyzed Veterans of America.[75,76] There has been documented lower mortality, atelectasis and need for MV.[77]

Care of the Associated Issues

All these issues need thorough attention in the patients of SCI.

Nutrition and metabolic factors: Proper nutrition prevents neuromuscular deconditioning and atrophy of muscles. Certain metabolic factors as hypokalemia, hypomagnesemia, hypocalcemia, and alkalosis can all lead to functional neuromuscular deficiency and they can prolong and increase the need of mechanical ventilation. Apart, there is immune dysfunction in inappropriate nutrition which may predispose to infection.

Treatment of OSA, traumatic fat embolism, etc.: OSA has been discussed as more prevalent in SCI patients. It requires proper attention whenever required. Traumatic fat embolism is a situation.

Care of skin, mouth, eye, wounds and other organs: This has been discussed elsewhere.

Care of mental well-being: This is very important to ensure the patients positive outlook to life and a maximum cooperation in the rehabilitation of the patients.

Care of the comorbidities: Comorbidities like diabetes mellitus, renal failure, COPD, etc. need proper attention since they can compound the respiratory care.

Respiratory care and patient education: Patient education should be an integral part of physical therapy. "Shoulder Air" classes stresses on the need for patients to learn to balance shoulders and breathe efficiently.[78] Because of the complications from smoking, smoking cessation efforts for SCI patients should be given to prevent long-term complications.[79] It has been found that on self-reported respiratory problems with patients with chronic SCI, the current smokers with paraplegia have more frequent episodes of phlegm and wheezing.[80]

References

1. DeVivo MJ, Black KJ, Stover SL. Causes of death during the first 12 years after spinal cord injury. Arch Phys Med Rehabil. 1993;74(3):248-54.
2. DeVivo MJ, Krause S, Lammertse DP. Recent trends in mortality and causes of death among persons with spinal cord injury. Arch Phys Med Rehabil. 1999;80:1411-9.
3. Berkowitz M, O'Leary PK, Kruse DL, et al. Spinal cord injury: An analysis of medical and social costs. New York: Demos, 1998.
4. Johnson RL, Brooks CA, Whiteneck GG. Cost of traumatic spinal cord injury in a population-based registry. Spinal Cord. 1996;34(8):470-80.
5. Fishburn MJ, Marino RJ, Ditunno JF Jr. Atelectasis and pneumonia in acute spinal cord injury. Arch Phys Med Rehabil. 1990;71(3):197-200.
6. Jackson AB, Groomes TE. Incidence of respiratory complications following spinal cord injury. Arch Phys Med Rehabil. 1994;75(3):270-5.
7. DeVivo MJ, Black KJ, Stover SL. Causes of death during the first 12 years after spinal cord injury. Arch Phys Med Rehabil. 1993;74(3):248-54.
8. VanBuren RL, Wagner, FC Jr. Respiratory complications after cervical spinal cord injury. Spine. 1994;20:2315-20.
9. Villanueva PA, Ruben BH, Greenberg J. Neurologic injury: prevention and initial care. In: Civetta JM, Taylor RW, Kirby PR (Eds). Critical Care, 3rd edn. Lippincort Raven, Philadelphia PA. pp. 1212.
10. Ayas, N, Garshick, E, Lieberman, SL, Brown, R. Breathlessness in spinal cord injury depends on injury level (abstract). Am J Respir Crit Care Med. 1997;155:A173.
11. Bach JR. Pathophysiology of paralytic-restrictive pulmonary syndromes. In: JR Bach (Ed). Pulmonary rehabilitation: The obstructive and paralytic conditions. Philadelphia: Henley and Belfus; 1996. pp. 275-83.
12. Eger RJ, Turba EM, Yarkony GM, Roth EJ. Cough in spinal cord injured patients: comparison of three methods to produce cough. Arch Phy Med Rehabil. 1993;74:1358-61.
13. Voelker KG, Chetty KG, Mahutte CK. Resolution of recurrent atelectasis in spinal cord injury patients with administration of recombinant Dnase. Intensive Care Med. 1996;22(6):582-4.

14. Jackson AB, Groomes TE. Incidence of respiratory complications following spinal cord injury. Arch Phys Med Rehabil. 1994;75:270-5.
15. Stinneford JG, Keshavarzian A, Nemchausky BA, Doria MI, Durkin M. Esophagitis and esophageal motor abnormalities in patients with chronic spinal cord injuries. Paraplegia. 1993;31(6):384-92.
16. Hsu S, Dreisbach JN, Charlifue SW, English GM. Glottic and tracheal stenosis in spinal cord injured patients. Paraplegia. 1987;25(2):136-48.
17. Euler AR, Ament ME. Gastrophageal reflux in children: clinical manifestations, diagnosis, pathophysiology, and therapy. Pediatric Gastroenterol. 1976;22: 678-89.
18. Britto J, Demling RH. Aspiration and lung injury. New Horiz. 1993;1(3):435-9.
19. Wolff RK, Dolovich MB, Obminski G, Newhouse MT. Effect of exercise and eucapnic hyperventilation on bronchial clearance in man. J Appl Physiol. 1977;43(1):46-50.
20. Clarke SW, Rationale of airway clearance. Eur Resoir J Suppl. 1989;7:599S-603S.
21. Green D, Twardowski P, Wei R, Rademaker AW. Fetal pulmonary embolism in spinal cord injury. Chest. 1994;105(3):853-55.
22. Short DJ, Straddling Jr, Willams SJ. Prevalence of sleep apnoea in patients over 40 years of age with spinal cord lesions. J Neurol Neusurg Psychiatry. 1992;55(11):1032-6.
23. Bach JR, Alba AS, Saporito LR. Intermittent positive pressure ventilation via mouth as an alternative to tracheotomy for 257 ventilator users. Chest. 1993;103(1):174-82.
24. Mckinley WO, Jackson AB, Cardenas DD, et al. Long-term medical complications after traumatic spinal cord injury: a regional model systems analysis. Arch Phys Med Rehabil. 1999;(80):1402-10. (PubMed)
25. Ashba J, Garshick E, Tun CG, et al. Spirometry—acceptability and reproducibility in spinal cord injured subjects. J Am Paraplegia Soc. 1993;16(4):197-203. (PubMed)
26. Roth EJ, Lu A, Primack S, et al. Ventilatory function in cervical and high thoracic spinal cord injury. Relationship to level of injury and tone. Am J Phys Med Rehabil. 1997;76(4):262-7. (PubMed)
27. Ryan M, Klein S, Bongard F. Missed injuries associated with spinal cord trauma. Am Surg. 1993;59(6):371-4. (PubMed)
28. Bain G, Bodley R, Jamous A, et al. A comparison of the chest radiograph and computerised tomography in assessing lung changes in acute spinal injuries: an assessment of their prevalence and the accuracy of the chest X-ray compared with CT in their assessment. Paraplegia. 1995;33(3):121-5. (PubMed)
29. Cahan C, Gothe B, Decker MJ, et al. Arterial oxygen saturation over time and sleep studies in quadriplegic patients. Paraplegia. 1993;31(3):172-9. (PubMed)
30. Kirshblum S, Johnston MV, Brown J, et al. Predictors of dysphagia after spinal cord injury. Arch Phys Med Rehabil. 1999;80(9):1101-5. (PubMed)
31. Spungen AM, Grimm DR, Lesser M, et al. Self-reported prevalence of pulmonary symptoms in subjects with spinal cord injury. Spinal Cord. 1997;35(10):652-7. (PubMed)
32. Fein ED, Grimm DR, Lesser M, et al. The effects of ipratropium bromide on histamine-induced bronchoconstriction in subjects with cervical spinal cord injury. J Asthma. 1998;35(1):49-55. (PubMed)
33. DeLuca RV, Grimm DR, Lesser M, et al. Effects of a beta-2-agonist on airway hyperreactivity in subjects with cervical spinal cord injury. Chest. 1999;115(6): 1533-8. (PubMed)

34. Meschino A, Devitt JH, Koch JP, et al. The safety of awake tracheal intubation in cervical spine injury. Can J Anaesth. 1992;39(2):114-7. (PubMed)
35. Bellamy R, Pitts FW, Stauffer ES. Respiratory complications in traumatic quadriplegia: analysis of 20 years' experience. J Neurosurg. 1973;39(5):596-600. (PubMed)
36. Claxton AR, Wong DT, Chung F, et al. Predictors of hospital mortality and mechanical ventilation in patients with cervical spinal cord injury. Can J Anaesth. 1998;45(2):144-9. (PubMed)
37. Myllynen P, Kivioja A, Rokkanen P, et al. Cervical spinal cord injury: the correlations of initial clinical features and blood gas analyses with early prognosis. Paraplegia. 1989;27(1):19-26. (PubMed)
38. Bach JR. New approaches in the rehabilitation of the traumatic high level quadriplegic. Am J Phys Med Rehabil. 1991;70(1):13-9. (PubMed)
39. Bach JR, Alba AS. Noninvasive options for ventilatory support of the traumatic high level quadriplegic patients. Chest. 1990a;98:613-9.
40. Bach JR, Saporito LR. Criteria for extubation and tracheostomy tube removal for patients with ventilatory failure: a different approach to weaning. Chest. 1996;110(6):1566-71.
41. DeVivo MJ, Ivie CS 3rd. Life expectancy of ventilator-dependent persons with spinal cord injuries. Chest. 1995;108(1):226-32. (PubMed)
42. Tromans AM, Mecci M, Barrett FH, et al. The use of the BiPAP biphasic positive airway pressure system in acute spinal cord injury. Spinal Cord. 1998;36(7): 481-4. (PubMed)
43. Bach JR, Alba AS. Intermittent abdominal pressure ventilator in a regimen of noninvasive ventilatory support. Chest. 1991;93(3):630-6.
44. Bach JR, Rajaraman R, Ballanger F, et al. Neuromuscular ventilatory insufficiency: effect of home mechanical ventilator use vs. oxygen therapy on pneumonia and hospitalization rates. Am J Phys Med Rehabil. 1998;77(1):8-19. (PubMed)
45. Miller HJ, Thomas E, Wilmot CB. Pneumobelt use among high quadriplegic population. Arch Phys Med Rehabil. 1988;69(5):369-72. (PubMed)
46. Gross D, Ladd HW, Riley EJ, et al. The effect of training on strength and endurance of the diaphragm in quadriplegia. Am J Med. 1980;68(1):27-35. (PubMed)
47. Lane CS. Inspiratory muscle weight training and its effect on the vital capacity of patients with quadriplegia. Cardiopulmonary Q. 1982;10:5.
48. Derrickson J, Ciesla N, Simpson N, et al. A comparison of two breathing exercise programs for patients with quadriplegia. Phys Ther. 1992;72(11):763-9. (PubMed)
49. Huldtgren AC, Fugl-Meyer AR, Jonasson E, et al. Ventilatory dysfunction and respiratory rehabilitation in post-traumatic quadriplegia. Eur J Respir Dis. 1980;61(6):347-56. (PubMed)
50. Walker J, Cooney M. Improved respiratory function in quadriplegics after pulmonary therapy and arm ergometry [letter]. N Engl J Med. 1987;316(8):486-7. (PubMed)
51. DiPasquale PA. Exhaler class: a multidisciplinary program for high quadriplegic patients. Am J Occup Ther. 1986;40(7):482-5. (PubMed)
52. Glenn WL, Holcomb WG, McLaughin AJ, et al. Total ventilatory support in a quadriplegic patient with radiofrequency electrophonic respiration. N Engl J Med; 1972. pp. 286-513.
53. Elefteriades JA, Hogan JF, Handler A, Loke JS. Long-term follow-up of bilateral pacing of diaphragm in quadriplegia. N Engl J Med. 1992;326:1433-4.
54. Elefteriadeo JA, Quin JA. Diaphragm pacing. Ann Thoracic Surg. 2002;73(2):691-2.

55. Montero JC, Feldman DJ, Montero D. Effects of glossopharyngeal breathing on respiratory function after cervical cord transection. Arch Phys Med Rehabil. 1967;48(12):650-3. (PubMed)

56. Fugl-Meyer AR. Effects of respiratory muscle paralysis in tetraplegic and paraplegic patients. Scand J Rehabil Med. 1971;3(4):141-50. (PubMed)

57. Estenne M, De Troyer A. Mechanism of the postural dependence of vital capacity in tetraplegic subjects. Am Rev Respir Dis. 1987;135(2):367-71. (PubMed)

58. Hart GB, Strauss MB, Riker J. Vital capacity of quadriplegic patients treated with hyperbaric oxygen. J Am Paraplegia Soc. 1984;7(1):8-9. (PubMed)

59. Spungen AM, Grimn DR, Strakhan M, et al. Treatment with an anabolic agent is associated with improvement in respiratory function in persons with tetraplegia: a pilot study. Mt Sinai J Med, 1999.

60. Segal JL, Brunnemann SR. 4-Aminopyridine improves pulmonary function in quadriplegic humans with longstanding spinal cord injury. Pharmacotherapy. 1997;17(3):415-23. (PubMed)

61. Ferguson GT, Khanchandant NN, Lattin CD, Nieshoff E, Goshgarian HG. Clinical effect of theophylline on inspiratory muscle drive in tetraplegia. J Spinal Cord Medicine. 1998;21(4):362.

62. Brokowski C. A comparison of pulmonary complications in spinal cord injured patients treated with two modes of spinal immobilization. J Neurosci Nurs. 1989;21(2):79-85. (PubMed)

63. Lemons VR, Wagner FC Jr. Respiratory complications after cervical spinal cord injury. Spine. 1994;19(20):2315-20. (PubMed)

64. Green BA, Green KL, Klose KJ. Kinetic Nursing for acute spinal cord injury patients. Paraplegia. 1980;18(3):181-6. (PubMed)

65. Jaeger RJ, Turba RM, Yarkony GM, et al. Cough in spinal cord injured patients: comparison of three methods to produce cough. Arch Phys Med Rehabil. 1993;74(12):1358-61. (PubMed)

66. Kirby NA, Barnerias MJ, Siebens AA. An evaluation of assisted cough in quadriparetic patients. Arch Phys Med Rehabil. 1966;47(11):705-10. (PubMed)

67. Lin KH, Lai YL, Wu HD, et al. Effects of an abdominal binder and electrical stimulation on cough in patients with spinal cord injury. J Formos Med Assoc. 1998;97(4):292-5. (PubMed)

68. Sugerman, B, Brown D, and Muscher D. Fever and infection in spinal cord injury patients. JAMA. 1982;248:66-70.

69. Craven DE; Steger KA; Barber TW. Preventing nosocomial pneumonia: state of the art and perspectives for the 1990s. Am J Med. 1991;91(3B):44S-53S.

70. Craven DE. Steger KA. Epidemiology of nosocomial pneumonia. New perspectives on an old disease. Chest. 1995;108(2 Suppl):1S-16S.

71. Scheld WM. Developments in the pathogenesis, diagnosis and treatment of nosocomial pneumonia. Surg Gynecol Obstet. 1991;172 (Suppl):42-53.

72. Guidelines for Prevention of Nosocomial Pneumonia Summary This document updates and replaces CDC's previously published "Guideline for Prevention of Nosocomial Pneumonia" (Infect Control. 1982;3:327-33, Respire Care. 1983;28:221-32, and Am J Infect Control. 1983;11:230-44).

73. Waites KB, Canupp KC, Edward K, Palmer P, Gray BM, Divivo MJ. Immunogenicity of pneumococcal vaccine in spinal cord injury. Arch Med Rehab. 1998;79(12):1504-09.

74. Grean D, Twardowski P, Wei R, AW Rademaker. Fatal pulmonary embolism in spinal cord injury. Chest. 1994;105(3):853-5.

75. Guidelines by Paralyzed Veterans of America/Consortium for spinal Cord Medicine. Prevention of thromboembolism in spinal cord injury. Washington DC: Paralyzed Vaterans of America (PVA). 1999. p. 29.

76. Prevention of thromboembolism in spinal cord injury. J Spinal cord Med. 1997; 20(3):259-83.

77. McMichan JC, Michel L, West Brook PR. Pulmonary dysfunction following traumatic quadriplegia: Recognition, prevention and treatment. JAMA. 1980;243:528-31.

78. Druin E and Planter K. Shoulder Air Class: a prospective approach to shoulder problem and respiratory insufficiency in patients with spinal cord injuries. J Spinal Cord Med. 1999;22(1):18.

79. Linn WS, Adkins RH, Gong H, Waters R. Pulmonary function in a large southern California outpatient population with chronic spinal cord injury. J Spinal Cord Med. 1999;22(1):27-28.

80. Spungen AM, Grimm DR, Lesser M, Bauman WA, Almenoff PL. Self-reported prevalence of pulmonary symptoms in subjects with spinal cord injury. Spinal Cord. 1997;35(10):652-7.

26

Nutritional Management in Spinal Cord Injuries

Shrabani Sanyal Bhattacharya

Spinal cord injury (SCI) causes traumatic damage to the spine and the cord. But the post-SCI sequel is not limited to the spine only. The complex nature of changes that occur in the body, includes various metabolic and nutritional issues which should be monitored properly.

Metabolic and Endocrine Changes after Spinal Cord Injury

The immobilization and sedentary lifestyle of an SCI patient results in a state of insulin resistance, hyperinsulinemia, and high adiposity, which may precipitate HTN, lipid abnormalities and coronary heart disease.

The dyslipidemia is compounded with the decreased concentration of anabolic endogenous hormones. Reduced testosterone and growth hormone results in changes of body composition. Due to prolonged inactivity, patients undergo osteoporotic changes in the bones which may be associated with low vitamin D and calcium level, reduced anabolic hormones and secondary hyperparathyroidism. These changes of altered body composition, high adiposity and bony structural decline are also associated with altered carbohydrate and lipid metabolism.

Carbohydrate and Lipid Metabolism in Chronic Spinal Cord Injury

Compared to able-bodied population, people with SCI are more likely to have oral carbohydrate intolerance, insulin resistance, elevated low-density lipoprotein cholesterol, and reduced high-density lipoprotein cholesterol, associated with increased prevalence of diabetes mellitus and cardiovascular disease. To reduce mortality and morbidity associated with these risk factors, periodic screening for carbohydrate and lipid abnormalities is recommended, with appropriate therapeutic interventions.

It is also seen that people with SCI having high HDL and high C-reactive protein levels, are more at risk for cardiovascular disease. It is also evident that visceral adipose tissue is more than the subcutaneous adipose tissue in adults with SCI than those without SCI, despite matching waist circumference.

It is seen that adolescents with SCI has higher prevalence of components of 'metabolic syndrome' in comparison to normal individuals and obese SCI patients has higher prevalence than nonobese ones. Metabolic syndrome is defined as having more than or equal to three of the following components (a) Obesity, (b) ADL <45 mg/dL for males and <50 mg/dL for females, (c) Triglyceride 2100 mg/dL, (d) Systolic or diastolic BP more than or equal to 95th percentile for age/height/gender, (e) insulin resistance defined by serum glucose 100–125 mg/dL, fasting insulin more than or equal to 20 micro U/mL.

In acute phase, immediately after SCI the metabolic scenario is a bit different. Usually the patient faces a negative balance status due to high-protein-energy demand for the rapid loss of muscle bulk, infections, bedsore, etc. This hypermetabolic state in early phase justifies the prescription of high protein feeds, to achieve a positive nitrogen balance. Though it is till debatable, because, some experts believe that more than 1.5 g/kg body weight of protein is sufficient and any extra amount is simply oxidized, as acute SCI patients are usually catabolic, a protein rich dietary regime is usually of till, suggested. But after stabilization of trauma when acute events are settled, the factors like adiposity (obesity), high lipid state, etc. are taken into consideration and the nutritional guidelines are suggested accordingly.

Weight Management

The dietary management for preventing overweight, focuses on the balance of energy expenditure and intake of calories. A patient on active rehabilitation, with regular energy consuming exercise has low chances of, developing high adiposity. But patients with reduced physical activities should be recommended a low calorie but high nutrient foods. A lower muscle mass and a decrease in activities cause lower metabolic rate. This means the patient needs fewer calories each day in order to maintain a desirable weight. After rehabilitation, the ideal body weight of a person with SCI is lower than for a non-disabled individual. In figuring the numbers of calories needed by an individual with SCI, dieticians normally decrease the amount of food by 5% for those with paraplegia and 10–15% for those with tetraplegia (quadriplegia).

Basic guidelines for weight control after a spinal cord injury are to:
- Eat foods high in nutrients.
- Balance the calories the patient takes with the calories he burns.
- Choose foods moderate in calories.
- Maintain normal activities without tiring easily.

Understanding Calories, Grams and Nutrients

It is important to know how to get the recommended amount of each nutrient to maintain a patient's desired weight. Before suggesting the menu of a SCI patient, one should design daily food plan based on the recommended daily amounts for each nutrient. This amount is based on a percentage of the total daily calories.

- Carbohydrates—50–60% of total calories
- Protein—20% of total calories
- Fat—30% or less of total calories.

Each nutrient also contains a specific number of calories per gram.

- Carbohydrates = 4 calories/g
- Protein = 4 calories/g
- Fat = 9 calories/g

Fat grams are the most important to count in a weight control program. Using the following formula we can determine the proper amount of fat grams to include in daily food plan.

For example, supposing that a patient can eat 1800 calories each day to maintain the weight. To determine the amount of fat grams each day figure:

- 1800 calories × 0.3 (30%) = 540 calories
- 540 calories/9 g = 60 g or less of fat a day.

We can also adjust this formula to figure the amount (grams) of protein and carbohydrates that a patient needs to eat each day.

Nutritional Management for Cardiac and Urinary Problems after Spinal Cord Injury

Individuals with SCI are at greater risk for cardiovascular and heart problems, since their life span has been increased:

- Too much cholesterol can increase the risk of heart disease. Calculating the amount of cholesterol that the patients eat each day, and checking the cholesterol level during annual medical check-up is mandatory.
- One should need to limit the amount of salt in the daily food plan. Too much salt is a hazard if the person has high blood pressure or heart problems.
- Individuals with spinal cord injuries may be prone to develop renal calculi. Certain beverages can cause crystals to form in the urine. It is better not to eat or drink an excess of dairy products (milk, cheese, yogurt, ice cream).
- The best way to avoid renal or bladder stones is to make water the beverage of choice.

The loss of normal bladder function after SCI increases risk for urinary tract infection (UTI). A high fluid intake everyday reduces the problem of infections and stone forming. The fluids that pass through the kidneys help keep the bladder and catheter relatively clear. We need to understand how much fluid to drink each day to manage the bladder program.

Drinking carbonated beverages like soda pop, orange juice, and grapefruit juice can cause the urine to become alkaline. When urine becomes alkaline it can have a strong, unpleasant odor. Alkaline urine is a breeding ground for bacteria that can cause UTI. It is better to limit the number of these beverages patient drinks each day.

Bowel Management

The neurogenic bowel problem after SCI is a common phenomenon and this results in constipated hard stool formation. A bowel management program including a high fiber diet is an integral part of rehabilitation, the effect of a high fiber diet on large bowel function in SCI requires further classification. The time required for food to move through the gut is slower in neurogenic hypomotile intestine. If the bowel is not emptied on a regular basis, hard stools, and impaction may occur. Sometimes diarrhea occurs with impaction. This type of diarrhea may be incorrectly treated with an antidiarrheal medication.

Drinking water and eating highfiber foods such as fruits, vegetables, whole grains and legumes may help to soften the stool, making it easier for them to pass through the intestines. They also make the stool bulkier, which stimulates movement of the bowel. In addition, peristalsis can be stimulated with vegetables, fruits (especially dried fruits), caffeine and warm fluids with lemon juice.

If high fiber foods are eaten only on occasion, loose stools and incontinence may occur. Therefore, fibrous foods should be gradually increased in the diet until the stools are soft and formed. Adequate fluid in the diet is also essential to help prevent impaction. Once the bowel program and diet are established, eating habits should not be radically altered so that the extremes of constipation and incontinence can be avoided. Although no definitive studies have been done in SCI people, a change of only 25% in the amount of fiber in the diet could cause a significant change in stool consistency. A starting goal of at least 15 g of fiber each day is advised as part of a healthy diet. **Table 26.1** gives a general idea of how much fiber is in different types of food.

Certain foods may cause excessive gas, so substitutions or decreased intake may be necessary. To increase the intake of fiber action of the following factors may be taken under consideration:

- Eating whole meal bread, buns and rolls, not white
- Having a high fiber breakfast, e.g. bran flakes, porridge, oat bran or soya bran
- Cooking potatoes in their skins and eating the skins
- Eating more vegetables, salads and fruits (dried fruit is good)
- Using more pulses (peas, lentils, etc.). Adding to stews, casseroles and salads
- Eating more seeds (linseeds, sunflower seeds, pumpkin seeds).

Table 26.1: Availability of fiber in different types of food		
	Quantity	*Grams of fiber*
Vegetables		
Beans, baked	½ cup	8.8 g
Beans, cooked	½ cup	5.0 g
Dried peas, cooked	½ cup	4.7 g
Fruits		
Apple (with skin)	1 medium	3.5 g
Prunes	3 medium	3.0 g
Orange	1 medium	2.6 g
Banana	1 medium	2.4 g
Cereals		
Bran flakes	1/3 cup	8.5 g
Raisin–bran type	¾ cup	4.0 g
Shredded wheat	2/3 cup	2.6 g
Breads		
Bran muffins	1 muffin	2.5 g
Whole wheat bread	1 slice	1.4 g
Bagels	1 bagel	0.6 g
Milk, Dairy Products	Any amount	0.0 g
Meat, Fish, Seafood	Any amount	0.0 g

Any increase in fiber should be gradually done over a 4–6 week period to prevent bloated feeling and too much gas. Everyone responds a bit differently to different foods and beverages.

It is important to note that:

• Particular foods and beverages are disturbing to a SCI patient.
• Onions, cabbage and beans are gas forming and can induce bloating and excessive flatus.
• Spices and alcohol can be responsible for diarrhea and bowel accidents.
• Coffee and tea are bowel stimulants and can contribute to diarrhea or fecal incontinence.
• Cold carbonated beverages can cause loose motion and bloating.

Proper maintenance of a food record shows that some of these foods or beverages cause problems, it is better to eliminate them from the diet.

Strategies for the Prevention of Osteoporosis

Osteoporosis is a well-known complication of a person with SCI. Strategies for the prevention of osteoporosis include: a balanced diet which provides a calcium intake of at least 800 mg/day; encouragement of a physically active lifestyle; avoidance of smoking and alcohol and caffeine intakes; minimization of glucocorticoid use; promotion of intake of vitamin D, protein, vitamin K, vitamin C and potassium.

Skin Care

Proper nutrition prevents skin from pressure sore development, especially when malnutrition is present. Lack of sufficient nutrients can be the reason that a wound does not heal completely. Nutrients particularly necessary for the health of skin include protein, vitamin C, vitamin A, and zinc.

Protein is primarily found in meat, fowl, fish, eggs, milk and milk products, nuts, and in dried peas and beans. Citrus fruits, tomatoes, peppers, greens, raw cabbage, strawberries, pineapple, and potatoes are a rich sources of vitamin C. Vitamin A is found in dark green and dark yellow vegetables and fruits, egg yolks, liver, and dairy products.

Zinc is primarily found in meat, fish, turkey, whole grain products, sunflower seeds, and dried beans, so food should be balanced containing all these nutrients for SCI patients with high risk of pressure sore, dried and cracked skin.

Adequate fluid intake is also necessary for keeping the skin healthy. In healing, the work of the vitamins and minerals depend upon the presence of water in the body. Water strengthens the skin, making it less susceptible to breakdown.

Bibliography

1. Blissitt PA. Nutrition in acute spinal cord injury. Critical Care Nursing Clinic of North America. 1990;2(3):375-84.
2. Cameron, et al. Assessment of the effect of increased dietary fibre intake on bowel function in patients with spinal cord injury. Paraplegia. 1996;34(5):277-83.
3. Cruse, et al. Facilitation of immune function, healing of pressure ulcers, and nutritional status in spinal cord injury patients. Experimental and Molecular Pathology. 2000;68(1):38-54.
4. Cox, et al. Energy expenditure after spinal cord injury: An evaluation of stable rehabilitating patients. Journal of Trauma-Injury Infection and Critical Care. 1985;25(5):419-23.
5. Donna JR. Obligatory negative nitrogen balance following spinal cord injury. Journal of Parenteral and Enteral Nutrition. 1991;15(3):319-22.
6. Maggioni, et al. Body composition assessment in spinal cord injury subjects. Acta Diabetologica. 2003;40(Suppl 1):183-6.
7. Nuhlicek, et al. Body composition of patients with spinal cord injury. European Journal of Clinical Nutrition. 1988;42(9):765-73.
8. Patrick JK. Nutritional and metabolic response to acute spinal cord injury. Journal of Parenteral and Enteral Nutrition. 1992;16(1):11-5.
9. Perkash A, Brown M. Anemia in patients with traumatic spinal cord injury. Journal of American Paraplegia Society. 1986;9(1-2):10-5.
10. Rodriguez, et al. The metabolic response to spinal cord injury. Spinal Cord. 1997;35(9):599-604.
11. Robabeh, et al. Serum levels of vitamins A, C, and E in persons with chronic spinal cord injury living in the community. Archives of Physical Medicine and Rehabilitation. 2003;84(7):1061-7.
12. Suparna, et al. Clinical Assessment and management of obesity in individuals with spinal cord injury: A review. Journal of Spinal Cord Medicine. 2008;31(4):361-72.

27

Wheelchair Selection and Training in Spinal Cord Injury Patients

Amit Pathak

Introduction

Wheelchair is the primary means of ambulation for the spinal cord injury patient facilitating participation in home, work and community settings.

Wheelchair selection has a functional orientation that considers the users':
1. Needs and goals
2. Home, work, recreational and other community environments
3. Physical and oriental status
4. Financial and community resources
5. Views about social acceptability.

Evaluation

When evaluating, the therapist must consider the patient's immediate as well as long-term needs. The therapist can best assist in wheelchair selection by understanding the clients, personal and medical status.

Personal Status

It includes:
- Age and stature
- Living environment
- Educational or work planning
- Recreational persuits.

The factors, which should be considered in context of private and public environments are:
- Floor surfaces
- Outdoor terrain
- Climate
- Hall spaces
- Doorways

- Workspace design
- Transportability and parking.

Medical Status

- Level of injury
- Type of injury—complete/incomplete
- Neuromuscular status, e.g. muscle tone, postural control and reflexes
- Musculoskeletal status, e.g. range of motion, deformity, strength and endurance
- Sensory status, e.g. skin integrity and anesthetic skin
- Physiological status, e.g. temperature regulation, cardiopulmonary needs and respiration.

Seating Needs

It is important for selection of a wheelchair is attention given to seating and postural needs of the patient.

Goals of Effective Sitting

1. *Prevention of deformity:* By providing a symmetrical base of support and proper skeletal alignment.
2. Accommodation of existing deformity.
3. *Tone normalization:* By providing proper body alignment and bilateral weightbearing, tone normalization can be maximized.
4. *Maximum sitting tolerance:* Wheelchair sitting tolerance will increase as support comfort and symmetrical weightbearing are provided.
5. *Optimal respiratory function:* Support in an erect, well-aligned position can decrease compression of the diaphragm and thus contribute to a vital capacity.
6. *Promotion of function:* Pelvic and trunk stability is necessary to free the upper extremity for participation in the functional activities including wheelchair mobility and daily living skills.
7. *Pressure management:* Pressure sores can be caused by improper alignment and an inappropriate sitting surface.

Proper seat cushions can provide comfort, assist in pelvic and trunk alignment and create a surface that minimizes pressure, heat and shearing, the primary cause of skin breakdown.

Wheelchair Types (On the Basis of Mobility)

Manual

Indications:
- User having sufficient strength and endurance to propel chair
- If manual mobility enhance functional independence
- If user require manual mobility as exercise mobility.

Manual Recline

Indications:
- If the patient is unable to sit upright secondary to hip contractures, poor balance, fatigue
- If a caregiver is available to assist with weight shifts and position changes
- Low socioeconomic status.

Electric

Indications:
- Patient having insufficient strength and endurance to propel manual wheelchair
- Powered mobility as an energy conservation option
- If it is required to increase independence at work and the community.

Power Recline

Indications:
- Patient having potential to operate independently
- If independent weight shifts and position changes indicated for skin care and increased sitting tolerance
- If there are resources for care and maintenance of the equipment
- If patient require quick position changes in the event of hypotension and dysreflexia.

Ergonomic Consideration in Wheelchair Selection

Sizing

Measurement should be determined with user in an optimally seated position. If the patient will wear a brace or body jacket or require any additional devices in the chair, these should be in place during the measurement.

Seat Width

Aims:
- To distribute the patient's weight over the widest possible area
- To keep the overall width as narrow as possible.

Measurement

Widest part across the hips and thighs and typically adds a total of two inches for adequate clearance on the sides **(Fig. 27.1)**.

Seat Depth

From the rare of buttocks to inside of bent knee and 5 cm is subtracted to allow as much weightbearing through the thigh as possible.

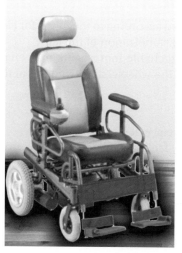

Fig. 27.1: Measurement of wheelchair
(For color version, see Plate 14)

Seat Height

Seat height is based on the positioning of the individual such that footrests have at least 5 cm clearance from the floor. Measurements are taken from under the distal thigh to the heel of the individual's commonly used footwear or shoe.

Back Height

For full trunk support measure from top of the seat post to top of the shoulders. For minimum trunk support, top of back upholstery should permit free arm movement and no skin irritation while providing good total body alignment.

Arm Rest Height

From under each elbow to the cushioned seating surface with shoulder in neutral, the arms hanging at the sides and the elbows flexed to 90°.

Common Components

In addition to overall sizing, user should consider selection of head and neck rests, arm rests, leg rests and other option.

Arm Rest

- User should consider arm rest stability for performing wheelchair push ups for pressure release
- Detachable or swing away types may allow greater ease in sideways transfer
- Attachment of lap tray may require full-length arm rests.

Leg Rests and Foot Plate

- Options are selected according to the needs for elevation of calf and foot, ankle position and stabilization of the leg
- Swing away or detachable foot rigging may enable easy transfers and transportability of the wheelchair in and out of the vehicles.

Castars

- As either front or rear wheels
- Small ones usually facilitate maneuverability.

Seat Belt, Safety Vests and Harness

Vary in design and are used for both safety and positioning.

Other Accessories

- Lap trays can be used for postural support of the upper limbs and serve a variety of purposes related to functional activity
- Other accessories include mounting bags for storage and carrying, bottle holders for taking fluids, etc.

Rim Projections

Patient having insufficient hand grip may use adapted hand rim projection for propulsion of wheelchair.

Wheelchair Safety Measures

1. Brakes should be locked during all transfer.
2. It is advantage to have swing away footrests during most of the transfer.
3. Footplates should never be stood on and during most of the transfer.
4. If the caregiver wishes to push the patient up a ramp, he/she should move in a normal, forward direction.
5. If the caregiver wishes to push the patient down a ramp, he/she should tilt the chair backward by pushing the foot down on the tipping levers.

Wheelchair Maneuvers by Tetraplegic Patient without a Grip

To Manipulate the Brakes

To reach the right brake:
1. Hook the left elbow behind the left chair handle.
2. Lean forward and to the right, allowing the left biceps to lengthen as the trunk movement occurs.

   To release the brake, use flexion of the elbow and shoulder to push the lever forward with the palm of the hand or the lower part of the supinated forearm. To apply the brake, pull the lever back using the right biceps and either the extended wrist (lesion at C6) or the supinated forearm (lesion at C5).

To remove the armrests:
1. Release the catch by pushing down with the base of the thumb over the catch.
2. Hook the right elbow behind the right chair handle.
3. Place the left hand at front and the right hand at the back of the right armrest. Using the wrist extension grip, lift the armrest out of its socket with both hands.
4. Hold the armrest with the left hand and balance it on supinated forearm.
5. Place the armrest on the floor beside the rear wheel or hook it over the left chair handle.

To reach down the footplates:
This position will be necessary to adjust the footplates, to empty the urinal or for adjustment while dressing.
1. Lean forward on the elbows on the armrests.
2. Change the position of the arms one by one and lean on the forearm on thighs.
3. Put one hand at a time down to the foot, leaning the chest on thighs.

To regain the upright position patients without triceps must:
1. Throw the stronger arm back over the backrest and hook the extended wrist behind the chair handle, and
2. Pull the trunk upright by strongly extending the wrist and flexing the elbow.
Patients with good functioning of triceps pull the trunk upright by hooking one or both extended wrist underneath the upper, outer edge of the armrests.

To Lift the Buttocks Forward

Patient with Cervical Lesions with Triceps

To lift the right buttock forward:
1. Lean over the forearm, which is placed well forward on the armrest.
2. Lift with the right hand on the armrest.
3. At the same time, throw the head back and wriggle the right buttock forward.
Repeat this procedure to lift the left buttock forward.

Wheelchair Maneuvers by Paraplegic Patient

To push on the flat: When wheeling on the flat, the push forward with the arms is reinforced if accompanied by strong flexion of the head and shoulder girdle. Momentum is gained due to general forward thrust with the upper part of the body.

To use the Chair on Stopping Ground

To push up a slope:
1. Leaning forward, place the hands towards the back of the top of the tyre.
2. Push forward using flexion of the elbows and flexion and adduction of the shoulders.

To turn the chair to the right

1. Place the right hand towards the back of the tyre with the arm over the backrest behind the chair handle.
2. Laterally, rotate the right arm and with the body weight over the hand push backwards on the inner side of the wheel.
3. Push forward with the left hand.

Wheelchair Prescription on the Basis of Level of Injury

Table 27.1 lists the prescribed types of wheelchair depend on the levels of spinal injury.

Table 27.1: Wheelchair prescription based on type of injury		
Level	*Pattern of weakness*	*Wheelchair prescription*
C1-3	Total paralysis of trunk, upper extremities and lower extremities Dependence on respirator	Propel power wheelchair equipped with portable respirator and chin or breath control
C3-4	Paralysis of trunk, upper extremities and lower extremities Difficulty in breathing and laughing	Power wheelchair with chin or breath control
C5	Absence of elbow extension, pronation and all wrist and hand movements	Indoors—wheelchair with hand rim adaptation Outdoors—power wheelchair
C6	Absence of elbow extension and ulnar wrist extension	Independent in propelling wheelchair on level terrain and minimum grade inclines with plastic or foam coated rims
C7-8	Lack of trunk muscles comprises full shoulder stability	Can propel manual wheelchair (may needs friction tap on hand rims)
C8-T1	Paralysis of lower extremity Endurance reduced	Manage manual wheelchair on all surface Independent wheelchair transfers
T4-9	Partial paralysis of trunk and paralysis of lower extremity	Manual wheelchair with independent transfer and mobility
T10-L2	Paralysis of lower extremities	Wheelchair is chosen for speed, energy conservation and sports
L3-L4	Partial paralysis of L/E hip extension, knee flexion and ankle and foot movements	May use a wheelchair for convenience, energy conservation and sports

28

Orthotic Management in Stroke and Spinal Cord Injury

Mouli Madhab Ghatak, Tanmay Sengupta

Orthotics plays are important role in the process of rehabilitation. An orthosis is an external apparatus worn to restrict or assist movement. Some are prescribed to prevent deformity, some are to improve functional limitation and restoration of the power. So, orthosis or splints are administrated to treat a specific problem.

Types of Splints

Orthosis can be classified according to 2 primary categories.

According to American Society of Hand Therapist (ASHT)

Dynamic Splints

These are designed to augment active motion by assisting a joint through its range or to substitute for lost functions. It includes a resilient component (elastic, rubber band, springs) and a static base on which the movable, resilient component is attached.

Static Splint

It has no resilient component and immobilizes a joint or body part. This type of splint is applied to rest, to protect or to reduce pain or to prevent muscle shortening and contracture.

1. *Serial static:* It achieves a slow, progressive increase in ROM by repeated remoulding. Each remoulding positions the joint at its end ROM.
   It has no movable resilient component, e.g. cylindrical cast designed to reduce PIP joint flexion contracture through frequent removal and remoulding.

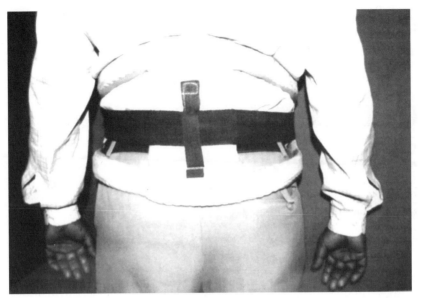

Fig. 28.1: Lumbosacral brace
(*For color version, see Plate 15*)

2. *Static progressive:* It has a static mechanism that adjusts the amount/angle of traction acting upon a part. It includes turnbuckle, nylon line or buckle, e.g. web strap adjusts with Velcro closure.

According to Splint Classification System (SCS) (Fig. 28.1)

Splints

1. Restrictive
2. Immobilizing
3. Mobilizing.

1. *Restrictive:* It limits a specific aspect of ROM but does not completely stop joint motion fully, e.g. Murphy ring splint which blocks PIP joint hyperextension while allowing unlimited pip joint flexion.
2. *Immobilizing:* It may be fit for several reasons including protection to prevent further injury, rest to reduce inflammation or pain and positioning to facilitate proper healing, e.g. resting pan splint to prevent wrist and finger contracture.
3. *Mobilizing:* It is designed to increase limited ROM or to restore or augment a patient's function.

   Upper extremity: Stroke and seg patients may require orthosis of any type as mentioned above for maintaining a body part in position or for functional reactivation for trunk, upper limbs and lower limbs.

Shoulder orthosis: Spasticity can develop slowly after stroke or brain injury. The extremity initially stay in a flaccid state. The weight of hanging arm can cause the shoulder to sublux inferiorly because the supporting muscles are weak. So in order to prevent subluxation the following orthosis are generally prescribed.

1. *Lap board:* Board placed over the arm of the wheelchair can serve as a support for the upper extremity and also erect spinal posture can be maintained.
2. *Arm support:* This is to be done in wheelchair where a string from the overhead bar supports the arm.
3. *Sling:* It is the most common in use to position the arm. The lightweight hemisling is the choice for ambulatory patients.

Elbow orthosis: In elbow region flexor spasticity is very common. This spasticity may lead to contracture if untreated. This is treated by different types of 'casting'. But in recent development turn-buckle with some modification are also used widely.

Wrist and hand orthosis: Spastic forearm flexor muscles causing wrist and finger flexion contractures are very common. Orthosis are used to correct residual contracture or position the wrist and hand or both. Dynamic splints are generally used to correct IP flexion contracture. The splints generally administrated are listed below **(Fig. 28.2)**:

a. *Resting pan splint:*
   - It is single surface static splint.
   - It helps maintain hand in 20°–30° wrist extension, 45°–60° MCP flexion, 15°–30° PIP/DIP flexion.
   - It helps prevent contracture of wrist, web space and PIP and DIP joints.

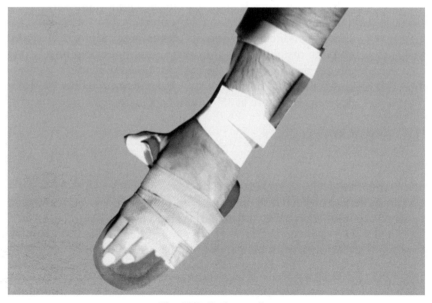

Fig. 28.2: Cock up splint
(For color version, see Plate 15)

- It also maintains hand in functional position.
- It provides rest and helps reduce pain.

b. *Gutter splint:*
  - It is a static splint.
  - It prevents flexion contracture of PIP and DIP joint of finger and maintains proper position of digit.
  - It provides support and relieves pain.

c. *Cock-up splint:*
  - It is also a static splint.
  - It is applied to the volar aspect of the forearm and extends from proximal to distal palmar crease up to the mid forearm.
  - It allows full flexion of fingers.

d. *Short opponens splint:*
  - It is called thumb stabilization splint.
  - It may be used with median nerve injury.
  - It maintains the thumb in opposition and in the position of pinch.
  - It helps achieve normal pinch when there is a paralysis of thumb musculature predominantly in median nerve injury involvement.

e. *PIP–DIP splints:*
  i. Loop splint:
     - It is a dynamic splint.
     - It is made up of lamp wick, elastic, a finger nail loop and rubber band traction.
     - This is used to increase flexion of both PIP and DIP joints.
     - Tension can be adjusted with Velcro closure.
  ii. Three point finger splint:
     - In this splint, force is applied to three points of pressure.
     - It is used to correct PIP and DIP contracture.
     - This designs include two points of pressure, one proximal to joint and one distal and the third or central opposing force acting directly over or close to the joint as shown in figure.
     - This is made up of spring wire, which helps to reduce PIP joint flexion contracture of 35° or less.

Lower Extremity

Below Knee

1. Permanent devices are prescribed once the patient's status stabilizes.
2. An ankle-foot orthosis (AFO) is commonly prescribed to control impaired ankle-foot function. AFO with posterior leaf is used to control drop foot. Solid AFO provide maximum strength and restrict all untoward motion. Dual channel AFO is for patients with sensory impairment.

Above Knee

Knee instability can be stabilized by AFO by placing 5° dorsiflexion or 5° plantarflexion whichever is required but extensive bracing such as knee-

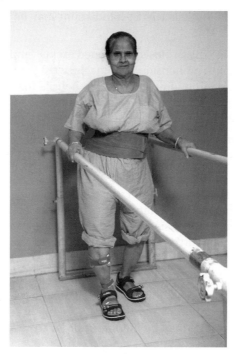

Fig. 28.3: Knee-ankle-foot orthosis
(*For color version, see Plate 16*)

ankle-foot orthosis (KAFO) are also administered in particular cases. In paraplegics having power in hip muscles around 3/5, KAFO is of help for mobility purposes. Usually an elbow crutch gait with KAFO is achieved in these cases. An AFO can be modified according to the patient need. Say, a patient with mediolateral instability of ankle and hyper-extension of knee, we should modify the AFO, so that it can serve both as Swidish Knee Cage and AFO **(Fig. 28.3)**.

Levelwise Orthotic Management of Spinal Cord Injury

C4 motor level: The patient with a complete C4 motor level injury loses the power in elbow and wrist and cannot use any dynamic orthosis. Static wrist hand orthosis is generally prescribed to maintain functional position of hand and wrist by placing the wrist in 20° extension and holding the thumb in abduction along with support on palmar arc. The patient is benefited, as it is effective to prevent contracture especially in case of possibility of neurological return distal to the injury. Another orthosis that can be recommended to some energetic patients is a mouth stick, through which some special work like page turning, etc. can be performed after proper training.

C4 motor level with some C5 return: The C4 patient may develop some C5 return. A mobile arm support can be attached with the wheelchair to obtain horizontal movement. OT makes the patient able to place the hand for functional activities. A ratchet-wrist-hand splint may be useful when used in conjunction with MAS.

Ratchet-W-H orthosis: This orthosis is designed exclusively for the patient with the level to accomplish prehension. It holds the wrist joint in a static position while thumb, index and middle finger in prehensile manner. Prehension is possible by motion of the contralateral hand against the finger pieces to flex the fingers against the thumb.

C5 motor level with some C6 return: Here the wrist extensors will attain some power, so a wrist-action wrist-hand orthosis (WAWHO) may be used for a short period.

C6 motor level: At the C6 motor level, the patient has intact radial extensors, which helps the individual to harness the tenodesis action of the wrist to accomplish dynamic prehension for feeding and hygiene. The tenodesis or wrist-driven wrist-hand orthosis (WDWHO) transfers the power of the wrist extensors to finger flexors to attain prehension.

C7 motor level: At the C7 motor level the patient has intact triceps, which may help in many ADL activities. Though there may be some strength in finger extensors or flexors or both still proper hand function remains a problem. Again tenodesis orthosis may be helpful in order to strengthen remaining muscle power and restrict radial deviation.

C8 motor level: At C8 motor level, the patient has intact finger flexion. Thus, a static WHO is prescribed. It holds thumb in opposition and middle and index fingers in prehension. An extra lumbrical bar is provided for the intrinsic minus hand to prevent clawing. If clawing is already exists, then a Knuckle–Bender may be useful.

T1–L5 motor level: Patients with thoracic or lumbar spinal cord injuries are paraplegics. It is found that useful walking can be achieved in patients with complete lesion below T12. Above T12, due to excessive energy consumption, it is practically not possible for the patient to walk for a prolong time. But it must be firmly noted that orthosis assisted standing can prevent joint contracture, lowering osteoporosis and enhance all physiological and metabolic process.

L1 motor level: At L1 motor level though hip flexors return but patient may not have the power to stabilize his/her hip. Hip-knee-ankle-foot orthosis (HKAFO) may be the choice to ambulate the patient with the help of crutch in swing through manner. A para walker or Hip guidance orthosis can be given for free functional operation and support lower thoracic region.

L2 motor level: At this level, patient is lacking adequate power of quadriceps. Therefore, bilateral KAFO with soft padding can make the patient ambulatory.

L3–S1 motor level: As the knee extensor are intact, bilateral AFO can be sufficient if there is no other sign of knee instability or Genu recurvatum. AFO with different types such as 90° stop, D/F assist, P/F assist, etc. are prescribed according to the patient's need **(Figs 28.4 and 28.5)**.

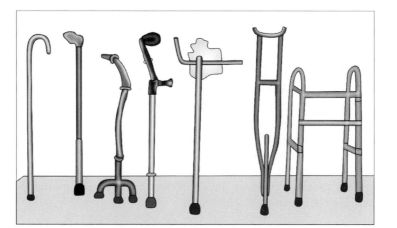

Fig. 28.4: Different types of crutches, canes, walker, etc.

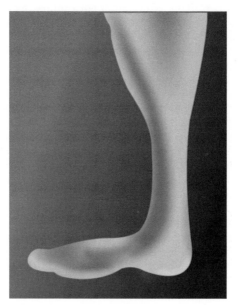

Fig. 28.5: Ankle-foot orthosis (with foot drop prevention)

Advanced Orthosis

With the time and advancement of medical science, many orthosis are being invented day to day, which offer remarkable progress and better compliance. Reciprocal gait orthosis or RGO is one of such orthosis, which is now widely seen, in clinical practice to ambulate paraplegic. It gives structural support to the lower trunk and limbs while allowing walking by means of cable coupling system. It is designed in such a manner so that flexion of one limb transmits external power to the opposite limb. In some RGOs, a push-pull cable is used to increase the efficiency of locomotion. Those patients who have weak extensors are getting benefited from this.

Conclusion

To improve the outcome and results of stroke and seg rehab orthotics plays a great role if it is correctly applied. For application of an orthosis, the proper time and stage of the disease and the exact nature of the disabling condition should be identified. With the modern advancement of the science of orthotics especially with the introduction of electrically powered materials a new horizon of rehab is now rapidly growing up and the more the electronic science with develop, the more advanced technologies will gradually come up to replace the conventional orthotics.

Bibliography

1. Barbecue, et al. Walking after spinal cord injury: Evaluation, treatment and functional recovery. Archive of Physical Medicine and Rehabilitation. 1999;80(2):225-35.
2. Behrman, et al. Locomotor training progression and out comes after incomplete spinal cord injury. Phys Ther. 2005;85:1356-71.
3. Buurke, et al. The effect of an ankle foot orthosis on walking ability in chronic stroke patients: A randomized controlled trial. Clin Rehabil. 2004;18:550-7.
4. Buurke, et al. Usability of thenar eminence orthoses: Report of comparative study. Clin Rehabil. 1999;13:288-94.
5. Dunning, et al. A four week, task specific neuroprosthesis program for a person with no active wrist or finger movement because chronic stroke. Phys Ther. 2008;88:397-405.
6. Engen. Development of externally powered upper extremity orthotic system. J Bone Joint Surg Br. 1965;47B:465-8.
7. Farmer, et al. Dynamic orthoses in the management of joint contracture. J Bone Joint Surg Br. 2005;87B:291-5.
8. Jaeger, et al. Rehabilitation technology for standing and walking after spinal cord injury. Am J Phys Med and Rehabil. 1989;68(3):111-59.
9. Jan Bruckner. Design for a soft orthosis, suggestion from the field. Phys Ther. 1985;65:1522-3.
10. Jhon D Stewart. Foot droop, where, why and what to do? Pract Neurol. 2008;8:158-69.
11. Lobley, et al. Orthotic design from the New England regional spinal cord injury center: Suggestion from the field. Phys Ther. 1985;65:492-3.
12. Marsolaiset, et al. Orthoses and electrical stimulation for walking in complete paraplegia. Neurorehabil Neural Repair. 1991;5:13-22.
13. Mayr, et al. Prospective, blinded, randomized crossover study of gait rehabilitation in stroke patient using the locomat gait orthosis. Neurorehabil Neural Repair. 2007;21(4):307-14.
14. Mulcahey MJ. Upper limb orthoses for the person with spinal cord injury, Chapter-15, 203-212, AAOS Atlas of Orthoses and Assistive Devices, 4th edn. MOSBY, Elsevier.
15. Opera, et al. Effect of selected assistive device on normal distance gait characteristics. Phys Ther. 1985;65:1188-91.

16. Page, et al. Resistance-based, reciprocal upper and lower limb locomotor training in chronic stroke: Randomized cross over study. Clin Rehabil. 2008;22:610-7.
17. Roy, Blamire. The functional shoulder orthosis in hemiplegic shoulder subluxation: A pilot study. Clin Rehabil. 1989;3:107-09.
18. Schmeisser, Seamone. An upper limb prosthesis-orthosis power control system with multi-level potential. J Bone Joint Surg Am. 1973;55:1493-501.
19. Shu, Mirka. A laboratory study of the effect of wrist splint orthosis on forearm muscle activity and upper extremity posture. Human Factors. 2006;48:499-510.
20. Winchester, et al. A comparison of paraplegic gait performance using two types of reciprocating gait orthosis. Prosthet Orthot Int. 1993;17(2):101-06.

Section 3

Brain Injury Rehabilitation

Traumatic brain injury (TBI), results a wide spectrum of disability out of damage to the central nervous system in a dissimilar and variable manner and highly dependable on the nature, extent and site of brain damage. In contrary to cerebrovascular accident, it is frequently associated with epileptic attacks, endocrinal disturbance and a variety of neurobehavioral changes, etc. Moreover, the paralytic, dystonic and focal neurodisability complicates the whole scenario. And so the rehabilitation of TBI demands a highly specialized and individualistic service with multidisciplinary approach. Rehab approach and outcome in TBI varies widely. The outcome is definitely different from a person with a vegetative state to a near normal disable individual out of TBI.

29

Consequences of Traumatic Brain Injury

Indrajit Roy

Traumatic brain injury (TBI) is such a common accompaniment of spinal injuries and may produce that it devastating consequences but it is natural to be included in a book dealing with spinal injuries. It is usually for the sequelae of TBI to be grouped under *neurophysical sequelae* and *neurobehavioral sequelae*. The former refers to focal neurological deficits like cranial nerve defects, hemiparesis, post-traumatic seizures, etc. Neurobehavioral sequelae, on the other hand, include impairments of memory, attention, language, perception, and changes in behavior. Obviously, both the groups greatly influence the quality of life and the final outcome of the injury. It is also important to bear in mind the fact that both the groups can, and often do, co-exist and profoundly affect the management of each other. The patient with post-traumatic epilepsy will very often exhibit behavioral changes, while attention and language deficits can make the task of rehabilitating a hemiplegic person much more complex. Hart and coworkers asked a group of patients to rate themselves in the three domains of physical cognitive and behavioral functioning following TBI and compared the results with those made by physicians. They found that patients rated themselves highest in the behavioral domain and lowest in the physical, irrespective of their physicians' assessment. The lack of awareness of the neurobehavioral sequelae among the sufferers often delays and impedes treatment of this group of conditions.

In order to bring uniformity in the assessment of global disability following TBI the Glasgow Outcome Scale is frequently used. It is a five-point scale which comprises (1) Death; (2) Persistent vegetative state; (3) Severe disability-dependent with physical or psychological disabilities or both; (4) Moderate disability-disabled but independent; (5) Good recovery-normal or near normal recovery. The outcome, however, is significantly affected by the time of assessment after injury. It has been found that one third of patients in group-3 at three months post injury will improve to group 4 if seen one year after injury. Similarly, one third of patients in group 4 at three months will show good recovery in a year. Most patients will have maximal recovery in six months to one year, after which very few will have any major improvement in neurological status. If the Glasgow outcome scale is divided into favorable, i.e. 4 and 5, and unfavorable, i.e. 1,2,3, groups, the score at six months is 94% accurate in predicting the long-term prognosis.

Consequences of TBI are not always directly proportional to the severity of the injury. Kraus et al. classified all TBI into severe, moderate, and mild according to the following criteria. Patients having a Glasgow coma scale of 8 and below were categorized as severe. Moderately injured patients were those who had a hospital stay of at least 48 hours and any one of the followings: abnormal CT scan findings, or brain surgery, or Glasgow coma scale between 9 and 12. All other patients were classified as minor. None of the groups, however, were immune from long-term debilitating and devastating consequences of brain trauma.

Neurophysical Sequelae

Post-traumatic epilepsy may be considered to be one of the most common sequelae among the survivors of moderate to severe TBI. Within the first year of TBI the incidence of seizures exceeds 12 times the population risk. It has been assessed to be present in a frequency of 5–18.9% of civilian and 32–50% of military patients. Temkin has shown that subgroups with significantly elevated risk of developing post-traumatic seizures include those with evacuation of a subdural hematoma; surgery for an intracerebral hematoma; Glasgow coma scale in the severe range of 3–8; early seizures, especially delayed early seizures; time to follow commands of a week or more; depressed skull fracture that was not surgically elevated; dural penetration by injury; at least one non reactive pupil; and parietal lesions on CT scan.

Cerebrospinal fluid fistulae may be detected immediately after injury but may be revealed from months to years after the accident. It is possible that a small leak may have been missed during the management of acute TBI and is detected only when the patient develops florid meningitis. (*See* case reports-SB). More likely, however, the bony defect is produced by the original trauma and pulsation of the meninges causing enlargement of the defect and rupture of the arachnoid at a later date. Fractures of the frontal bone involving the paranasal sinuses produce CSF rhinorrhea, while fractures of the petrous bone involving the mastoid air cells usually give rise to CSF otorrhea. Both fractures can give rise to a posterior nasopharyngeal leak that is perceived by the patient as a salty tasting posterior nasal drip. Frontal orbital injury can cause a leak through the orbit producing the so called "CSF tears".

Cranial nerve injuries are frequently diagnosed late due to the difficulty of performing a thorough neurological examination in an unconscious and critically ill patient. The cranial nerves I, VII and VIII are more frequently involved, followed by II and III. The trunk of the trigeminal and the lower cranial nerves are injured least frequently. Loss of smell, when it occurs is usually complete and permanent. The condition is not as trivial as it may seem as it greatly interferes with taste by removing all flavors from food. Facial nerve injury, apart from being cosmetically unacceptable, also puts the cornea at risk. Fortunately, the last condition is often treatable with fairly good results. Compared to the last two injuries a unilateral deafness interferes less with the patient's day to day living and may be more acceptable. Injuries to the optic nerves may result in permanent loss of vision on the affected side and is not amenable to treatment. Third nerve injuries can interfere with vision by producing ptosis. If the ptosis is corrected the even greater problem of diplopia results. Malfunctioning of the lower cranial nerves, though not a frequent sequel of TBI, can be life-threatening when present. Swallowing difficulty is a serious finding in the pediatric age group and the importance of clinical observation is paramount in this condition. Recently some Australian authors have attempted to correlate post-TBI dysphagia in children with cognitive defects thereby suggesting a multifactorial etiopathology for the condition.

Endocrine dysfunction has been reported to be present in 53% of patients with moderate to severe TBI, and hypogonadism and cortisol hyporesponsiveness were the most common abnormalities found. Bondanelli et al found that TBI might be associated with impairment of pituitary hormone secretion, which may contribute to long term physical, cognitive, and psychological disability. They found pituitary dysfunction in 54% of their patients and also suggested that the condition was directly related to the severity of the injury. In their series, 37.5%, 57.1% and 59.3% of mild, moderate and severe cases of TBI were respectively associated with some abnormality of pituitary function. In another study, 17–36% of males with a history of TBI were found to have developed some kind of ejaculatory problem including premature ejaculation.

Motor paralysis and spasticity may be a direct result of damage to the motor cortex or the pyramidal pathways in the brain caused by the injury. It may also be caused by post-traumatic infarction resulting from vasospasm due to carbon dioxide depletion, reduced perfusion pressure due to raised intracranial tension, or brain herniation. Although, the paralysis may be incomplete the accompanying spasticity or render the affected part quite useless. Intervening early in the course of the disease can only prevent such profound functional impairment. Formation of contractures can further complicate the management of TBI patients. Ankle contractures, in particular, can make walking impossible. Fortunately recent reports suggest that its incidence is far lower than previously estimated.

Cerebellar symptoms, extrapyramidal features and ataxia may all be present as a consequence of TBI depending on the site of the injury. They not only make ambulation and self-care extremely difficult but also may make independence and return to gainful employment impossible.

Hydrocephalus may result from blockage of the cerebrospinal fluid pathways by blood. Hypoxic insults to the brain have also been held responsible for third ventricular dilation. Approximately 50% of severely brain injured patients develop hydrocephalus and some of them require surgical treatment. Hydrocephalus may contribute to behavioral changes and post-traumatic epilepsy.

Heterotopic calcification and ossification may occur within a month of the injury, but is also known to have appeared after years. The condition is more common in spinal injuries and the cause is not yet known. It commonly develops around the hip, knee and elbow. Swelling, redness and increased local temperature may be early signs of this complication.

Post-traumatic glioma developing in the scar of an old TBI is now accepted as a possibility. It has been demonstrated to occur at the site of an old injury to the brain in patients without any evidence of tumor being present in the immediate post injury CT scan. Moorthy and Rajsekhar have proposed a new criterion for the radiological diagnosis of these tumors.

Neurobehavioral Sequelae

Post-traumatic syndrome is a group of symptoms commonly seen among survivors of mild TBI. The consistency of its symptomatology has convinced most people of its actual existence. Patients suffering from this condition may present with any of the following complaints: headache, emotional laibility, sleep abnormalities and dizziness. They may also have problems with concentration and memory, personality changes, and anxiety or depression. About 93% of patients with uncomplicated TBI will have one or more of these symptoms ten days after the injury and most of them will be symptom-free within three months. A small number will, however, have persistent complaints at one year or beyond. Clinical examination of a patient with this syndrome will not reveal any significant neurological abnormality and the nature of the complaints makes objective assessment impossible. The morbid anatomy of the condition remains unclear.

Memory and attention deficits have been assessed to be present in the form of impaired learning and retention of new information in about half of severely brain injured patients. It has also been postulated that presence of at least one nonreacting pupil after injury was a better predictor of subsequent memory defect than a low score on the Glasgow coma scale. Recovery of memory after severe injuries occurs during the first six months but the improvement is negligible. In contrast, memory returns to normal or near normal levels within three months of a mild injury. The memory deficits in post-TBI patients is disproportionate to any intellectual deficits and they exhibit impairment of visual and verbal memory even in the presence of intelligence levels comparable to the average normal population. Attention disorders may include cognitive defects involving phasic alertness or quickness of response, selective attention or ability of selecting appropriate data, sustained attention over a minimum of 20 minutes, focused attention, and the speed of data processing or divided attention. All types of attention defects are found in patients who survive TBI. Mildly injured patients usually recover within three months of injury, and moderately injured patients show near normal attention by two years. After severe TBI, attention defects may persist much longer and even be permanent. Spatial attention defects have been shown to recover in less than half the patients during the acute phase of TBI and neglect of the contralateral limb is a negative prognostic factor for functional motor recovery. Recent work suggests the involvement of basal forebrain, hippocampal formation, and regions of the neocortex, pointing to cholinergic dysfunction as the etiologic factor responsible for cognitive and memory defects. Ariza et al have described the effects of hypoxia and hypotension in TBI and suggested that these factors are of great importance in producing cognitive and memory disorders. (1) It has also been shown that age (>45), delay in starting enteral feeding, and pneumonia during the acute phase subsequently led to extensive, long-lasting cognitive, emotional and functional problems. Along with age, educational level, and lack of job qualification, cognitive impairment remains one of the most difficult impediments to adaptation and return to work following TBI.

Neuropsychiatric symptoms such as depression, mania, anxiety, psychosis, apathy, and sleep disturbance are common after TBI. Obsession, compulsion and obsessive compulsive disorder are other recognized sequelae. Both, moderate to severe and mild TBI are associated with an increased risk of subsequent psychiatric illness. While there is a higher initial risk in patients with moderate to severe TBI, persistent psychiatric illness is more common among those who suffer a mild injury. There is a great deal of disagreement regarding the exact area of the brain while it is injured to produce a particular psychiatric symptom. Functional imaging of the brain with positron emission tomography may provide more definitive information in the future.

Case Reports

RM. A 22-year-old, male sustained closed head injury and was hospitalized in September 2001 with a GCS score of 7. CT scan showed brain stem injury and he required ventilatory support for ten days. He went home with cognitive and speech defects, and right hemiparesis. He showed steady improvement with psychiatric care and intensive physiotherapy. By January 2005 he has become self-supporting and independent with mild, residual spasticity and moderate dysarthria. He is now employed as a computer operator **(Figs 29.1 to 29.3)**.

SB. A 25-year-old, male, engineering student was injured in a two-wheeler accident in March 2001. He underwent two craniotomies for SDH and left parietal contusion and had to be provided ventilatory support in the post-operative period. He was sent home with considerable cognitive and motor deficit. In January 2002, he started having convulsions and CT scan showed hydrocephalus which was treated with a ventriculo-peritoneal shunt. Soon after he developed shunt blockage and respiratory tract infection. He improved with shunt revision and antibiotics, but came back with CSF rhinorrhea and pyogenic meningitis. The meningitis was controlled with great difficulty and craniotomy was performed to repair the dural defect with fascia-lata. He remained drowsy after the operation, and CT scan showed hydrocephalus

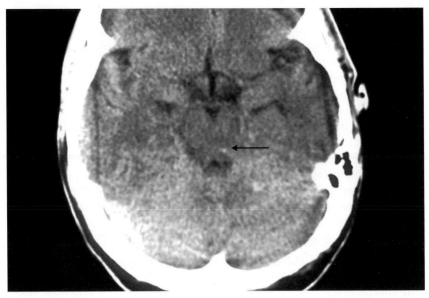

Fig. 29.1: CT scan RM September, 2001

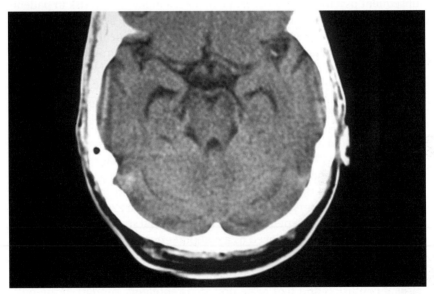

Fig. 29.2: CT scan RM February, 2002

necessitating a second ventriculo-peritoneal shunt, this time on the left side. Since then, he has gradually improved with the help of psychiatrist, physiotherapist and speech therapist. Although, he cannot resume his career in engineering. He is now self-caring and independently ambulant with intact mental faculties **(Figs 29.4 to 29.6)**.

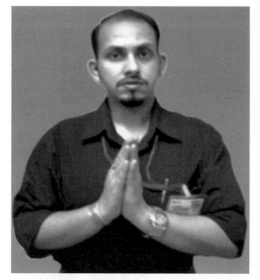

Fig. 29.3: RM January, 2005
(For color version, see Plate 16)

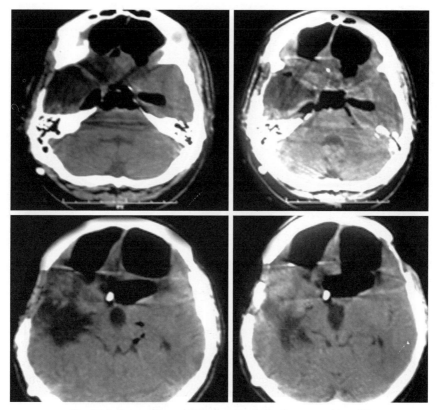

Fig. 29.4: Pneumoencephalocele with cerebral compression—SB

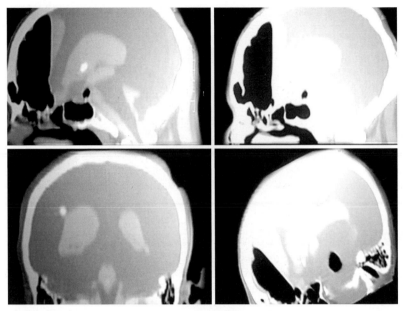

Fig. 29.5: Ventriculogram of same patient. Note defects in frontal and paranasal sinuses

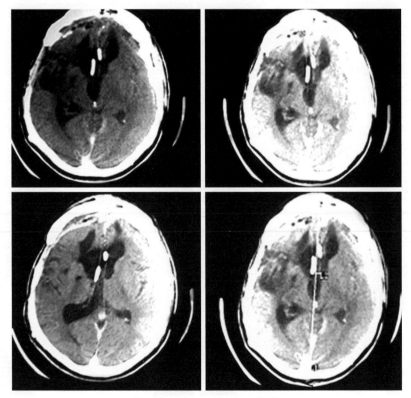

Fig. 29.6: CT scan in June, 2003

Conclusion

Traumatic brain injury can indeed have catastrophic consequences on the quality of life of the survivor. Proper diagnosis and adequate and timely treatment, however, can often provide major relief to the victim. This is one condition that severely tests the skills of the treating physicians as well as the patience and the perseverance of the caregivers at every stage. The rewards of such efforts can sometimes be very great, but one has to be prepared to face frustration and defeat at every step. In the final count, it is the cooperation of the patient and his will to win that really makes the difference between a helpless, pitiable cripple, and an independent dignified individual. The latter is one of the finest examples of the indomitable human spirit that no adversity can defeat.

Bibliography

1. Ariza M, Mataró M, Poca MA, Junqué C, Garnacho A, Amorós S, Sahuquillo J. Influence of extraneurological insults on ventricular enlargement and neuropsychological functioning after moderate and severe traumatic brain injury. J Neurotrauma. 2004;21(7):864-76.
2. Bohnen N, Twijnstra A, Jolles J. Posttraumatic and emotional symptoms in different subgroups of patients with mild head injury. Brain Inj. 1992;6:481.
3. Bondanelli M, De Marinis L, Ambrosio MR, Monesi M, Valle D, Zatelli MC, Fusco A, Bianchi A, Farneti M, degli Uberti EC. Occurrence of pituitary dysfunction following traumatic brain injury. J Neurotrauma. 2004;21(6):685-96.
4. Bushnik T, Englander J, Duong T. Medical and social issues related to posttraumatic seizures in persons with traumatic brain injury. J Head Trauma Rehabil. 2004;19(4):296-304.
5. Cairns H. Injuries of the frontal and ethmoidal sinuses with special reference to cerebrospinal rhinorrhea and aeroceles. J Laryngol. 1937;52:589.
6. Caveness WF. Epilepsy, a product of trauma in our time. Epilepsia. 1976;17:207-15.
7. Choi SC, Barnes TY, Bullock R, et al. Temporal profile of outcomes in severe head injury. J Neurosurg. 1994;81:169-73.
8. Dimopoulou I, Tsagarakis S, Theodorakopoulou M, Douka E, Zervou M, Kouyialis AT, Thalassinos N, Roussos C. Endocrine abnormalities in critical care patients with moderate-to-severe head trauma: incidence, pattern and predisposing factors. Intensive Care Med. 2004;30(6):1051-7.
9. Fann JR, Burington B, Leonetti A, Jaffe K, Katon WJ, Thompson RS. Psychiatric illness following traumatic brain injury in an adult health maintenance organization population. Arch Gen Psychiatry. 2004;61(1):53-61.
10. Farne A, Buxbaum LJ, Ferraro M, Frassinetti F, Whyte J, Veramonti T, Angeli V, Coslett HB, Ladavas E. Patterns of spontaneous recovery of neglect and associated disorders in acute right brain-damaged patients. J Neurol Neurosurg Psychiatry. 2004;75(10):1401-10.
11. Franulic A, Carbonell CG, Pinto P, Sepulveda I. Psychosocial adjustment and employment outcome 2, 5 and 10 years after TBI. Brain Inj. 2004;18(2):119-29.
12. Geisler WO, Jousse AT. Rehabilitation after central nervous system lesions, in Neurological Surgery. Youmans JR, WB Saunders Co, USA; 1996. pp. 3715-27.

13. Gissane W, Rank BK. Post-traumatic cerebrospinal rhinorrhoea with case report. Br J Surg. 1940;27:717.

14. Grados MA. Obsessive-compulsive disorder after traumatic brain injury. Int Rev Psychiatry. 2003;15(4):350-8.

15. Hart T, Sherer M, Whyte J, Polansky M, Novack TA. Awareness of behavioral, cognitive, and physical deficits in acute traumatic brain injury. Arch Phys Med Rehabil. 2004;85(9):1450-6.

16. Hugenholtz H, Stuss DT, Stethem LL, et al. How long does it take to recover from a mild concussion? Neurosurgery. 1988;22:853-8.

17. Jennett B, Bond M. Assessment of outcome after severe brain damage: A practical scale. Lancet. 1975;1:480-4.

18. Jennett B, Snoek J, Bond MR, et al. Disability after severe head injury: Observations on the use of the Glasgow Outcome Scale. J Neurol Neurosurg Psychiatry. 1981;44:285-93.

19. Joshi KK, Crockard HA. Traumatic cerebrospinal fluid fistula simulating tears. J Neurosurg. 1978;49:121.

20. Keane JR, Baloh RW. Post-traumatic Cranial Neuropathies, in Neurology and Trauma: Evans RW—ed., WB Saunders Co., USA, 1996.

21. Kraus JF, Fife D, Conroy C. Pediatric brain injuries: The nature, clinical course and early outcome in a defined US population. Pediatrics. 1987;79:501.

22. Lee HB, Lyketsos CG, Rao V. Pharmacological management of the psychiatric aspects of traumatic brain injury. Int Rev Psychiatry. 2003;15(4):359-70.

23. Levin HS, Eisenberg HM, Gary HE, et al. Intracranial hypertension in relation to memory functioning during the first year after severe head injury. Neurosurgery. 1991;28:196-200.

24. Levin HS, Gary HE Jr, Eisenberg HM, et al. Neurobehavioral outcome one year after severe head injury: Experience of the Traumatic Coma Data Bank. J Neurosurg. 1990;73:699-709.

25. Levin HS, Mattis S, Ruff RM, et al. Neurobehavioral outcome following minor head injury: A three-center study. J Neurosurg. 1987;66:234-43.

26. Lewin W. Cerebrospinal fluid rhinorrhea in closed head injuries. Br J Surg. 1954;42:1.

27. Mazzini L, Campini R, Angelino E, Rognone F, Pastore I, Oliveri G. Post-traumatic hydrocephalus: a clinical, neuroradiologic, and neuropsychologic assessment of long-term outcome. Arch Phys Med Rehabil. 2003;84(11):1637-41.

28. Mincy JE. Post-traumatic cerebrospinal fluid fistula of the frontal fossa. J Trauma. 1966;6:618.

29. Moorthy RK, Rajshekhar V. Development of glioblastoma multiforme following traumatic cerebral contusion: case report and review of literature. Surg Neurol. 2004;61(2):180-4.

30. Morgan A, Ward E, Murdoch B. Clinical characteristics of acute dysphagia in pediatric patients following traumatic brain injury. J Head Trauma Rehabil. 2004;19(3):226-40.

31. Morgan A, Ward E, Murdoch B. Clinical progression and outcome of dysphagia following paediatric traumatic brain injury: A prospective study. Brain Inj. 2004;18(4):359-76.

32. Raaf J. Post-traumatic cerebrospinal fluid leaks. Arch Surg. 1967;95:648.

33. Russell WR. The Traumatic Amnesias. New York, Oxford University Press. 1971.

34. Salmond CH, Chatfield DA, Menon DK, Pickard JD, Sahakian BJ. Cognitive sequelae of head injury: involvement of basal forebrain and associated structures: Brain. 2005;128(1):189-200.

35. Salvati M, Caroli E, Rocchi G, Frati A, Brogna C, Orlando ER. Post-traumatic glioma. Report of four cases and review of the literature. Tumori. 2004;90(4): 416-9.

36. Sibony PA, Anand AK, Keuskamp PA, et al. Posttraumatic cerebrospinal fluid cyst of the orbit. J Neurosurg. 1985;62:922.

37. Simpson G, McCann B, Lowy M. Treatment of premature ejaculation after traumatic brain injury. Brain Inj. 2003;17(8):723-9.

38. Singer BJ, Dunne JW, Singer KP, Jegasothy GM, Allison GT. Non-surgical management of ankle contracture following acquired brain injury. Disabil Rehabil. 2004;26(6):335-45.

39. Singer BJ, Jegasothy GM, Singer KP, Allison GT, Dunne JW. Incidence of ankle contracture after moderate to severe acquired brain injury. Arch Phys Med Rehabil. 2004;85(9):1465-9.

40. Stuss DT, Ely B, Hugenholtz H, et al. Subtle neuropsychological deficits in patients with good recovery after closed head injury. Neurosurgery. 1985;17:41.

41. Till JS, Marion JR. Cerebrospinal fluid masquerading as tears. South Med J. 1987;80:639.

42. Van Zomeren AH, Deelman BG. Long-term recovery of visual reaction time after closed head injury. J Neurol Neurosurg Psychiatry. 1978;41:452-7.

43. Vitaz TW, Jenks J, Raque GH, Shields CB. Outcome following moderate traumatic brain injury. Surg Neurol. 2003;60(4):285-91.

44. Zafonte R, Elovic EP, Lombard L. Acute care management of post-TBI spasticity. J Head Trauma Rehabil. 2004;19(2):89-100.

30

An Outline of Brain Injury Rehabilitation

Bhabani Kumar Chowdhury

Introduction

The admittance of cases with traumatic brain injury (TBI) to trauma centers or medical emergency departments are increasing day by day due to modernization of lifestyles. Most frequently admitted patients are children and babies but the mean age group in our country is 20–35. The average mortality rate is more than 30% of the cases admitted with TBI. Road Traffic Accidents (RTA), fall from tree or roof, alcoholism and less commonly sports activities are the most common causes of TBI.

Traumatic brain injury (TBI) describes a wide range of conditions and has in the past been used interchangeably with the term "Head Injury". The use of the prefix "Trauma" differentiates this group of patients from those who have sustained any disruption to the vascular supply of the brain. TBI may often accompany other types of injuries particularly of skull fracture, which may be simple or compound, undisplaced or depressed, etc. along with injury to other peripheral parts of body. The damage to the brain may be caused either at the time of injury which is termed as primary or as a result of other injuries or their complications (secondary).

The potential problems and complications of TBI includes hydrocephalus, epilepsy, cranial neuropathy (mostly I, III, IV, VI and VIII) neuroendocrinal and autonomic dysfunction, urinary incontinence, skeletal problems like heterotrophic ossification (HO), sexual dysfunction, motor and movement disorder including paralysis, hypertonicity, rigidity, dystonia, etc. cognitive and behavioral abnormalities, sensory disturbances and malnutrition. The mixed signs and symptoms psychophysical deficit, requires well-formulated rehabilitation programs following a thorough evaluation of the problem.

Rehabilitation of Cases with Traumatic Brain Injury

Before going for proper and scientific rehabilitative approach one must make proper assessment of a TBI patient in relation to prognostication as well as functional inabilities, capabilities and also the outcome.

As indicated earlier the prognostic indicators related to TBI includes the duration of coma in the Glasgow Coma Scale, length of the post-traumatic amnesia (PTA) or the results of a computed tomography (CT) or MRI.

The shorter the duration of amnesia, the better is the outcome. The duration of more than 11 weeks is inconsistent with dependent living. The site of lesion does not always associated directly or very powerfully with the outcome. Other prognosticate indicator include age of the patient. Patients under the age of 20 generally do better than those over 60, sustaining similar kind of injury. The exception is a patient under the age of 2.

Assessment Scale

The most frequently used assessment scales are:
- Glasgow Outcome Scale (GOS)
- Disability Rating Scale (DRS)
- Rancho Los Amigos Scale (RLAS)
- Functional Independent Measure (FIM)
- Functional Assessment Measure (FAM).

The Glasgow Outcome Scale includes five categories like:
- Dead
- Persistent vegetative state
- Severe disability
- Moderate disability
- Good outcome.

This scale is not very popular rather it was criticized by many as it is relatively insensitive.

The disability rating scale includes a reversed Glasgow Coma Scale with additional measurements of basic function skill, employability and total level of dependence. This scale has been correlated with somatosensory evoked potential (SSEP) and has been demonstrated to be scientifically valid. It is more sensitive than Glasgow Coma Scale.

The Rancho Los Amigos Scale has eight categories. Its utility is essentially to expedite communication. It is also unscientific and is not a valid scale.

Other scales include functional independent measures and functional assessment measures. FAM scale is more scientific for TBI as opposed to general disability.

Diaschisis

This term refers to one of the several general theories that concerns to the recovery of function following TBI. Diaschisis includes the concept that damage to one region of brain can produce altered function in the region adjacent to or distant from the site of damage as long as there is a connection between the two sites. That means there may be an altered function in the intact areas of brain that receives inputs from a damaged area.

Management in Context to Rehabilitation

The initial management after trauma involves primarily the life support measures and subsequent transfer of the patient to a hospital with adequate facilities.

The overall goals of management in the acute stage are:
1. Medical stability
2. Clearing of post-traumatic amnesia
3. Reduction of behavioral and physical dependence.

To keep a patient medically stable, following measures are to be undertaken. The very first approach should be towards keeping the airway open and hence endotracheal intubation is mandatory. Time to time suction is to be made to keep the air passage clear. The next step is to provide adequate oxygen to make the nerve cells alive and for this oxygen inhalation (40%) in proper humidified state is to be maintained. Hyperventilation or mechanically assisted ventilation may temporarily reduce intracranial pressure. But once this is withdrawn the intracranial pressure (ICP) may rise again.

Brain injury cases often encounter hypovolume shock for which maintenance of fluid intake, especially osmolar fluid, is very important. Once the patient is conscious oral nutrition, adequate in protein and electrolytes, can be instituted with nasogastric tube.

Next important factor is bladder and bowel function. Initially indwelling Foley's catheter is retained but later intermittent catheterization is to be practiced. Apart from the above measures, clinical assessment, laboratory investigations and overall neurologist or neurosurgeon's opinion regarding operative interference and management of other medical as well as surgical problems are to considered.

Each patient of TBI has a complex combination of physical, cognitive and behavioral deficit that presents a unique rehabilitation problem and hence the rehabilitation program must be individualized.

Traumatic brain injury (TBI) patients with many complex neurological complications are best managed by an experienced interdisciplinary team, using a patient centered and goal oriented approach. TBI patients can a wide variety of impairments depending on the site of damage. Early rehabilitative measures make things easier. Residual problems like cognitive impairments, disruption of executive function and the resultant psychological deficit can lead to significant limitation in social interaction and retuning to independent living (Lezak 1986, Brooks and McKinley 1983).

In rehabilitating a patient with TBI, multifocal attention must be given. The role of physiotherapeutic management in acute stage though not very much significant, is important. Proactive management in preventing postural secondary complication sometimes and usually enhance patient's outcome.

The main physiotherapeutic approaches are:
a. To preserve the integrity of neuromuscular system and to prevent or to minimize adapting shortening and contracture by the application of passive movement, corrective measures in positioning, postural managements and prophylactic serial plastering.
b. To provide an appropriate level of sensory stimulation by careful handling and use of sensory stimulation regime.
c. To provide early family education, support and counseling by discussing about the course, involvements of family members, friends, etc. and the potential outcome of the interventions.

In subsequent phases, true rehabilitation comes into focus. The cognitive abilities and behavioral presentation of the patient with TBI will have an impact upon their level of function. So, it is very much necessary to assess the patients of their capability as well as their incapability after which the goal of interaction can be built up. Otherwise, most efforts later turn out to be futile.

The main goals of rehabilitation at this stage are:
a. To encourage the return of active movement that carries over to function.
b. To take measures to prevent secondary deformity.
c. To prevent unnecessary and potentially damaging compensatory movements strategies.
d. To enhance respiratory function.
e. To encourage social and vocational reintegration.
f. To provide advice to the family, caretakers and the other members of the team on aspects of patient management.

Rehabilitation of brain injury cases can be done during the hospital stay (IBR) or at home (Community-based Program). Rehabilitation can be active or preventive. Active rehabilitation increases adaptive recovery to best functional outcome whereas preventive rehabilitation incorporates early intervention, prevention, treatment of complication and modification of risk factors.

Active Rehabilitation

Here, proper positioning of the body parts is maintained to prevent tightening of tendon or contracture of muscles. Frequent change of posture is maintained to prevent formation of pressure sores. Adequate maintenance of hygiene is stressed. Simple ROM exercises are done to paralytic limb to keep the muscles viable. Simple occupational therapy for activities of daily living (ADL) is instituted. Once medical stability is achieved physical therapy can be started.

The traditional exercise programs are done to prevent complications of prolonged immobilization and to regain ADL skills. The techniques are FRPM, joint mobilization exercise, isometric and isotonic exercises. Multiple

repetitions help in motor relearning. The basic principles of neurophysiologic approaches are:
- Application of sensory stimuli to facilitate or inhibit an activity
- Patient's evaluation and treatment plans should be based on milestone of development
- Utilization of reflexes to facilitate or inhibit motor activity
- Utilization of concept of motor relearning, e.g. repetitions
- Close interaction between the patient and therapist
- Focus should be made on the patient "As a Whole".

Functional Electrical Stimulation

Electrical stimulation of nerves results in contraction of muscles supplied by them. The functional electrical stimulation (FES) helps in improvement of muscle strength, bowel and bladder function and functional activities. Walking is assisted by correction of foot drop. Walking prevents muscle atrophy, bone demineralization and joint contracture.

Electromyography Biofeedback

In this method, the activity of muscle are picked up using surface or needle electrode and are converted into audio and/or visual signal for the patient by which the patient can be taught to relax or contract his muscles. Thus, it can be used to teach joint motion and coordinated movement patterns. Each session lasts for 40–60 minutes. And about 20–30 such sessions are needed to regain function.

Gait Training

This is done on a farm mat where full range of movement exercise (FROM) is done including turning, side lying, limb movement, sitting balance, standing balance, parallel bar walking and cane walking. Cane should be grasped by the healthy hand and it should be moved fast followed by the effected leg. Similarly, stair climbing and getting down should be practiced. Bicycle ergometer drill and trademill walking can be practiced for better gait training. Use of orthosis and braces gives additive effect in normal walking. Patients having failure in functional ambulation may be advised to use wheelchair. So, wheelchair training and adequate transfer techniques are to be trained.

ADL Training

The importance of ADL training is unquestionable in the rehabilitation of brain injury patients. This is conducted jointly with principles of physiotherapeutic as well as occupational therapeutic approach. Here the unaffected limb is trained to be used first then volitional effort is given to the affected limb. Sometimes assistive devices or modified devices like special type of knife, fork, comb, etc. are utilized to help the patients.

Speech Therapy

Difficulty in communication is often a problem to post-brain injury patients, who feel handicapped. Based upon individual patient's deficit and their neurophysiologic basis, speech therapy are carried out. In nonfluent aphasia, word association, word approximation and melodic information are stressed. Many a time singing helps aphasic patients in overcoming their disabilities and facilitates natural recovery of spoken language. Pictographic communication boards, visual and gesturing program for communication help in overcoming speech disorders. Even use of computers, body language, facial expression and voice output systems are of immense value.

Cognitive Rehabilitation

As mentioned earlier altered behavior often causes problems in the rehabilitation of brain injured patient. Features which affect very much are memory deficit, behavioral dyscontrol, disturbances in level of arousal, speed of processing of information, memory, abstract reasoning, flexibility, self-awareness, distractibility and limitation to attention span. For cognitive rehabilitation, an intact sensory system is needed. The very first step is the documentation of cognitive impairments and residual capabilities. Cognitive retraining is a systematic attempt aimed at improving intellectual deficits. Functional adaptation is encouraged in daily life to overcome the impairments. Patients are subjected to copy simple to complicated tasks in cases of constructional apraxia. In visual neglect, Fresnel's prism or wide angle lenses are used.

Sexuality Rehabilitation

Patients with brain trauma often face apprehension well as difficulties in physiologic urge for sexual gratification. As such physical causes are to be looked for and adequate pharmacotherapy and physical therapy are to be undertaken. Regular counseling of the patient and also the opposite partner gives effective result.

Outcome of Brain Injured

The outcome of recovery varies widely. Most of the patients can return to work because 80% of TBIs are of mild variety. However, people having moderate to severe brain injuries, the prospect of returning to work is considerably less.

Bibliography

1. Adams JH. Diffuse axonal injury in head injury: definition, diagnosis and grading. Histopathology. 1989;15(1):49-59.
2. Batchelor JS, et al. Minor head injuries in adults: A review of current guidelines. Trauma. 2003;5:191-8.

3. Boto GR, et al. Severe head injury and the risk of early death. J Neurol Neurosurg Psychiatry. 2006;77:1054-9.
4. Clausen T. Medical treatment and neuroprotection in traumatic brain injury. Curr Pharm Des. 2001;7(15):1517-32.
5. Ginsberg, et al. Classification of mild and severe head injury. Archive of Clinical Neuropsychology. 1995;10:332-333.
6. Greenwood, et al. Effects of case management after severe head injury. BMJ. 1994;308:1199-205.
7. Heiden JS, et al. Severe head injury: Clinical assessment and outcome. Phys Ther. 1983;63:1946-51.
8. Jamshid, et al. Traumatic brain injury. The Lancet. 2000;356(9):923-9.
9. Kreutzer JS, et al. Primary caregivers' psychological status and family functioning after traumatic brain injury. Brain Inj. 1994;8(3):197-210.
10. Levin, et al. Aphasic disorder in patients with closed head injury. J Neurol Neurosurg Psychiatry. 1976;39:1062-70.
11. Mary AR. Considerations for functional training in adults after head injury. Phys Ther. 1983;363:1975-82.
12. Mathew, et al. Brain monitoring in severe head injury: a practical guide. Trauma. 1999;1:105-14.
13. Moppett, et al. Traumatic brain injury: assessment, resuscitation and early management. Br J Anaesth. 2007;99:18-31.
14. Morton, Wehman. Psychosocial and emotional sequelae of individuals with traumatic brain injury: a literature review and recommendations. Brain Inj. 1995;9(1):81-92.
15. Oddy, et al. A comprehensive service for the rehabilitation and long-term care of head injury survivors. Clinical Rehabilitation. 1989;3:253-9.
16. Olver JH, et al. Outcome following traumatic brain injury: a comparison between 2 and 5 years after injury. Brain Inj. 1996;10(11):841-8.
17. Pentland, Michael. Staffing provision for early head injury rehabilitation. Clinical Rehabilitation. 1988;2:309-13.
18. Pentland B. Rehabilitation needs after severe head injury. BMJ. 1994;309:129.
19. Pickard JD, et al. Mapping rehabilitation resources for head injury. J R Soc Med. 2004;97:384-89.
20. Ponsford, et al. Traumatic Brain Injury: Rehabilitation for Everyday Adaptive Living Psychology Press, 1995.
21. Salmond, et al. Cognitive sequelae of head injury: involvement of basal forebrain and associated structures. Brain. 2005;128:189-200.
22. Stambrook, et al. Effects of mild, moderate and severe closed head injury on long-term vocational status. Brain Inj. 1990;4(2):183-90.
23. Wilson, et al. Neuropsychological consequences of two patterns of brain damage shown by MRI in survivors of severe head injury. J Neurol Neurosurg Psychiatry. 1995;59:328-31.
24. Workman, et al. Physical abilities after head injury: a retrospective study. Phys Ther. 1983;63:2010-17.

Section 4

Integration and Extension

With the advancement of rehabilitation science, stroke and spinal injury patients have been blessed by the opportunity of comprehensive and multidimensional rehabilitation treatment starting from the acute phase and extending to a long-term rehabilitation with various scientific models and modern updates of theories which are being practically implemented in various newer rehabilitation units. The path of modern rehabilitation is never narrow but spreads its branches day by day with options of regular and modern experiments. With the aim of generating the maximum functional reactivation of such patients, this science has developed newer approaches, fruitful models and productive instruments and profiles that may establish an open, broad and scientific pathway.

31

Models of Rehabilitation in Spinal Cord Injury and Stroke

Mouli Madhab Ghatak

Introduction

Rehabilitation may be called a support system or encouraging instrument to reactivate the lost functions, by generating the lost areas or by a sustained growth of the residual sound areas to supplement the lost areas.

A person when loses his functional capacity after stroke or spinal cord injury (SCI) needs proper scientific back up to rejuvenate him up to the highest possible level through a continuous, long-term group management programs which is called medical rehabilitation. Such a scientific rebirth and regrowth requires a group of medical persons to form the rehabilitation team. It consists of physiatrist (neurologist, orthopedician at times), physical therapist, occupational therapist, cognitive behavioral therapist/psychologist, orthotist, social worker, vocational counselor, nutritionist, speech and language therapist and trained skilled rehabilitation nurse. Recently, recreational therapists are also being included in the team and a responsible family member should always be in the rehabilitation team. The role and responsibilities of these specialities are described below **(Fig. 31.1)**.

The physician: Physiatrist should be in charge of managing or coordinating the rehabilitation programs. Where physiatrists are not available, a physician with sound knowledge on this subject or a neurologist or an orthopedician may take the primary responsibility. The initial and successive medical and rehabilitative evaluation is performed by the physiatrist. The associated medical management including taking care of blood pressure, diabetes, bed sore, urinary infections, respiratory problems or other various comorbid conditions are to be properly monitored, controlled and treated so that such medical problems cannot be barriers for smooth progression of rehabilitation. In case of any other serious comorbid conditions, the related specialist should be referred.

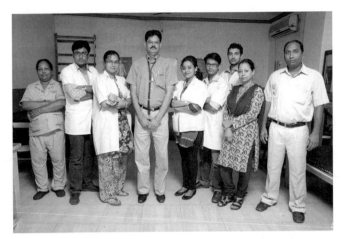

Fig. 31.1: A group discussion session with a stroke patient
at Medical Rehabilitation Center, Kolkata
(For color version, see Plate 17)

After proper assessment and examination, the physiatrist formulates the goals and procedures of rehabilitation of a particular patient based on the individual need. A group discussion is usually preferred among all sub specialities of the team under the leadership of the physiatrist. During such discussion, the physiatrist should make aware about the complicating factors, any serious medical problem which may arise from any particular therapeutic procedure and ensures that a goal-oriented rehabilitation process can be implemented smoothly. A regular and serial check up or investigations with necessary medical treatment related to rehabilitation should be continued by the physiatrist. An experienced physiatrist or the physician can organize the whole program intelligently, taking proper measures against medical complications and can guide such programs effectively with a positive zeal and inspiring instructions. In fact the physiatrist is the prime driving force of the whole team.

1. *Rehabilitation nurse:* Rehabilitation of a patient is not limited to only a few hours a day. All the 24 hours of a day is to be devoted for the proper care and rehabilitation. Constant watch and monitoring of the patient's physical, mental and cognitive conditions and taking decisions regarding changes in the care systems or informing the doctors are the primary responsibility of a rehabilitation nurse. Infact the rehabilitation nurse plays a role of full-time coordinator and observer of a patient with stroke or spinal injury. A rehabilitation nurse is not restricted to the job of noting blood pressure, pulse and temperature, intake-output chart, serving the medicines at times but she is a round-the-clock responsible scientific caregiver with a soft and sympathetic touch. She should be aware of medical problems including autonomic problems, hypoglycemia, bedsores, etc. the usual complications in a rehabilitation ward. The nurse notes all relevant happenings and serves all these information to the

physician and participates actively in the discussion. Actually the role of a well-trained, sincere nurse reinforces the basic foundation of the rehabilitation services in a rehabilitation ward.

2. *Physical therapist:* Physical therapists are the backbone for providing the principal therapeutics of neuromuscular disabilities and locomotor abnormalities in stroke and spinal injury patients. A physical therapist engages himself in the processes for development of tone, strength, endurance of the muscles, improving range of motion of joint, tone-spasticity-synergy modification programs, cardiopulmonary endurance training and standing and gait training of stroke and SCI patient. Physical therapists should have sound knowledge of neuromuscular pathology and must be oriented with the modern updates of motor training procedures and should know the preventive ways on special issues like spasticity-synergy-joint stiffness and the autonomic and vasomotor complications arising from stroke and spinal cord injury.

   The application of role of various electrotherapies like FES, TENS, US therapy and modern biofeedback and motor training equipment should be properly guided and performed by the physical therapist. Physical therapist should emphasize on practicing isolated muscular movements, reversing complex and mass movements, repeated training and retraining. They should frequently employ selective sensory stimulation to encourage use of impaired limbs and help survivors regain awareness on the neglected side of the body. Physical therapists should handle the people with proper care and scientific techniques even to a patient too weak to bear exercise strains or having gross cognitive problems or different medical complications. They should constantly keep in touch with the Physiatrist for the sake of a smooth and enhanced recovery program, maintaining proper coordination among team members **(Fig. 31.2)**.

3. *Occupational therapist:* Occupational therapists are essential part of a rehabilitation team for treating stroke and SCI patient. The development of various motor skills through repetitive task specific activity programs related to the brain plasticity are the major concern of this speciality. The modern concept of rehabilitation of stroke and seq emphasizes on motor relearning through repetitive functional training and goal directed activities. The activity of daily living and return to the community and the profession through proper functional training is the prime concern of an occupational therapist. With the advancement of civilization, while the people expect a more productive life, various functional rehabilitation programs are of immense importance. Different complex movements and activity schedules are trained with an individualistic view and repeated practice initiates relearning in a better way.

   Various hand therapies in a hand unit including peg board activities, buttoning, unbuttoning, holding and unholding of objects and different finer activity programs are trained by the occupational therapist. In the functional gym, they also train standing; walking and how to prevent fall during walking or how to get up from the ground when

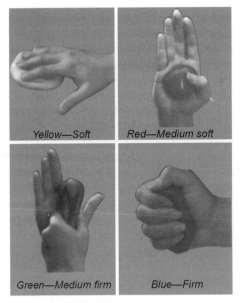

Fig. 31.2: Hand exercises
(For color version, see Plate 17)

the patient falls down, how to cross a barrier and how to tackle various situations which may appear during outdoor mobility and professional activities. Paraplegics with possibility of poor return of limb function or quadriparetics and hemiplegics with impaired hand function are given wheelchair training based on the specific disability by the occupational therapist **(Fig. 31.3)**.

4. *Speech and language pathologist:* A good number of stroke survivors, specially patients with left-brain involvement are frequently sufferers of speech disorder. Speech and language pathologist evaluates the exact nature and type of speech pathology and disorders related to communication through history, clinical examination and use of diagnostic tools. They use various specialized therapeutic techniques including intensive exercises, repetitive practice of their specific directives, reading, writing exercises, conversational coaching and rehearsal along with development of prompts or cues to help the people remember specific words, etc. The language disabilities are also dealt by these therapists. Recent advances in computer technologies have spurred the development of new types of equipment to enhance communication.

Swallowing difficulty is another important area of intervention of speech-language pathologists, who by the use of noninvasive imaging techniques study swallowing patterns of stroke survivors, identifying the exact source of impairment. After determining the exact cause, like delayed swallowing reflex, inability to detect remainings, lodged in the cheeks, inability to manipulate food with tongue, etc. The therapist formulates strategies to overcome or minimize the deficit, recommends

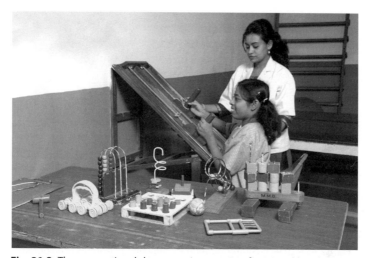

Fig. 31.3: The occupational therapy unit operating functional hand training
(For color version, see Plate 18)

the changes of eating habits (say like taking small bites, chewing slowly, etc.) or the texture of foods or changing the body position during eating, etc.

A patient with dysarthria and dysphagia is solely managed by this speciality, something taking the views of an ENT specialist. It is to be noted that the overall rehabilitation is affected by such communication and deglutition disorder because of poor interaction, which aggravates psychological and mood disturbances. Nutrition also gets hampered in presence of dysphagia and all these factors are modified by the scientific techniques and therapeutic intervention of a speech and language therapist **(Fig. 31.4)**.

5. *Psychobehavioral and cognitive therapists:* Stroke survivors with gross cognitive impairment usually has a poor rehabilitation outcome because of lack of following instructions and performing higher motor regulated activities. Here lies the role of a cognitive therapist who apply various modern techniques and training to combat the difficulties related to higher functions like agnosia, apraxia, body skill disturbance, hemi neglect and so many psychobehavioral issues. The speech and language dysfunction related to the cognitive problems is jointly dealt by a speech therapist and a cognitive therapist.

Stroke and spinal injury patients may suffer from various types of psychological disturbances including mild to moderate depression, anxiety disorders that may be either organic or functional. Proper psychological therapies are regularly given to these patients by the psycho-cognitive therapists. Before starting the therapeutic sessions, they usually need a meticulous evaluation using various modern scales, which provides a clear idea over the requirement of exact therapeutic interventions are decided. Psycho-cognitive therapists also guide the

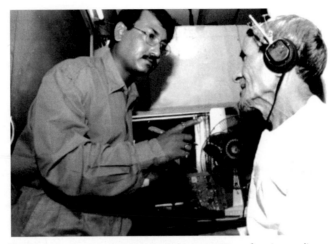

Fig. 31.4: A speech communication therapy unit performing audiogram
(For color version, see Plate 18)

rehabilitation team regarding the way of behaving towards a particular patient during a rehab process. The therapists also explain the family members their role. Training a patient to develop a positive motivation towards life is of immense importance because the training and learning motor skills are greatly related to the patients internal motivation, initiation and efforts. In an indoor rehabilitation unit, a psychotherapist can better perform by counteracting anxiety and depression through a group therapy where examples of the improvements of disabling factors of the other patients admitted in the same set up, can be represented.

6. *The vocational counselor and social workers:* When the long-term rehabilitation of stroke and SCI patients is concerned, the proper return and placement of the patient in the society and the profession becomes a major issue specially for those on whom the other family members depend for their monitory and social support. These two specialities after assessing the patient's disabilities, premorbid job status, and environmental factors of job site, formulates a possible professional attachment and social adjustment guidelines.

The vocational counselor sometimes acts as a mediator between employers and employees to negotiate the provision of modification of job and a reasonable accommodation near by the work place. They also help the patient search specific jobs considering the patient's interest, educational and financial background.

Usually a support group is formed by the social worker for continuous psychological, social and even financial support to the stroke survivors. The support group consists of near friends and relatives as per the patient's choice. The patient is really benefited by a good social rehabilitation when he gets back the lost confidence of life force within himself. The acceptance of the patient in the society fruitfully is a great task of a social worker and through such a well-organized social guideline, patient ultimately identifies the ultimate essence of rehabilitation.

7. *Orthotist and prosthetist:* The orthotists play an important role by supporting the rehabilitation process by fabricating splints, calipers, braces, belts, collars and various other aids for structural stabilization or functional assistance of any body part. They should have sound knowledge on different body mechanics with a strong base of structural anatomy.

8. *Nutritionist:* Nutritionist helps in a successful rehabilitation through maintenance of proper metabolic parameters by scientific supply of required nutritional materials. Stroke survivors with parenteral nutritional status or Ryle's tube feeding having frequent dyselectrolytemia, diabetes or uremia, dyslipidemia all require specialized nutritional prescriptions. The requirement of total calorie including essential nutrients in a particular case is to be recommended and guided and the servings are to be supervised, by the nutritionist.

SCI patients in need of high protein dietary regime also need scientific guidelines. Unscientific and improper nutrition in SCI and stroke patients lead to medical complications as well as poor growth of musculature which delays the rehabilitation. Nutritionists are also important for coordinating the patient and the cook.

The secondary prevention of stroke also requires a good nutritional guideline to keep various biochemical and metabolic factors (lipid, sugar, urea, etc.) under good control.

Systems of Rehabilitation in Stroke and Spinal Cord Injuries

Rehabilitation services may be offered to a patient with stroke or seq in the following ways:

A. *Daycare rehabilitation:* The patient having mild to moderate degree of disability and not inflicted by other medical complications may opt for daycare or home rehabilitation program. A secured ambulation and transport of the patient must be assured before taking the option of daycare rehabilitation. However, daycare rehabilitation in a well-equipped rehabilitation center is always a superior choice as the patient can avail the full rehabilitation team and equipment and rejuvenated by an inspiring group rehabilitation program which accelerates the positive motivational factors to achieve maximum functional independence.

B. *Home rehabilitation:* The choice of home rehabilitation should be concentrated for stroke survivors or SCI patients who have minimal disability, poor transportability due to far distance, lack of assistance of family members, etc. or poor affordability of day care rehabilitation. Few patients having reduced psychological adaptability, who cannot accommodate clinical setup and comfortable with only home environment for constant support of family members, also choose home rehabilitation program.

C. *Integrated, indoor team rehabilitation:* It is the best choice in early phase and also for long-term provision of a critically ill patient. The indoor rehabilitation has got special advantages because of the following criteria:
- Using different gadgets and instruments like stand-in-frame, multiple exerciser, balancing board, specially made plinths, low height chairs, mats, slings, wheels, support systems, tilt table, ladders, hand gym kits, lots of evaluation kits, instruments, upgraded biofeedback and electrotherapy instruments, updated motor training kits, psychotherapy and speech therapy kits, bed and bedside modifications and so many other equipment. These cannot be shifted to home and if at all some are shiftable, providing required qualified group of persons to execute the programs with these instruments is a difficult task.
- Regular check up by the doctor (Physiatrist/Rehabilitationist) and necessary change in programs and controlling other medical problems by a group of qualified specialists is possible in indoor set ups.
- *Full day intervention:* A patient registered for all programs, gets double session (about 6–8 hours) intervention of different programs in every working day.
- Grand discussion among all doctors, therapists and persons involved in different programs—helps in modification of programs regularly, the rehab becomes more scientific and accurate.
- Specialized trained manpower for proper positioning, postural care, bedsore care, urinary measurement and care, dysphagia management, bedside therapies, vocational interventions, etc. are available in an indoor set up. All these are guided by a consultant doctor **(Fig. 31.5)**.

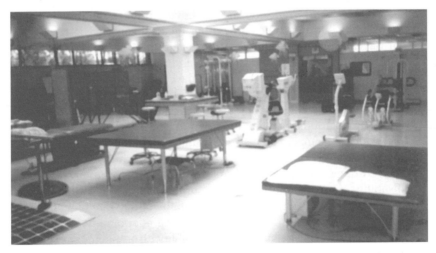

Fig. 31.5: Part of a rehabilitation gym
(For color version, see Plate 19)

- Monitoring and diagnostic advantages, including regular blood pressure, blood sugar, cardiac, respiratory and neuromuscular examinations like EMG, NCV, CT scan and other pathological tests are available easily in indoor set ups.

However, wherever may be the place of rehabilitation, a stroke and SCI rehabilitation system must have a mechanism for reviewing the quality of services.

It is important to notice and record, the quality of assessment, and the rehab services provided to any patient, related to the goal.

Regular updation through scientific seminars, meetings and discussions are of immense importance for developing the services. The monotony and willful neglect of the team members may restrict the rehabilitation outcome. A good rehabilitation outcome always requires proper scientific goal directed intervention of the positive minded rehabilitation team members.

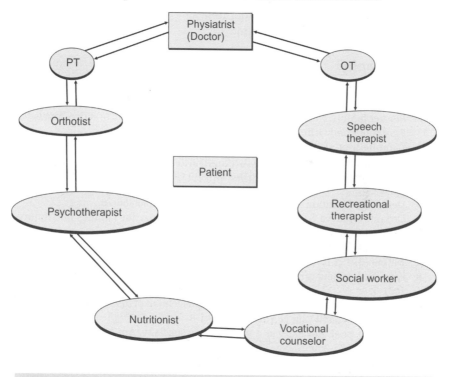

Specialized Units in a Spinal Cord Injury and Stroke Rehabilitation Center

Primary Units

1. Diagnostics CT/MRI/EMG/NCV/Pathology/Urodynamics, etc.
2. Brain and spinal surgery clinic (Spine Surgeon).
3. Spinal and stroke rehabilitation clinic (Physiatrist).
4. Interventional pain management unit (Anesthetist or Pain Doctor).

5. Spasticity clinic (Surgeon, Anesthetist, Physiatrist, Physical therapist).
6. Gait analysis and training unit (Physiatrist, Physical therapist, Electrophysiologist).
7. Wheelchair clinic (Occupational therapist).
8. Functional training unit (Occupational therapist).
9. Physical therapy gym and Electrotherapy unit (Physiotherapist).
10. Orthosis/Prosthesis unit (Orthotist and prosthelist).
11. Urinary rehabilitation unit (Urologist or a trained nurse).
12. Speech and communication unit (Speech therapist).
13. Psycho-cognitive and behavioral rehabilitation unit (Psychotherapist).
14. Nutrition and dietetics unit and clinic (Dietitians).

Supportive/Secondary Units

1. Cardiac/hypertension unit.
2. Diabetes and metabolic disorder unit.
3. General and plastic surgery unit.

Bibliography

1. Bilssitt PA. Nutrition in acute spinal cord injury. Crit Care Nurs Clin North Am. 1990;2(3):375-84.
2. Bowker Jhon H. Neurological aspects of prosthetic/Orthotic practice. Journal of Prosthetics and Orthotics. 1993;5(2):40/52-42/54.
3. Campbell, et al. Report of research and experimentation in exercise and recreational therapy. Am J Psychiatry. 1940;96:915-33.
4. Dauphinee, et al. A randomized trial of team care following stroke. Stroke; 1984. pp. 864-72.
5. Dennis M. Nutrition after stroke. Br Med Bull. 2000;56:466-75.
6. DeSanto-Madeya S. Adaptation to spinal cord injury for families post-injury. Nurs Sci Q. 2009;22(1):57-66.
7. Devivo MJ, et al. Employment after spinal cord injury. Arch Phys Med Rehabil. 1987;68(8):494-8.
8. Ernst E. A review of stroke rehabilitation and physiotherapy. Stroke. 1990;21: 1081-5.
9. Fowler, et al. The role of physiatry in the management of neuromuscular disease. Phys Med Rehabil Clin N Am. 1998;9(1):1-8.
10. Fransisco, et al. Physiatry as a primary care specialty. Am J Phys Med Rehabil. 1995;74(3):185-256.
11. Gill, et al. Psychosocial impaction of spinal cord injury. Crit Care Nurs Q. 1999;22(2):1-7.
12. Hatfield, et al. Characterizing speech and language pathology outcomes in stroke rehabilitation. Arch Phys Med Rehabil. 2005;86(12 Suppl 2):61-72.
13. Indredavik, et al. Benefit of a stroke unit: a randomized control trial. Stroke. 1991;22:1026-31.
14. Indredavik, et al. Medical complication in a comprehensive stroke unit and an early supported discharge service. Stroke. 2008;39(2):414-20.
15. Indredavik, et al. Treatment in a combined acute and rehabilitation stroke unit, which aspects are more important? Stroke. 1999;30:917-23.

16. Jum Kimura. Electrodiagnosis in disease of nerve and muscles, principles and practice, 3rd edn. Oxford University Press, US, 2001.
17. Lincoln, et al. Cognitive behavioral psychotherapy for depression following stroke. A randomized controlled trial. Stroke. 2003;34:111-5.
18. Lincoln, et al. Effectiveness of speech therapy for aphasic stroke patient: a randomized controlled trial. Lancet. 1984;2(1):1197-200.
19. Long AF, et al. The role of the nurses within the multi-professional rehabilitation team. J Adv Nurs. 2002;37(1):70-8.
20. Manns PJ, Chad KE. Components of quality of life for person with a quadriplegic and paraplegic spinal cord injury. Qual Health Res. 2001;11(6):795-811.
21. Merletti, Pinelli. A critical appraisal of neuromuscular stimulation and electrotherapy in neurorehabilitation. Eur Neurol. 1980;19(1):30-2.
22. Ron Seymour. Orthoses for spinal conditions, clinical decision making, Chapter-17, Prosthetic and orthotics, Lower Limb and spinal. Lippincott Williams and Wilkins; 2002. pp. 427-50.
23. Saeki S. Disability management after stroke: its medical aspect for workplace accommodation. Disabil Rehabil. 2004;22(13):578-82.
24. Tomassen PC, et al. Return to work after spinal cord injury. Spinal Cord. 2000;38(1): 51-5.
25. von Koch L. Rehabilitation at home after stroke: a descriptive study of an individualized intervention. Clin Rehabil. 2000;14(6):574-83.
26. Wilmore, et al. Exercise prescription: role of the physiatrist and allied health profession. Arch Phys Med Rehabil. 1976;57(1):315-9.
27. Yerxa EJ. An introduction to occupational science. A foundation for occupational therapy in the 21st century. Occup Ther Health Care. 1990;6(4):1-17.
28. Zasler, et al. The role of medical rehabilitation in vocational recovery. Head Trauma Rehabil. 1997;12(5),vii-ix:1-101.

32

Recreational Therapy in Rehabilitation

West E Ray

Inclusion of recreational therapists as members of rehabilitation teams adds an important dimension to the rehabilitation care and services provided to patients. Qualified and competent recreational therapists compliment and expand the rehabilitation care and services provided by other members of the rehabilitation team by designing interventions to address specific aspects of patients' physical, cognitive, emotional and social functioning during rehabilitation. In addition, recreational therapists teach patients to adapt to activity limitations and restrictions in participation in life situations to enhance patients' adjustment to disability and to increase their independence and quality of life after discharge. Simply stated, recreational therapists assist the rehabilitation team to provide patients with opportunities to improve functioning and independence during rehabilitation, and also assist the team with efforts to provide patients with the opportunity to have a meaningful life after rehabilitation. The purpose of this chapter is two-fold: (1) to provide an understanding of recreational therapy as a professional discipline to be included in the team of rehabilitation specialists responsible for the provision of rehabilitation services and (2) to provide an understanding of recreational therapy practice and of interventions that may be used by a recreational therapist in the rehabilitation of persons who have had strokes or spinal cord injuries. In order to develop an understanding of the value of recreational therapy in rehabilitation an introduction to recreational therapy practice will be provided. The introduction to recreational therapy will be followed by content that describes applications of recreational therapy practice in treating and rehabilitating persons and includes specific content about recreational therapy interventions for patients who have had strokes and spinal cord injuries.

Introduction to Recreational Therapy

Recreational therapy has been practiced by professionals, with degrees in therapeutic recreation or recreational therapy, in the United States for over fifty years, but in other parts of the world recreational therapy is often not well understood or distinguished from leisure and general recreation services. In the following content, definitions of recreational therapy service will be used to describe recreational therapy as a service separate and distinct from general recreational services. A definition of qualified and competent recreational therapists will be used to describe the basic qualifications and credentials of a recreational therapist. Academic preparation, practice competencies and standards that guide the practice of recreational therapy will also be reviewed to provide a basic understanding of the qualifications, competency and practice parameters of recreational therapists.

Definition of Recreational Therapy

The United States Department of Labor estimates that approximately 27,000 recreational therapists were employed in the U.S. in 2002.[1] The American Therapeutic Recreation Association (ATRA), a national professional association for recreational therapists in the United States, uses the following definition to define therapeutic recreation and recreational therapy[2]:

"Therapeutic Recreation is the provision of Treatment Services and the provision of Recreation Services to persons with illnesses or disabling conditions. The primary purposes of Treatment Services, which is often referred to as Recreational Therapy, are to restore, remediate, or rehabilitate in order to improve functioning and independence as well as reduce or eliminate the effects of illness or disability. The primary purposes of Recreation Services are to provide recreation resources and opportunities in order to improve health and well-being. Therapeutic Recreation is provided by professionals who are trained and certified, registered, and/or licensed to provide Therapeutic Recreation."

In this definition two distinct services are described as components of therapeutic recreation services. The first service described is treatment, often referred to as recreational therapy, and the second service described is recreation. The purpose of treatment or recreational therapy is to restore, remediate or rehabilitate specific aspects of patients' physical, cognitive, emotional or social functioning in order to improve overall functioning and independence. The purpose of recreation, provided as an aspect of therapeutic recreation service, is to provide resources and opportunities for the patient to engage in recreation in order to improve or maintain health and well-being. Different from the concept of participating in recreation simply for pleasure, diversion or entertainment, this goal-oriented approach recognizes that a purpose of participation in recreation activities is not only a means of self-expression, but, perhaps as important from a rehabilitation perspective, a means to exercise abilities (e.g. physical, cognitive, social and emotional) in order to improve functioning and maintain health.

The World Health Organization (WHO), in its recent International Classification of Functioning, Disability and Health, defines terms in the context of health that assist in understanding the contributions of recreational therapy to improving the health and functioning of persons with disabilities. WHO defines an activity as an execution of a task by an individual and defines activity limitations as difficulties an individual may have in executing activities.[3] WHO also defines participation restrictions as problems an individual may have in involvement in life situations.[3] Integrating these terms into an example adds some clarity to the definition of therapeutic recreation service and how the service may be used in a rehabilitation setting. For example, when blood flow to the brain is disrupted, as happens during a cerebral vascular accident (CVA), the body function of circulation of blood flow to the brain is disrupted. As a result, parts of the brain are without oxygen and neurological impairment, such as hemiparesis or hemiplegia may result. The patient may experience the impairment as a weakness (paresis) or complete loss of motor function (paralysis) on one side of their body. The ATRA definition states the purpose of recreational therapy is to restore or rehabilitate to improve functioning and independence and to reduce or eliminate the effects of illness or disability. Using the WHO terms to add clarity and context to the definition of recreational therapy, recreational therapy interventions are designed to improve patients' functioning and to reduce the activity limitations and restrictions in participation in life situations caused by an illness or disabling condition. In addition to the value of recreational therapy as a treatment service, by using goal-oriented recreation patients assume responsibility for engaging in opportunities to maintain their functioning and health. For example, as a result of the impairment (e.g. weakness or paralysis) the patient may experience activity limitations such as the inability to use the affected arm and leg in personal care activities (e.g. dressing, feeding, etc.) or restrictions to participating in work or leisure activities due to the need for and limited availability of transportation opportunities that will accommodate those who use a wheelchair for mobility. As an aspect of rehabilitation services, recreational therapists address specific impairments in physical, cognitive, emotional and social functioning in the context of activity limitations that may restrict participation in life situations. By using interventions designed to restore or rehabilitate functioning and by teaching patients to use adaptations to activities to reduce restrictions in life situations (e.g. participation in recreation and leisure activities), recreational therapists enhance patient's independence in life activities after rehabilitation.

In a rehabilitation program, various disciplines (e.g. physicians, nurses, psychologists, speech therapists, physical, occupational and recreational therapists) apply a variety of treatment interventions and techniques to address the patient's impairment in body function or structure and activity limitations in order to improve the patient's participation in life activities. Initially the cause of the impairment is medically corrected or stabilized, to the extent possible, to prevent additional impairment in body functions or structure. Following medical stabilization, treatment is used to improve and restore, to the extent possible, physical, cognitive and emotional functioning. In addition, the patient is taught to adapt to physical, cognitive, emotional and social limitations, so he/she can return to participation in life activities (e.g. self-care, work, recreation, etc.) with as much independence, choice and control as possible, sometimes with the use of activity adaptations or adaptive equipment necessary for successful participation. When the patient not only learns to adapt to limitations and environmental factors they must overcome as a result of the disability, but returns to independent participation in life activities, including recreation, he/she has a means to live as independently as possible, contribute to society and to continue to improve or maintain their health. A recreational therapist uses a patient and family-centered approach to empower the patient to take responsibility for his/her health and well-being. In the initial stages of illness or disability, such as immediately following a CVA or spinal cord injury, the recreational therapist will establish a therapeutic or helping relationship with a patient and will design and use recreational therapy interventions, such as exercise, cognitive retraining, or coping skills training to improve specific aspects of physical, cognitive, emotional and social functioning, complimenting interventions provided by other rehabilitation disciplines. As the patient becomes more independent, the recreational therapist teaches and encourages the patient to assume responsibility to choose activities that may reach therapeutic goals during hospitalization, but also have potential for the patient to use after discharge to continue to improve or maintain functioning and health. For example, a recreational therapist, working collaboratively with physical and occupational therapists, may use exercise with a patient to strengthen or improve function in a weak arm or leg, but as the patient improves in strength and functioning to where he/she can function safely and more independently, a recreational therapist may help the patient determine how and where the patient may participate in an activity of inherent interest to continue to improve or maintain strength or function after discharge from rehabilitation. Sometimes this might involve a continuation of exercises learned during rehabilitation that can be done in the patient's home, but it may also involve identifying community resources such as a health club, exercise facility or wellness center where a patient can continue a daily exercise routine to improve or maintain strength and cardiovascular functioning as an aspect of general health. The recreational therapist may also help the patient to find alternative activities to reach treatment goals and improve functioning, such as swimming as a means to exercise weak muscles and improve conditioning. In this type of situation, the recreational therapist uses the helping or therapeutic relationship to counsel and encourage the patient to take a more independent role in planning for discharge and in selecting activities of intrinsic interest for participation after discharge to continue to improve functioning and to achieve and maintain maximum independence. As an aspect of counseling the patient and planning for discharge, the recreational therapist will teach the patient about adaptations (e.g. adaptive equipment and activity adaptations) to overcome limitations and environmental barriers (e.g. transportation, attitudinal barriers towards people with disabilities, etc.) the patient will encounter after discharge in order to assist the patient and family to prepare for the patient's integration into normative life routines and involvement in community activities after discharge.

Qualifications, Credentials and Competencies of Recreational Therapists

It is important to understand the basic qualifications, credential and competencies of recreational therapists in order to understand how recreational therapists may be qualified and competent to use recreational therapy interventions to achieve patient outcomes. The Joint Commission on Accreditation of Health Care Organizations (JCAHO), an organization that accredits healthcare organizations around the world, has defined a *qualified recreational therapist* as an individual who, at a minimum, is a graduate of a baccalaureate degree program in recreational therapy, accredited by a nationally recognized accreditation body, and is currently a Certified Therapeutic Recreation Specialist by the National Council for Therapeutic Recreation Certification and meets current legal requirements of licensure, registration, or certification.[4] In their definition JCAHO also stated that a qualified recreational therapist has the documented equivalent in education, training, and experience and is currently competent in the field.[4]

In this definition of a *qualified* recreational therapist, JCAHO describes minimum qualifications of a recreational therapist (e.g. specialized bachelors level degree) and minimum credentials (e.g. Certified Therapeutic Recreation Specialist™) of a qualified recreational therapist. In addition to the listing the minimum qualifications of a degree in recreational therapy (therapeutic recreation is the degree title in many colleges and universities) from an accredited college or university, national certification as a Certified Therapeutic Recreation Specialist™ (CTRS™) and state credentials where required, JCAHO also states that the qualified recreational therapist must be currently *competent* in the field. Competence is usually defined as having the knowledge, skills and abilities necessary to perform the required duties of the position. The degree and certification as a CTRS™ are generally considered minimal qualifications for employment. JCAHO requires accredited agencies to assess the competency of staff to perform the required duties of their position during the staff's initial orientation after hiring to assure that, in addition to requiring minimal qualifications of a degree and credentials, the competency to perform required job functions is also assessed.

A Certified Therapeutic Recreation Specialist™ is defined by the National Council for Therapeutic Recreation Certification (NCTRC), a national credentialing organization in the United States, as an individual who has met the eligibility requirements, including standards for certification that include education, experience and has passed the national therapeutic recreation specialist examination of NCTRC.[5] **Table 32.1** provides the Standards of Minimal Knowledge, Skills and Abilities that serve as a foundation for the NCTRC certification examination.[5] These standards are based upon the 1997 National Job Analysis conducted by NCTRC and are used as the basis for developing the NCTRC certification examination. NCTRC requires relevant continuing education for recertification at five-year intervals. NCTRC has certified over sixteen thousand therapeutic recreation specialists in the United States and has also certified four therapeutic recreation specialists from Puerto

Rico, eighty-seven from Canada and twenty-seven from other countries, as verified by NCTRC (Bob Riley, personal communication, November 15, 2004) **(Table 32.1)**.

Table 32.1: National Council for Therapeutic Recreation Certification Standards of Minimal Knowledge, Skills and Abilities
A minimally acceptable, entry level Certified Therapeutic Recreation Specialist (CTRS) must:
1. Possess knowledge of the theories and concepts of therapeutic recreation, leisure, and human development as related to the nature and scope of human service delivery systems, and the ability to integrate these in a variety of settings.
2. Possess an essential knowledge of the diversity of populations including cultural and diagnostic groups served within the therapeutic recreation process, including etiology, symptomatology (cognitive, physical, social, sensory and communication and psychiatric impairments), prognosis, treatment of conditions and related secondary complications. Have a basic command of medical terminology.
3. Have a thorough understanding of the assessment process utilized within therapeutic recreation practice including, but not limited to, purpose of assessment, assessment domain (including cognitive, social, physical, emotional, leisure, background information), assessment procedures (including behavioral observation, interview, functional skills testing, a general understanding of current TR/leisure assessment instruments, inventories and questionnaires and other sources of commonly used multidisciplinary assessment data) selection of instrumentation, general procedures for implementation and the interpretation of findings.
4. Have a basic understanding of the published standards of practice for the profession of therapeutic recreation and the influence that such standards have on the program planning process.
5. Possess detailed knowledge of the intervention planning process, including program or treatment plan design and development, programming considerations types of programs, nature and scope of interventions, selection of programs to achieve the assessed needs and desired outcomes of the person served and the impact of social issues on programming.
6. Possess basic knowledge related to the implementation of an individual intervention plan, including theory and application of facilitation styles, intervention techniques, and methods for behavioral change.
7. Have a fundamental knowledge of the processes of documentation and evaluation as incorporated in all phases of the intervention process.
8. Possess a broad understanding of organizing and managing therapeutic recreation services including, but not limited to, the development of a written plan of operation and knowledge of external regulations, personnel practices, and components of quality improvement.
9. Be able to identify and understand the components of professional competency within the realm of therapeutic recreation practice, including requirements for certification, ethical practice, public relations, and the general advancement of the profession.

The American Therapeutic Recreation Association (ATRA) in its publication *Guidelines for Competency Assessment and Curriculum Planning in Therapeutic Recreation: A Tool for Self-Evaluation*[6] has defined competency at a somewhat higher level than the knowledge skills and abilities NCTRC **(Table 32.1)** uses as a basis for the national certification exam. In this publication, ATRA defines the knowledge, skills and abilities that a therapeutic recreation specialist, in this context also known as a recreational therapist, should be able to demonstrate for safe and effective practice. The competencies are developed around specific content areas (e.g. subject, topic or focus) of the national job analysis conducted by the NCTRC as a basis for the national certification examination and also follow the parameters of practice defined in the ATRA Standards for the Practice of Therapeutic Recreation. Competency is viewed as an educational taxonomy where *knowledge* is the basis of understanding the concepts or basic factual information and constructs of practice, *skill* represents the application of the knowledge in performance of skills in practice and *ability* represents the analysis, synthesis, and evaluation of information to reach intended patient outcomes.[6] An example would be that a recreational therapist must have basic *knowledge* to understand how to individually assess patients using a variety of techniques, methodologies and assessment instruments. A recreational therapist must also have *skill* to efficiently and effectively conduct individualized patient assessments and they must have the *ability* to analyze the results of the assessment in order to determine treatment goals and specific interventions to be used to reach intended patient outcomes. The ATRA publication *Guidelines for Competency Assessment and Curriculum Planning in Therapeutic Recreation* includes a self-assessment tool that lists knowledge, skills and abilities by content areas and provides a very useful means to assess the competency of those who will practice as recreational therapists.

Table 32.2 lists the content areas (e.g. subject, topic or focus) from *Guidelines for Competency Assessment and Curriculum Planning in Therapeutic Recreation* that ATRA defines as necessary for effective practice as a therapeutic recreation specialist.[6] For each content area identified there are detailed lists in the publication of specific knowledge, skills and abilities necessary to develop adequate competency in the given content area. The contact hours (e.g. class contact time) listed for each content area are those usually used by U.S. colleges and universities to determine course credit hours. Twelve–fifteen contact hours usually equal a one-credit course, thirty contact hours usually translates into a two-credit course and forty-five contact hours usually translates into a three-credit course. The support content (e.g. biological and behavioral science requirements for the recreational therapy degree such as anatomy, physiology, abnormal psychology, etc.) provides an understanding of basic human functioning and provides the foundation necessary for effective practice as a recreational therapist. Generally recreational therapists have somewhat less course content in their academic preparation in the biological sciences than do physical and occupational therapists, but recreational therapists often have somewhat more

Table 32.2: Guidelines for curriculum planning in therapeutic recreation: a tool for self-evaluation	
Content area	*Contact time*
Foundations of Professional Practice	45 hours
Assessment for Therapeutic Recreation	45 hours
Therapeutic Recreation Intervention/Program Planning	45 hours
Leadership and Group Dynamics	45 hours
Helping/Counseling Skills	45 hours
Evaluation of Therapeutic Recreation	45 hours
Management of Therapeutic Recreation Services	45 hours
Healthcare Organization and Delivery	45 hours
Legal Aspects of Health Care	45 hours
Human Growth and Development	45 hours
General Psychology	45 hours
Educational/Cognitive Psychology	45 hours
Abnormal Psychology	45 hours
Anatomy and Physiology	45 hours each
Kinesiology	45 hours
Motor Skill Learning	45 hours
Survey of Medical/Disabling Conditions	45 hours
Pharmacology	30 hours
Introduction to Recreation and Leisure Services	45 hours

From Guidelines for Competency Assessment and Curriculum Planning in Therapeutic Recreation: A Tool for Self-Evaluation. © American Therapeutic Recreation Association, 2000.

course content in their academic preparation in the behavioral sciences. This understanding of basic human development and functioning, understanding of how people learn and understanding of influences on human behavior prepares the recreational therapist to work in a holistic manner with patients, integrating a focus on human development and functioning with a focus on how people integrate functioning into life activities to develop and maintain life satisfaction.

Table 32.3 provides a list of modalities, identified by Kinney and Witman in the ATRA publication *Guidelines for Competency Assessment and Curriculum Planning in Therapeutic Recreation: A Tool for Self-Evaluation*,[6] that are used by recreational therapists in treatment interventions with patients. The modalities listed are documented in professional literature and are used by recreational therapists as interventions to reach treatment goals and patient outcomes. Based upon their personal interests as well as patient and agency needs for specialized interventions, recreational therapists will develop competencies to use selected modalities or activities as interventions to meet patient

Table 32.3: Guidelines for competency assessment in therapeutic recreation: a tool for self-evaluation	
Modality skills:	
Adventure experiences/initiatives	American sign language
Arts/crafts	Behavior modification/management
Animal facilitation interventions	Cognitive retraining
Assertiveness training	Family interventions
Athletics/sports	Grief and loss counseling
Aquatics	Group interventions
Bibliotherapy/storytelling	Games
Camping/outdoor recreation	Guided imagery
Community integration	Humor
Dance/movement	Leisure education/counseling
Drama	Play therapy/skills
Empowerment/self-esteem exercises	Prepostoperative/procedural training
Exercises/fitness/aerobics	Remotivation
Horseback riding	Resocialization
Horticulture	Reality orientation
Meditation	Reminiscence
Music/singing	Sensory stimulation
Parties/special events	Social skills training
Problem solving	Stress management/relaxation
Projects/service activities	Therapeutic community
Weight training	Values clarification
Biofeedback	

From Guidelines for Competency Assessment and Curriculum Planning in Therapeutic Recreation: A Tool for Self-Evaluation. © American Therapeutic Recreation Association, 2000.

treatment goals. Some employers require certifications of competency in some modalities, such as exercise or biofeedback, by independent organizations, as a measure of competency to use the intervention safely and effectively.

Standards of Practice

In addition to understanding professional definitions of recreational therapy, as well as qualifications and competencies of recreational therapists, it is also important to understand that qualified and competent recreational therapists who practice in accordance with professional standards of practice are more likely to consistently reach valued patient outcomes. In its publication *Standards for the Practice of Therapeutic Recreation and Self-Assessment*

Guide, ATRA outlines standards for direct practice in therapeutic recreation including[2]:

Standard 1. Assessment
Standard 2. Treatment Planning
Standard 3. Plan Implementation
Standard 4. Reassessment and Evaluation
Standard 5. Discharge and Transition Planning
Standard 6. Recreation Services
Standard 7. Ethical Conduct

The publication has establishes standards for the management of direct practice including[2]:

Standard 8. A Written Plan of Operation (e.g. policies and procedures)
Standard 9. Staff Qualifications and Competency Assessment
Standard 10. Quality Management
Standard 11. Resource Management
Standard 12. Program Evaluation and Research.

A unique aspect of the *Standards for the Practice of Therapeutic Recreation* is that for each standard there are structure, process and outcome criteria and a rating scale to be used by recreational therapists in the self-assessment of compliance with the standards of practice.[2] *Structure criteria* focus on structural parameters of practice such as policies and procedures, facilities, and resources. *Process criteria* focus on the key aspects of the actual provision of services such as therapist-patient interaction or interventions used to reach treatment goals. *Outcome criteria* focus on the key aspects of outcomes of service provision, including measured improvement in functioning or progress towards patients' treatment goals, patients' understanding and compliance with the treatment process and patients' satisfaction with the treatment process and services provided. The *Standards for the Practice of Therapeutic Recreation* is a document built upon the national consensus of recreational therapists and educators and the self-assessment process has been field tested for its value in assessing compliance with the standards and criteria. Since the revision in 2000, the publication also has data collection instruments (e.g. Documentation Audits, Management Audits, Outcome Assessment, Competency Assessment and Clinical Performance Appraisal) with an explanation of how to use the instruments in the data collection process to systematize the collection of data to be used in the self-assessment of compliance with the standards of practice. Use of the self-assessment process has proven effective in field tests as a means to determine opportunities to improve compliance with the standards as a means to improve the quality of services for patients.

In review, definitions of recreational therapy and therapeutic recreation have been described along with the JCAHO definition of a qualified recreational therapist. In addition, a description of minimal competencies (knowledge, skills and abilities) that serve as the basis for the national certification examination of the NCTRC, a national certification organization in the United States that also certifies growing numbers of recreational therapists from other countries, have been provided (*see* **Table 32.1**). Content areas and modalities that serve as the basis for practice competencies described in the publication *Guidelines for Competency Assessment and Curriculum Planning in Therapeutic Recreation: A Tool for Self-Evaluation* published by the American Therapeutic Recreation Association have also been reviewed (*see* **Tables 32.2 and 32.3**) as an example of a higher level of competencies for effective practice as a recreational therapist than the basic competencies required by for certification. Finally, the *Standards for the Practice of Therapeutic Recreation* have been reviewed to provide a reference for the essential aspects of practice as a recreational therapist. This content is intended to provide an understanding of recreational therapy services provided by qualified and competent recreational therapists as an introduction to understanding how recreational therapy may contribute to the rehabilitation of persons with cerebral vascular accidents and spinal cord injuries.

Recreational Therapy for Spinal Injury and Stroke Rehabilitation

Previous chapters of this text have described the basic anatomy of the brain and the spinal cord as well as evaluation and rehabilitation of patients with spinal cord injuries and strokes so that information will not be repeated in this chapter. This section of the chapter on recreational therapy will initially describe the therapeutic recreation processes of individualized assessment, treatment planning, plan implementation and discharge and transition planning that will be provided by qualified and competent recreational therapists and will follow these sections with a description of the benefits of recreational therapy with a focus on the benefits of recreational therapy in the rehabilitation of patients with strokes and spinal cord injuries.

Individualized Assessment

Like other members of the rehabilitation team, the recreational therapist will conduct an individualized assessment of the patient upon receiving a physician's order or consult for evaluation and treatment of a patient. Consistent with professional standards of practice,[2] the assessment process by the recreational therapist will be a structured process that includes a review of medical record information, a structured interview of the patient and family, if possible, observation of the patient in functional activities and performance or standardized testing of the patient. The purpose of the individualized assessment is to gather culturally appropriate and relevant baseline data that describes the patient's strengths and limitations in the following functional areas: physical, cognitive, social, behavioral, emotional and leisure/play.

The recreational therapist reviews the patient's medical record to determine the patient's diagnosis, medical history, limitations in functioning, nutritional needs, history of substance use/abuse, physical or emotional abuse, precautions and prognosis and social history (hometown, education level, occupation, family history, language spoken, religious/spiritual/cultural practices, etc.) and, in addition, any assessments of physical, cognitive, emotional and social functioning conducted by members of the rehabilitation team will be reviewed.

The recreational therapist will seek the patient's collaboration in the assessment process, to the extent the patient is able to participate, and will seek to involve the family of the patient, if available and as appropriate. The role of the patient and family in the assessment process is to identify information of particular importance to the patient and family such as patient goals for rehabilitation, stressors, coping skills, support available during and after hospitalization, previous interests and participation patterns (e.g. type of recreation interests, frequency and duration of participation, etc.) and plans for accommodations after discharge from rehabilitation. In addition to interviewing the patient and family, the recreational therapist will also involve the patient in a functional assessment (e.g. performance testing and/ or, observation in functional activities) to determine strengths and limitations in physical (e.g. mobility, balance, muscle strength, flexibility, gross/fine motor functioning and coordination, range of motion, sitting or standing tolerance, endurance, cardiovascular fitness, etc.), cognitive (e.g. memory, attention span, orientation judgment, problem solving, comprehension, communication skills, sequencing, etc.), social (e.g. appearance/grooming, social skills/ interaction, activity interests and participation patterns, personality type preferences such as introverted or extroverted, etc.) and emotional functioning (affect/emotions displayed, awareness of emotional response, etc.) as well as motivation and initiative to participate in rehabilitation and life activities after discharge.

The recreational therapist will analyze the results of the assessment to formulate clinical impressions and priorities for treatment interventions that will compliment the treatment plan formulated by the treatment team and will meet patient goals for rehabilitation and discharge. The recreational therapist may choose goals that other members of the team are also addressing to provide more intensive intervention, training or re-training for the patient, or may choose to address different goals to assure that a holistic approach to improving all aspects of patient functioning is employed by the team. The recreational therapist will document a summary of the assessment findings and clinical impressions.

Treatment Planning

Consistent with standards of practice[2] and based upon the results of the assessment and the overall rehabilitation treatment plan, the recreational therapist prioritizes patient problems or limitations to be addressed and identifies short- and long-term rehabilitation goals to be achieved by the patient prior to discharge. Once goals are determined, the recreational therapist will determine treatment interventions (e.g. modalities, **Table 32.3**) that will be implemented to achieve the planned functional patient outcomes. The recreational therapist will also consider any unique aspects of the particular patient (e.g. age, limitations, socioeconomic background, cultural practices and preferences, etc.), as well as facilitation techniques and strategies, activity adaptations and/or adaptive equipment needed, to determine effective methods of involving the patient to assure a successful intervention and achievement of goals. The recreational therapist will not only determine the type of intervention to be used to achieve treatment goals, but will also determine the frequency, duration and intensity of intervention (e.g. individualized or group intervention) needed to achieve the treatment goals, considering the patients functional level, endurance and overall treatment schedule. In planning treatment interventions, the recreational therapist will consider ways to involve the patient in the intervention to the extent possible, providing the patient with as much involvement and control as possible, while assuring success of the activity. Recreational therapists plan to involve the patient in assuming increasing amounts of choice, control and direction of the intervention as the patient improves functioning and progresses in his/her rehabilitation, to prepare the patient for discharge when he or she will need to assume responsibility for choosing and initiating activities that will continue rehabilitation improvement or maintain functional levels. The individualized recreational therapy treatment plan is documented in the patient's medical record, consistent with agency policies, and is shared with members of the treatment team.

Initially, when the recreational therapy program is being developed for a particular rehabilitation agency, interventions are selected from the list of modalities typically used by recreational therapists and a written description is developed to describe and tailor the specific aspects of the intervention to be used in the particular rehabilitation program for the patient populations served. **Table 32.4** provides an example of a format used for a written intervention description. Often, after the recreational therapist has established a program for the rehabilitation agency, written intervention descriptions have been developed for the patients served and will only need to be modified to match a particular patient's functional level and needs. This planning will consider the roles and functions of members of the rehabilitation team, interventions used by specific disciplines and whether any interventions will be provided as a co-treatment by different disciplines. For example, a recreational therapist and an occupational, physical or speech therapist may choose to cofacilitate an intervention in an interdisciplinary manner, capitalizing upon the specialized competencies each specialist may be able to use in the intervention.

In rehabilitation programs serving patients with strokes and spinal cord injuries typical recreational therapy interventions might include coping skills training (activities to facilitate expression of emotions and adjustment to disability, use of relaxation techniques to reduce stress, etc.), exercise, fitness, mobility or motor skills training, community re-entry (e.g. activities to adjust to re-entry into the community, including transportation, architectural barriers and attitudinal barriers towards persons with disabilities, adaptations needed

Table 32.4: Policy format for treatment intervention descriptions		
UNC™ HEALTH CARE *Excludes Rex Healthcare	Name of Policy	Approved Format for Treatment Interventions
	Policy Number	Tx-2
	Date Effective	07/07/94
	Date Last Reviewed	07/06/04
	Department Responsible for Review	Department of Recreational Therapy

Policy

All Recreational Therapy treatment interventions are to be written in the department approved format described in this policy and have necessary approvals prior to implementation.

Procedures

1. The following format will be used to describe recreational therapy treatment interventions:

   Title: Format for Writing Treatment Intervention Descriptions

   Purpose: Describe the intervention's purpose in terms of expected patient outcomes.

   Goals: Describe the specific patient outcome goals to be addressed through the application of the intervention.

   Procedures:

   Referral Criteria:

   Describe the criteria for referring the patient for the intervention. Relate to problems identified by the assessment and any patient competencies or abilities necessary for successful involvement in the intervention.

   Intervention Format:

   Describe the format for the intervention including:

   a. Frequency by which the intervention will be provided.
   b. Whether the intervention will be provided on a group or individual basis.
   c. Duration of the intervention.
   d. Specific activities to be used to reach patient outcome goals.
   e. Competency requirements for those conducting the intervention.
   f. The method of evaluation to be used to determine outcomes produced by the intervention.
   g. Resources necessary to effectively conduct the intervention.
   h. Provisions made for patient supervision, safety/risk management, and infection control.
   i. Medical documentation of the patients' responses, reactions, and outcomes reached as a result of the implementation of the intervention.
   j. If the intervention is conducted in a group, identify the following:
      - The group leader
      - Minimum and maximum number of patients to be included.
      - Location where the group will be conducted.
      - Session by session description of structure and content.

2. Written descriptions of treatment interventions are approved by Assistant Directors to determine resource allocation/cost effectiveness and that the activities are appropriate, medically necessary, and would reasonably produce the intended outcomes.

Approval - Director, Department of Recreational Therapy Date

for community trips, etc.), or cognition skills training (activities to improve communication skills, memory, sequencing, judgment, problem solving, organizational skills, etc.). Separate descriptions of the interventions will be developed for patients with strokes and patients with spinal cord injuries to address specific problems or limitations particular to strokes or spinal cord injuries. For example, there would be different content of the coping skills training intervention for patients with spinal cord injuries and patients with strokes taking into consideration the unique and different impairments and limitations in functioning resulting from each disabling condition.

Plan Implementation

According the professional standards of practice[2] the recreational therapist implements an individualized recreational therapy treatment plan, consistent with the overall rehabilitation plan of care for the patient, using appropriate interventions to restore and rehabilitate specific aspects of patient functioning to improve independence in life activities. When the patient's discharge destination (e.g. home, another treatment facility, residential facility, etc.) is considered along with available support systems and community resources, the plan should include discharge plans including equipment and resources necessary to reduce or eliminate, to the extent possible, the activity limitations and restrictions to participation in life activities in the home and community environment. The recreational therapist implements the treatment interventions according to the treatment plan, including the frequency, duration and intensity of intervention necessary to achieve patient treatment goals and reach desired patient outcomes. Patient involvement, response, reaction and progress is monitored, documented on the patient's medical record and shared with members of the treatment team.

Reassessment and Evaluation

The recreational therapist, in compliance with professional standards of practice[2] systematically reassesses, evaluates and compares the patient's progress relative to the recreational therapy treatment plan. The recreational therapist revises the plan or interventions, as needed, based upon changes in the patient's condition or response to the treatment plan to achieve treatment goals and reach planned patient outcomes. Changes to the treatment plan are documented on the medical record and shared with the rehabilitation team.

Discharge and Transition Planning

The recreational therapist, in compliance with professional standards of practice and in collaboration with the patient, family and members of the treatment team, plans and prepares the patient for discharge from the rehabilitation agency and transition to home or other living arrangement.[2] In this stage of service delivery the recreational therapist summarizes the patient's response to treatment interventions, including current functional level and treatment goals and outcomes achieved. The recreational therapist will also recommend any continued services or aftercare needed by the patient in consideration of specific needs related to cultural adaptations, living arrangements, support systems, leisure interests, financial considerations, adaptive equipment or activity modifications needed, community resources and any agency referrals needed. The discharge and transition plan is documented in the patient's medical record and shared with the patient and family to prepare them for discharge and transition. When the treatment plan is effectively implemented and the patient goals and outcomes are achieved, the patient should be prepared for discharge from the rehabilitation agency. The preparation for discharge actually begins with the initial assessment and continues through each phase of the treatment process so when the time for discharge or transition arrives, all should be prepared for the transition to the next living situation. If the recreational therapist and other members of the team have been successful, the patient and family are prepared to transition whether that means the patient will return home or to another treatment or living situation. When rehabilitation is successful, the patient has reached maximum functional improvement and is prepared and motivated to be as independent as possible in life activities in the least restrictive living situation. If the community re-entry interventions provided by the recreational therapist and members of the rehabilitation team have been successful, the patient is prepared for what he/she may encounter in the transition from the rehabilitation setting and has developed the coping skills needed to assume responsibility for participation in life activities to the maximal extent possible to maintain health, well-being and a satisfactory quality of life.

Benefits of Recreational Therapy

Like many other health care and allied health disciplines, efficacy of recreational therapy interventions, as determined by randomized controlled trials, has not been demonstrated. Effectiveness of recreational therapy and therapeutic recreation interventions are most often documented in the literature as a result of research studies, case studies, and anecdotal reports of successful outcomes of patient interventions. Much of what is documented in literature published in the United States describes the effectiveness of services provided in the United States or Canada. Much of what is documented in international literature refers to the effectiveness or benefits of recreation or sports for persons with disabilities. This is a reflection of the differences between the United States and other countries in the development and practice of the therapeutic recreation or recreational therapy. A search of web sites indicates that various forms of recreation, adapted recreation or therapeutic recreation services, not usually recreational therapy as defined in this chapter, are provided in Canada, United Kingdom, Japan, British Columbia, Thailand, Korea, Australia and New Zealand.[7] Therapeutic recreation degree programs are available in Canada and New Zealand.

ATRA's web site lists a Summary of Health Outcomes in Recreational Therapy that were identified in a national grant received by Temple University's program in Therapeutic Recreation and funded by the United States Department of Education's National Institute on Disability and Rehabilitation Research. Proceedings from a national consensus conference were described in a grant publication entitled Benefits of Therapeutic Recreation: A Consensus View. Studies described in this publication documented positive health outcomes in rehabilitation resulting from exercise, fitness and relaxation interventions.[8] Specific outcomes of recreational therapy interventions in physical medicine identified the following benefits[8]:

- *Improvement in physical health status:* Participation in various exercise and fitness activities resulted in significant improvements in cardiovascular and respiratory functioning, and increased strength, endurance, and coordination for persons with disabilities including paraplegia, cystic fibrosis, and asthma.
- *Reduction in complications related to secondary disability:* Physical activity has been demonstrated to reduce secondary medical complications arising from spinal cord injury and other physical disabilities. For example, decubitus ulcers and urinary tract infections were significantly reduced in a group of wheelchair athletes, as compared to nonathletes.
- *Improvement in long-term health status and reduction in health risk factors:* Lowered cholesterol levels, reduced heart disease risk, and improved ability to manage chronic pain were reported for persons with physical disabilities. Further, in a group of individuals with spinal cord injury, activity level was found to be significantly related to survival rate.
- *Improvement in cognitive functioning:* Enhanced attention, memory, perception, and organization skills were documented for persons with traumatic head injuries who participated in recreational activities and tasks focused upon using and developing these skills.
- *Improvement in psychosocial health and well-being:* Decreased depression, improved body image, and increased acceptance of disability have been reported for physically disabled participants in fitness and athletic activities.
- *Reduction in reliance upon the healthcare system:* Participation in exercise and other physical recreation interventions by persons with physical disabilities resulted in reduced use of asthma medication, and in decreased anxiety and stress of a magnitude equal to or greater than that accomplished through medication. A group of wheelchair athletes demonstrated a re-hospitalization rate which was one-third that of a matched group of nonathletes.
- For individuals with spinal cord injuries, active involvement in recreation postinjury was positively related to life satisfaction, high-quality social relationships, and low levels of depression.
- Participants in various adapted adventure activities including hiking and camping demonstrated significantly increased self-efficacy, self-confidence, and acceptance of disability.
- Recipients of individualized recreational therapy services in an inpatient rehabilitation setting demonstrated significantly greater self-esteem

at discharge, as well as ability to utilize activity to cope with stressors related to hospitalization, as compared to a group of matched controls not receiving recreational therapy services.

- A structured community transition intervention for physically disabled persons resulted in significant decreases in social isolation, and significant increases in perceived quality of life. These results support a related study of a structured community integration intervention which reported significant improvement in community functioning and barrier management.

The following outcomes of recreational therapy interventions with older adults were included[8]:

- *Reduction in symptom levels for chronic or degenerative disorders:* Older adults with arthritis or osteoporosis participating in physical activities demonstrated decreased pain and stiffness; increased mobility and muscular strength; and increased bone strength.
- *Improvement in physical health and reduction in health risk factors:* Participants in a variety of physical recreation, exercise, and fitness interventions experienced significantly increased cardiovascular fitness; decreased body weight and body fat; decreased blood pressure; and increased flexibility, strength, ambulation, and range of motion.
- *Improvement in cognitive functioning:* Cognitively impaired older adults participating in activities focused upon reality orientation, sensory simulation, and environmental awareness demonstrated significantly increased alertness and awareness of their surroundings; reduced confusion and disorientation; improved memory, attention span, and problem solving skills; and reduced reliance upon medication.
- *Improvement in psychosocial supports and psychological health:* Participants in a variety of social, expressive, artistic, or home- and nature-based activities demonstrated decreased loneliness and increased affiliation with others; increased verbal interaction; improved morale and life satisfaction; enhanced perceptions of personal control and competence; increased relaxation and ability to effectively manage stress; and reduced levels of depression.

Rehabilitation and Recreational Therapy for Persons with Strokes

Teasell, Foley, Bhogal and Speechley[9] in their review of evidenced-based stroke rehabilitation literature describe numerous findings at the moderate or strong level of evidence including that "greater intensity of therapy results in improved functional outcomes", "progressive strengthening exercises improve abilities to perform activities of daily living", "specific training programs can improve some elements of inattention", "specific treatment of visual neglect and perceptual disorders improves neglect functioning", "treatment utilizing primarily enhanced visual scanning techniques improves visual neglect post-stroke with associated improvement in function", "cognitive behavioral therapy may help alleviate post stroke depression in some patients", "music therapy improves post stroke depression", improved social support as an intervention improves outcomes" and "positive benefit of family education if it involves an active-educational-counseling approach". This evidenced-based review of rehabilitation literature also reports that prevalence of post stroke depression in the first two years post stroke ranges from 2 to 40% and lasts greater than six months[9] and that altered self-perception is associated with depression and social withdrawal.[9] Also reported is that deterioration in social and leisure activities is common post stroke and that perceptions of how others will view the disability and how they will be able to cope poststroke dictates how isolated patients will become.[9] It was reported that there was conflicting evidence regarding benefits of leisure therapy post stroke and following discharge.[9] While this research is not specific to recreational therapy practice it does indicate support for interventions that address strengthening exercises, inattention, visual neglect, perceptual disorders, social support, family education and counseling, all of which could addressed by recreational therapy interventions to compliment those provided by other members of the rehabilitation team. A striking outcome noted is the prevalence of depression poststroke and the relationship between altered self-perception, perceptions of coping poststroke, social withdrawal, social isolation and depression. Music therapy was noted to improve post stroke depression.[9] It was noted that there is conflicting evidence that leisure therapy alters functional outcomes, but it was noted that there was moderate evidence that outpatient social support interventions improve stroke outcomes.[9] The studies on leisure therapy appeared to be done using occupational therapists.

Support for Coping Interventions

The benefits of problem-focused and emotion-focused coping strategies, including relaxation exercises, to address stress associated with strokes are documented by Lyon.[10] The need for rehabilitation professionals to address and reduce stress as aspect of rehabilitation to reach the goal of wellness is supported by this author. Hood and Carruthers[11] have documented a coping skills intervention that involves problem-focused and emotion-focused coping strategies to be used by recreational therapists to assist people with disabilities to cope with various stressor associated with disabilities. McCraty and Tomasino[12] describe the value of Freeze-Framer, a new, computer-based heart rhythm coherence monitoring and feedback system. Evidence from studies conducted with diverse populations using HeartMath have demonstrated significant reductions in stress, anxiety and depression and increases in positive affect and attitudes. Unpublished and anecdotal results of the use of Freeze-Framer by a qualified and competent recreational therapist at UNC Hospitals in the United States has produced promising results of the value of this intervention in assisting patients to reduce stress and anxiety and cope with pain resulting from burns.

Support for Exercise Interventions

Motor recovery strategies after stroke documented by Stein[13] indicate that younger patients appear to have a greater ability to recover from strokes and there is some evidence, although not conclusive, that more intensive exercise programs provided when resources are available, with younger stroke patients, may result in better functional outcomes. Carr and Jones[14] document the value of exercise and strength training for stroke survivors including the ability to perform functional activities, including activities of daily living, with less fatigue. Wood, Murillo, Bach-y-Rita, Leder, Marks and Page[15] describe the value of a game-based intervention in improving patients' motor function. As a result of the intervention, patients demonstrated motor improvement and reported carry-over value to other activities such as gardening. Patients also expressed enjoyment and satisfaction as a result of participating in the intervention. While this particular study was done by occupational therapists it is supportive of game-based interventions to improve motor functioning. Recreational therapists frequently use a wide variety of game based interventions in their practice.

Role of Recreation and Therapeutic Recreation in Stroke Rehabilitation

Cowdell and Garrettt,[16] nurses in the United Kingdom, report that there is little evidence that recreational activity is viewed as an integral part of rehabilitation. Poststroke research by several authors investigates recreation in the community setting and concludes that a reduction in leisure activity is a result of strokes. They also report that there has been little research investigating the use of recreation in rehabilitation, but that recovery may be enhanced with the integration of recreation into the rehabilitation process.[16] MacNeil and Pringnitz[17] provide a review of the value of therapeutic recreation interventions used in stroke rehabilitation at a hospital and rehabilitation center in the United States. Interventions used include individualized recreational therapy, aquatics, unilateral skills class, evening activity program, community integration program and a family education program. The authors conclude that to reach the goal of continued patient involvement in social and leisure activities at the highest level of independence in his/her home environment it is helpful to have a therapeutic recreation specialist on the rehabilitation team. Nour, Desrosiers, Gauthier, and Carbonneau[18] describe a leisure educational program, with the components of self-awareness, leisure awareness and competency development, used in a research study to evaluate the value of the home leisure educational program in helping stroke patients adjust psychologically. The results indicated that the program did enhance the total and physical quality of life for participants, but the program did not reduce the level of depression. It was speculated that depression may have been less of a concern immediately after rehabilitation than it could be six months later and that a ten-week intervention at this stage may not have had the time to demonstrate impact upon depression. Field notes indicated that people perceived their life more positively as a result of the intervention even if their physical condition was poor. Participants resumed leisure activities and initiated participation in community activities. It was recommended that for the program to be maximally effective it should be initiated during inpatient of day rehabilitation.

*Rehabilitation and Recreational Therapy for Persons
with Spinal Cord Injuries*

Richter, Sherrill, McCann, Mushett and Kaschalk[19] describe the history of sports for people with disabilities, the risks and the benefits of recreation and sports for people with disabilities. An introduction to therapeutic recreation is provided and outcomes of therapeutic recreation interventions including "increasing personal awareness, increasing interpersonal or social skills, developing leisure skills, decreasing stress, improving physical fitness and functioning, developing feelings of positive self-regard, self efficacy perceived control, pleasure and enjoyment" are listed.[19] The authors conclude that, in most situations, the risks are outweighed by the significant benefits including physiological, psychological, social and existential.

Stass, Formal, Freedman, Fried and Read[20] describe the importance of recreation and sports for persons with spinal cord injuries as providing constructive use of leisure time and enhancing quality of life. The authors describe that, because of perception of leisure time as a problem and mobility concerns by those who have a new spinal cord injury, the program focus should be:
1. Education in the community's recreation resources.
2. Adaptations for previous leisure skills and interests.
3. Learning of new leisure skills.
4. Refinement of functional abilities related to specific leisure activities.[20]

Participation in sports and a general fitness program is described as an expression of well-being and a means to improved general health. Secondary benefits described include a more positive self-image, better interpersonal relationships, a decrease in secondary medical complications associated with inactivity and less likelihood of depression.[20]

Verbout[21] describes the value of recreational therapy in the rehabilitation of persons with spinal cord injuries. Outcomes of recreational therapy for persons with spinal cord injuries identified include: "improve short and long-term physical health, reduce secondary health issues such as skin breakdown and urinary tract infections, improve a person's mental and social health including decreased depression, improved body image and adjustment to disability, reduce reliance on health care, decrease social isolation, improve management of barriers to buildings and improve ability to get around the community, improve stress management and identify coping strategies and activities, increase self-assertiveness, and improve ability to develop social relationships and return to past recreational interests with new adaptive recreation skills and resources."[21] The publication also lists recreation/travel/ sports resources for persons with disabilities.

Humpage[22] describes a patient case study involving a community reintegration program designed to continue involvement in leisure activities, to develop community re-entry skills, and to integrate treatment with the patients overall rehabilitation program. The subject in the case study is a 24-year-old female with a C4-5 spinal cord injury involved in a series of goal directed community outings with her recreational therapist and, at times, the occupational therapist. As a result of the intervention, it was reported that the patient demonstrated the following benefits of the intervention: social interaction, social and emotional adjustment and initiative in accessing community resources.

In a case report involving a 34-year-old male with T-10-L-1 level spinal cord injury Wise and Hale[23] describe the benefits of a weight training intervention with designed to generalize self-efficacy from weight training to activities of daily living. As a result of the intervention, self-efficacy in weight training and activities of daily living increased during treatment and the increases were maintained for eight months post-treatment. Self-report from the patient indicated he was motivated to learn how to weight train after his injury and to use the opportunity to meet other people with spinal cord injuries. He also reported that the intervention helped him to realize he could have a life after the spinal cord injury. After rehabilitation he found a job, returned to school and joined a gym where he could continue his weight training.

Caldwell and Weissinger[24] studied a sample of patients with spinal cord injuries discharged from a hospital in Canada from 1982-1986 to determine psychological and demographical variables that influence perceptions of boredom in leisure. Caldwell and Weissinger[24] determined that while self-determination as a component of intrinsic motivation may be of significant importance to nondisabled persons, perceived skill or ability is more likely the cause of boredom for persons with spinal cord injuries. Other research reported indicated that in a study involving a sample of 790 adults with disabilities, 42% reported that a lack of physical ability was a barrier to leisure behavior and 32% reported that feeling unsure of abilities was a barrier to leisure behavior. An consideration for rehabilitation agencies from this study is that if the goal of rehabilitation is to return patients to independence and involvement in meaningful life activities, including recreation, more needs to be done to improve the skill and ability of persons with spinal cord injuries so the level of physical ability and lack of confidence in abilities are not a factor that limits involvement in leisure activities after discharge.

Patrick[25] compared ten novice, mobility impaired, athletes to veteran athletes and non-athletes prior to and after five, months after their first competitive wheelchair sports experience and compared self-concept and acceptance of disability. The results of the study supported that participation, as a novice, in wheelchair athletics has a powerful positive influence on self-concept and acceptance of disability. The results confirmed previous findings that athletes score higher than nonathletes in acceptance of disability.

Summary and Conclusion

As was stated in the beginning of this chapter, this purpose of this chapter was (1) to provide an understanding of recreational therapy as a professional discipline to be included in the team of rehabilitation specialists responsible for the provision of rehabilitation services and (2) to provide an understanding of recreational therapy practice and of interventions that may be used by a recreational therapist in the rehabilitation of persons who have had strokes or spinal cord injuries. As was also stated previously, efficacy of recreational therapy interventions, as determined by randomized controlled trials, has not been demonstrated. However, research studies, case studies, and anecdotal reports of program interventions demonstrate the value and benefits of recreation and therapeutic recreation in contributing to the rehabilitation of persons with strokes and spinal cord injuries. The prevalence of qualified and competent recreational therapists working in health care, rehabilitation and human service agencies in the United States demonstrate the emergence of a profession that can enhance rehabilitation outcomes for patient with strokes, spinal cord injuries and a variety of other disabling conditions. A review of the evolution of professionals working in recreation and therapeutic recreation, in not only the United States, but increasingly in other countries around the world and the benefits provided to persons with disabilities seems to indicate that this growth will continue. As academic programs preparing qualified and competent recreational therapists increase in countries around the world, recreational therapists will be better prepared to demonstrate the effectiveness of the interventions they use to improve the physical, cognitive, emotional and social functioning of patients in rehabilitation. Increased numbers of qualified and competent recreational therapists on rehabilitation teams will also contribute to patients' enhanced adjustment to disability, increased independence and quality of life after discharge from rehabilitation.

References

1. US Bureau of Labor Statistics. Occupational Outlook Handbook 2004-05 edition: Recreational Therapist, Available at: *http://www.bls.gov/oco/ocos082.htm.* Accessed November 8, 2004.
2. American Therapeutic Recreation Association. Standards for the Practice of Therapeutic Recreation and Self-Assessment Guide. Alexandria, VA; 2000.
3. World Health Organization. International Classification of Functioning, Disability and Health: ICF. Geneva, Switzerland; 2001.
4. Joint Commission on Accreditation of Healthcare Organizations. Comprehensive Accreditation Manual for Hospitals. Chicago, II: Joint Commission Resources, 2003.
5. National Council for Therapeutic Recreation Certification. Certification Standards, part v: nctrc national job analysis. Available at: *www.nctrc.org/certification/index.html* Accessed November 8, 2004.
6. Kinney T, Witman J (Eds). Guidelines for Competency Assessment and Curriculum Planning in Therapeutic Recreation: A Tool for Self Evaluation. American Therapeutic Recreation Association. Hattiesburg, MS, 1997.
7. Therapeutic Recreation and Adapted Recreation Around the World. Web Site. Available at: *http://www.recreationtherapy.com/rt.htm.* Accessed November 8, 2004.
8. American Therapeutic Recreation Association Web Site. Summary of health outcomes in recreation therapy. Available at: *http://www.atra-tr.org/benefitshealthoutcomes.htm.* Accessed on November 24, 2004.

9. Teasel RW, Foley NC, Bhogal SK, Speechley MR. An evidenced-based review of stroke rehabilitation. Top Stroke Rehabil. 2003;10:29-58.
10. Lyon BL. Psychological stress and coping: framework for poststroke psychosocial care. Top Stroke Rehabil. 2002;9:1-15.
11. Hood CD, Carruthers CP. Coping skills theory as an underlying framework for therapeutic recreation services. Ther Rec Journ. 2002;36:137-53.
12. McCraty R, Tomasino D. Heart rhythm coherence feedback. Proceedings of the First Baltic Forum on Neuronal Regulation and Biofeedback, 2004.
13. Stein J. Motor recovery strategies after stroke. Top Stroke Rehabil. 2004;11:12-22.
14. Carr M, Jones J. Physiological effects of exercise on stroke survivors. Top Stroke Rehabil. 2003;9:57-64.
15. Wood SR, Murillo N, Bach-y-Rita P, Leder RS, Marks JT, Page SJ. Motivating, game-based stroke rehabilitation: a brief report. Top Stroke Rehabil. 2003;10:134-40.
16. Cowdell F, Garrett D. Recreation in stroke rehabilitation part one: a review of the literature. Intern Journ of Ther and Rehabil. 2003;10:408-11.
17. MacNeil RD, Pringnitz TD. The role of therapeutic recreation in stroke rehabilitation. Ther Rec Journ. 1982;XVI:26-34.
18. Nour K, Desrosiers J, Gauthier P, Carbonneau H. Impact of a home leisure educational program for older adults who have had a stroke (home leisure educational program). Ther Rec Journ. 2002;36:48-64.
19. Richter KJ, Sherrill C, McCann CB, Mushett CA, Kaschalk SM. Recreation and sport for people with disabilities. In: Delisa JA and Gans BM (Eds). Rehabilitation Medicine Principles and Practices. Philadelphia, PA: Lippincott-Raven Publishers; 1998:853-71.
20. Staas WE Jr, Formal CS, Freedman MK, Fried GW, Read MES. Spinal cord injury and spinal cord injury medicine. In: Delisa JA and Gans BM (Eds). Rehabilitation Medicine Principles and Practices. Philadelphia, PA: Lippencott-Raven Publishers; 1998. pp. 1259-91.
21. Verbout JP. Recreational therapy. In: Spinal Cord Injury: You Do Have Choices [e-book], available at: *http://www.rtcil.org/choices/finalchoices.htm.* Accessed on November 9, 2004.
22. Humpage D. Community reintegration: getting back to life. Rehab Nurs. 2001;26:85-87.
23. Wise JB, Hale SB. Strengthening and generalizing self-efficacy in a male with a spinal cord injury. Ther Rec Journ. 1999;XXXIII:333-41.
24. Caldwell LL, Weissinger E. Factors influencing free time boredom in a sample of persons with spinal cord injuries. Ther Rec Journ. 1994;XXVIII:19-24.
25. Patrick GD. The effects of wheelchair competition on self-concept and acceptance of disability in novice athletes. Ther Rec Journ. 1986;XX:61-71.

33

Epilogue: Regeneration Research—A Hope for Future

Milind Deogaonkar

Introduction

There are some undisputed facts in life. It holds true for science and medicine. For decades, certain facts in medical science are accepted without question. One such fact was that brain cells are constant and are not regenerated. Medical doctors and scientists alike accepted as a matter of faith that the neurons, or brain cells, you were born with all the brain cells you would ever have. So, any damage to these brain cells and you lose the part of brain and its function. Then, Fred Gage, a neurobiologist at the Salk Institute for Biological Studies in La Jolla, California, showed in a groundbreaking experiment that brain cells are born even in adult brains.[1] This discovery forced scientists to rethink some of their most basic ideas about how the brain works. The cells, which are responsible for this, are not simple brain cells or neurons. They are progenitor cells or master cells able to take up any form and function of brain cells. These are called 'Neural Stem Cells' (NSC) and they are master cells with the ability to morph into any type of brain cell, depending on the chemical signals they receive as they grow. Researchers have shown that these cells are most commonly seen in the memory centers (called hippocampus) and in other deeper areas of brain called neurogenic areas. Gage and his team have shown that a part of the hippocampus contains actively developing neural stem cells. They can be pressed into function by a simple but timely addition or subtraction of a few key growth factors in the brain's chemical soup. In view of such modern miracles, it is essential to review the attempts made at regenerating the injured axons and nerve cells that constitute the spinal cord.

Nature of Spinal Cord Injury

The first step essential in the search for a cure of human spinal cord injury (SCI) is to appreciate the complexity of the disorder. Spinal cord injury is often viewed as an all-or-nothing event that is irreversible from the moment of injury. By this view, spinal cord injury is classified as either incomplete or complete. This dichotomy is not absolute, however, because some functional recovery occurs even after severe spinal cord injury. National Acute Spinal Cord Injury Study II (NASCIS II) revealed that patients with so-called complete loss of neurologic function recovered, on an average, 8% of the function they had lost, and patients with an incomplete injury recovered 59%.[2] An injury classified as complete does not necessarily involve loss of all connections. Several studies have demonstrated that many patients with a clinically complete lesion show evidence of residual connections.[3] A certain number of intact connections are probably necessary for functional recovery. The determinants of functional outcome are complex, however, and probably include not only the extent of axonal loss but also the level of dysfunction of the surviving axons and the plasticity of the spinal cord. Animal studies have shown that a small number of axons may be sufficient to support functional recovery.[4] Animals recover evoked potentials and the ability to walk with as few as 10% of their spinal axons. Nerve sprouting, one of the mechanisms of plasticity, allows a few nerves to carry out the function of many. Finally, animal studies have also shown that many of the axons surviving traumatic injury are dysfunctional and that many of these axons have lost part or all of their myelin sheath, which is the structural component that improves the reliability and speed of conduction. In this regard, it is not only the loss of ambulation but also the sensory and autonomic changes that are equally important in recovery. In addition, there are the serious social emotional psychological and lifestyle effects of SCI, which should also be taken into account. It is also true that no two SCI lesions are alike as each is the result of a SCI unique to that individual.

Spinal Cord Repair Research

Existing experimental methods are based on stimulating axonal regeneration by neutralizing inhibitory factors, adding positive tropisms and creating a permissive environment.[5] Better results are obtained by bridging the gap with grafts of peripheral nerves or transplants of Schwann cells and genetically engineered fibroblasts. Recently, the potential for stem cells to enhance this process has created great interest. This is because of the ability of pluripotential cells to differentiate into neural tissue. A cure based on the physiopathology of SCI requires pyramidal, extrapyramidal, sensory, cerebellar and autonomic pathways to be regenerated with their appropriate neurotransmitters restored and reflexes integrated physiologically and in synchrony. In human SCI, there is a very long distance anatomically for axonal regrowth to occur in order to reach their relevant nuclei. This is because of continuing Wallerian degeneration. It also presumes that the target neurons are intact and that there has been no transneuronal degeneration above or below the lesion. Alternatively, in place of regenerated long axons, a multisynaptic pathway may be constructed from stem cells that have developed into neurons. Whether such a pathway would restore useful neurological functions is unknown.

At present, the transplant and grafting research teams are exploring these possibilities in experimental animals. Moderate success in gaining axonal regeneration has been reported; however, it must be appreciated that the human lesion differs considerably from that of the experimental animal. In order to be successful, the neuropathology and neurophysiology of human SCI must be taken into account.

Cell Transplantation in Spinal Injury

There are a lot of newer treatment strategies aimed at transplanting the cells that can grow back into the spinal cord assisted by certain neurotrophic factors. Neural precursor cells (NPCs) are used by some researchers as a mode to recover injured spinal cord. They found that transplantation of NPCs into lesioned adult rat spinal cord results in only partial functional recovery, and most transplanted cells tend to differentiate predominantly into astrocytes. In order to improve functional recovery after transplantation, it is important that transplanted neural precursor cells appropriately differentiate into cell lineages required for spinal cord regeneration. In order to modulate the fate of transplanted cells, they advocated transplanting gene modified neural precursor cells. In their study, they demonstrated that gene modification to inhibit bone morphogenetic protein (BMP) signaling by noggin expression promoted differentiation of neural precursor cells into neurons and oligodendrocytes, in addition to astrocytes after transplantation. Furthermore, functional recovery of the recipient mice with spinal cord injury was observed when noggin expressing neural precursor cells were transplanted.[6] Another group of scientists used cryopreserved olfactory ensheathing cells (OECs) transplantation for axonal regeneration and functional recovery following spinal cord injury in adult rats. In their study at 12 weeks after transplantation, 2 rats (2/7) had lower extremities muscle contraction, 2 rats (2/7) had hip and/ or knee active movement, and MEP of 5 rats (5/7) could be recorded in the calf in the transplantation group. None of the rats (7/7) in the control group had functional improvement, and none had MEPs recorded. In the transplanted group, histological and immunohistochemical methods showed the number of transplanted OECs reduced and some regrown axons had reached the end of transected spinal cord. However, no regrown axons could be seen except scar formation in the control group.[7] Studies like this conclusively shows that transplanted cells could be integrated with the host and promotes regrowing axons across the transected spinal cord ends.

'Bridges' for Spinal Repair

One way to integrate different therapeutic strategies for SCI is to develop implantable scaffolds that can deliver therapies in a synergistic manner. Many investigators have developed implantable "bridges". An important property of such scaffolds is mechanical compatibility with host tissues. In a recent study, mechanically matched hydrogel-based scaffold are used to guide the axonal regrowth through the level of transection to treat SCI.[8] Biodegradable polymer implants for guidance and facilitation of axonal regrowth have recently been used.[9]

Electrostimulus Devices: Paraplegics Walk Again

In recent years, a variety of electrostimulus devices have been developed which help paralyzed individuals to gain control of their paralyzed limbs. In these devices, nerve cuffs are implanted around nerves in the body. These devices sense the signals generated by sensory receptors (like pain and pressure receptors) in the paralyzed limbs and covert them into electrical signals. These electrical signals are carried to a control unit. The control unit is programed to generate response to these stimuli and these are carried through similar nerve cuffs implanted over the motor nerves to the muscles. Once stimulated these muscles move in an orderly fashion for the individual to perform a useful movement.

In one such study, carried out at Case Western Reserve University in Cleveland, 11 paraplegics or low tetraplegics were fitted with Functional Electrical Stimulation system (FES). All the implant recipients at a 12 months review confirmed the ability to stand exercise and transfer.[10] All 11 implant recipients noted improved health and a reduced incidence of pressure sores, leg spasms, and urinary tract infections (UTIs). No incidents of deep-vein thrombosis, infection, cellulitis, or electrical burns because of the neuroprosthesis were noted. System recipients uniformly felt that the neuroprosthesis resulted in better overall health and general well-being. Subjects were moderately to very satisfied with the performance of the neuroprosthesis and unanimously expressed a willingness to repeat the surgery and rehabilitation to obtain the same clinical outcome. All implant recipients reported the system to be safe, reliable, and easy to use. The study concluded that the implanted standing neuroprosthesis appears to be a clinically acceptable and effective means of providing the ability to exercise, stand, and transfer to selected individuals with paraplegia or low tetraplegia.

This combined with advances in phrenic or diaphragmatic pacemakers and bladder pacemakers definitely are a ray of hope for SCI patients.

Epilogue

Once only a dream, researchers now are uncovering ways to repair spinal cord injuries. Current methods reduce the nerve cell damage or death that occurs in the hours following injury and increase the efficiency of surviving nerve cells. New evidence suggests that future treatments also may assist the regeneration of lost connections. Prospects include transplanting new nerve cells and supporting cells, delivering proteins that stimulate regeneration by the cells already in the spinal cord, and strategies to reduce inhibition of regeneration. Newer 'function accentuating implants' combined with regeneration research takes us nearer to the day when 'those without legs' will walk.

References

1. Gage FH. Neurogenesis in the adult brain. J Neurosci. 2002;22(3):612-3.
2. Young W, Bracken M. The second National Acute Spinal Cord Injury Study. J Neurotrauma. 1992;9:S429.
3. Dimitrijevic M, Dimitrijevic M, Faganel J, et al. Residual motor functions in spinal cord injury. Functional recovery in neurological disease. Waxman SE (Ed). Raven Press, New York, 1988.
4. Blight A, Young W. Axonal Morphometric Correlates of Evoked Potentials in Experimental Spinal Cord Injury. Humana Press, New York, 1990.
5. Kakulas BA. Neuropathology: The foundation for new treatments in spinal cord injury. Spinal Cord. 2004;42(10):549-63.
6. Setoguchi T, Nakashima K, Takizawa T, Yanagisawa M, Ochiai W, Okabe M, et al. Treatment of spinal cord injury by transplantation of fetal neural precursor cells engineered to express BMP inhibitor. Exp Neurol. 2004;189(1):33-44.
7. Shen HY, Yin DZ, Tang Y, Wu YF, Cheng ZA, Yang R, Huang L. Influence of cryopreserved olfactory ensheathing cells transplantation on axonal regeneration in spinal cord of adult rats. Chin J Traumatol. 200;7(3):179-83.
8. Bakshi A, Fisher O, Dagci T, Himes BT, Fischer I, Lowman A. Mechanically engineered hydrogel scaffolds for axonal growth and angiogenesis after transplantation in spinal cord injury. J Neurosurg Spine. 2004;1(3):322-9.
9. Friedman JA, Lewellyn EB, Moore MJ, Schermerhorn TC, Knight AM, Currier BL, et al. Synthes Award for Resident Research in Spinal Cord & Spinal Column Injury: Surgical repair of the injured spinal cord using biodegradable polymer implants to facilitate axon regeneration. Clin Neurosurg. 2004;51:314-9.
10. Agarwal S, Triolo RJ, Kobetic R, Miller M, Bieri C, Kukke S, et al. Long-term user perceptions of an implanted neuroprosthesis for exercise, standing, and transfers after spinal cord injury. J Rehabil Res Dev. 2003;40(3):241-52.

Appendix

K Venugopal, Indu Marium Jacob

Clinical Bedside Swallowing Assessment

Oral Motor Evaluation

1. *Structure:* Note any abnormalities (missing teeth, dentures)
2. *Jaw:* Open/close   Control
3. *Labial Function:*
   Lip spread   Lip round
   Lip closure at rest   Lip smacking
   Symmetry   Lip closure on "papa"
   Droop
4. *Lingual function:*
   Protrusion   Retraction
   Lick lips   Lateralization to corners
   Lateralization to buccal cavity   Elevation of tip
   Repetitive elevation of back
5. *Velar function:*
   Prolonged "a": Symmetry during elevation
   Resonance: Normal/hypernasal/hyponasal
6. *Dry swallow (swallow saliva):* +/–

Laryngeal Function

1. *Tracheostomy tube:*
   Cuffed
   Finger occluded
2. *Vocal quality:* Normal/hoarse/breathy/wet
3. *Voluntary cough:* Strong/weak/absent
4. *Throat clearing:* Strong/weak/absent

5. Pitch range
6. Volume control
7. Phonation time
8. Valving for speech.

Cognition/Communication

1. *Orientation:* Person	Time	Place
2. *Follows one-step directions:* +/–	with cues	without cues
3. *Follows two-step directions:* +/–	with cues	without cues
4. *Expressive language:* Gestures/points	single words	phrases
5. *Intelligibility:* Unintelligible confused speech	dysarthria	apraxia
6. Short-term memory		

Swallowing Assessment

1. *Ability to prepare bolus*
   a. Labial control
   b. Lingual elevation
   c. Lingual lateralization
   d. Mastication.

2. *Ability to manipulate bolus*
   a. Lingual function
   b. Oral transit time

3. *Ability to maintain bolus*
   a. Back of tongue control
   b. Labial closure
   c. Cheeks
   d. Lingual lateralization
   e. Clears oral cavity in one swallow
   f. # Swallows per bolus

4. *Pharyngeal phase*
   Initiate swallow/delay (secs)

5. *Laryngeal characteristics*
   a. Vocal quality
   b. Cough/throat clearing
   c. Elevation of larynx.

Index

Page numbers followed by *f* refer to figure and *t* refer to table.

A

Abdominal massage 317
Acetylcholine 313
Acromion 289
Adrenergic blockers, alpha 314
Adrenoreceptor blocker, alpha 314
Advance cardiac life support 58
Advanced interventional pain management
    systems 257
Agrammatism 19
Agraphia 19
Airway 242
  management 324
Alcoholism 372
Alexia 19
Alkaline urine 339
Alkalosis 330
Alveoli tend 322
American Society of Hand Therapist 349
American Spinal Injury Association 209, 241
American Therapeutic Recreation
    Association 393, 398
Anal fissure 316
Analgesia 197
Anemia 132, 172
Anesthesia 135, 197, 198
Anesthetic skin 343
Aneurysm, formation of 12
Ankle
  foot orthosis 352, 355*f*
  tendon 199
Anorectal reflexes 316
Antagonistic muscles, vibration of 276
Antibiotics 365
Anticholinergic therapy 313
Anticoagulant therapy 285
Antidromic recording 226
Antioxidants 176
Antipsychotics, typical 156
Antispastic medications 251
Anxiety 288, 364, 365
Aphasia 110, 111, 114, 115, 122
  comprehension battery for 116
  evaluation of 114
  fact chart 112*t*
  screening tests of 115
  severe 4
  severity of 118

syndromes 19
teaching 122
treatment of 117
types of 111
Apraxia 19, 163
  of speech 19, 114
Arachidonic acid 177
Areflexic bowel dysfunction 317
Arm rest 345
  full-length 345
  height 345
  stability 345
Arterial blood gas analysis 48
Arterial dissections 43
Arterial distribution of stroke 17
Arterial spin labeling 50
Arterial trunk
  anterior 196*f*
  posterior 196*f*
Artery 195
  of Adamkiewicz 195
Ashworth scale, modified 37
Aspiration
  care of 324
  prevention of 324
  risk of 150, 322
Assistive devices 261*f*, 317
Assistive technologies 258
Ataxia 363
Ataxic
  hemiparesis syndrome 20
  nystagmus 9
Atelectasis 319–323, 328
Atherothrombotic strokes 43
Atmosphere 319
Audiospinal facilitation 236
Auditory comprehension 110, 116
  task, functional 116
  test 116
Augmentative communication,
    alternative 122
Autonomic
  dysfunction 372
  dysreflexia 87, 312, 314, 316
  function, evaluation of 226
Autonomous neurogenic bladder 310
Awareness, loss of 199
Axial loading force 203

B

Babinski's extensor response 188
Baclofen 299
 pump 251, 300
Barium swallow, modified 145
Barthel index 36, 215
 modified 215
Basic life support 57
Beck depression inventory 219
Bedsore 251, 337
Behavior modification therapy 119
Behind chair handle 347
Benedikt syndrome 25
Biceps 305
Bite reflex 142
Bitemporal lower quadrantanopia 12
Bladder
 capacity 312
 dysfunction 309
 emptying 314
 expression techniques 312
 management techniques 312
 neck dysfunction 314
 outlet resistance 312, 314
 ultrasound of 253
Blood
 cord barrier 205
 pressure 33, 176
  management 53*t*
 supply of
  brain 3
  spinal cord 194
 test 47
Bobath approach 275
Bobath cuff 67*f*
Body weight 68, 69
Bolus scintigraphy 145
Bolus, maintain 422
Bone morphogenetic protein 418
Botulinum toxin 251, 277, 313, 314
Bowel care 317
 program 317
Bowel disorders 172
Bowel dysfunction 315
Bowel irrigation techniques 317
Bowel management 339
Bowel transit 316
Brain 153, 389
 electrical activity of 34
 functions, higher 94
 imaging of 34
 injury 138, 142, 350
  rehabilitation 359, 372
  severe 377
 motor control assessment 236
Brainstem auditory evoked response 223

Breathing 242
 deep 286
 diaphragmatic 287, 324
 pattern 286
 physiology of 319
Bronchiectasis 322
Bronchitis 322
Bronchospasm 323
Brown-Séquard syndrome 197, 240, 241
Brunnstrom approach 275
Brunnstrom stages of motor recovery 37

C

Calcium metabolism, disordered 81
Calf and foot, elevation of 346
Calorie, low 176
Canadian neurological scale 15
Canes, types of 355*f*
Carbohydrate 173, 336
Cardiac enzymes 48
Cardio-and atheroembolic strokes 43
Cardiopulmonary resuscitation 57
Cardiovascular
 accidents 91
 hazards 89
Carotid artery
 syndromes, internal 21
 internal 3, 10, 21
Carotid phonoangiography 34
Carotid stenosis 47
Catheterization 312
Catheters, external 312
Cauda equina 200, 315
 injuries 226
Cells
 of origin 193
 transplantation 418
Cerebellar infarction 23
Cerebellar symptoms 363
Cerebellum 199
Cerebral
 artery
  anterior 3-5, 10, 21
  bilateral anterior 159
  branches of posterior 7
  infarct, posterior 25
  posterior 4, 5, 7, 10, 21
  right middle 48, 49*f*
  syndromes, anterior 21
 blood flow test 34
 compression 367
 cortex 223
  role of 141
 ischemia 40
 model 269
 palsy 138
 vascular accident 394

Cerebrospinal fluid 363
    fistulae 362
Cerebrovascular accident 28, 152, 180
Cerebrum 12
    inferior surface of 5, 6f
    medial surface of 5, 5f
    superolateral surface of 4f
    supply of 3
Cervical cord 330
    injuries, high 320
Cervical enlargement 183
Cervical injuries, lower 320
Cervical myelopathy 232f
Cervical segments 327
Cervical spinal cord 315
Cervical spine 286
    extension injuries of 204f
    films 243
    stabilization 246f
Cervicomedullary syndrome 241
Chemical rectal agents 317
Chemodenervation 277
Chest 286
    excursion 286
    expansion 287
    injuries 290
    mobility 286
    muscle paralysis 286
    percussion 328
    physiotherapy 287
    wall tightness 286
    wall with paralysis 321
Chin-down posture 148
Chin-up posture 148
Cholesterol 178, 338
    emboli 43
    rich foods 178
Cholinergic dysfunction 365
Choroidal artery
    anterior 6, 10, 21
    posterior 6
Chronic pain, management of 254
Circle of Willis 3
Circulation infarct, posterior 15
Cisapride 318
Clinical stroke scale 25, 25t
Clonidine 314
Coagulation disorders 43
Cock up splint 351f, 352
Cognitive behavioral therapist/
        psychologist 381
Cognitive defects 167, 364
Cognitive deficits 159
    nature of 158
    prevalence of 159
Cognitive functioning 408, 409
Cognitive motor interference 161

Cognitive rehabilitation 377
Cognitive retraining, methods of 165
Cognitive therapy 119, 120
Collateral branches 193
Collateral sprouting 60
Colonic activity 318
Colonic transit 315
    time 317
Colonic wall 315
Coma, deep 9
Communication system
    alternative 263
    augmentation 263
Complete blood count 47
Complete transection 199
Complex regional pain syndrome 83
Compression neuropathies 93
Computer aided therapy 122
Congestive heart failure 46
Conscious muscle sense, loss of 197
Consciousness, loss of 87
Constipation 315, 316
Constraint induced movement therapy 69,
        70, 70f, 275
Conus medullaris 315
    maintain tone 315
    syndrome 241
Conus syndrome 198
Conventional orthotics 356
Conveys touch 186
Cool Calmy skin 87
Cordotomy 199, 258
Corpus callosum 4
Corpus cavernosum 235
Corpus of aphasia therapy 166
Cortical deafness 12
Corticonuclear fibers 10
Corticonuclear tracts 187
Corticospinal tract 187, 188, 194, 199
    anterior 187
Cortisol hyporesponsiveness 363
Cotton seed oil 177
Cough
    function 286
        chronic ineffective 321
    induction 324
    reflex 322
        absent 321
    stimulation 324
Cranial nerve 361, 362
    injuries 362
Cranial neuropathy 372
Craniotomy 365
Cricopharyngeal segment 143
Cricopharyngeous muscle 140
Cruciate paralysis, syndrome of 241
Crushing manner 203

Crutches, types of 355*f*
Cryoanalgesia 257
Cryotherapy 275
Cryptogenic stroke 44
Crystalline amino acids 175
Crystals 338
CSF rhinorrhea 362
Curriculum planning 398, 402
Cutaneous vasodilatation, segmental 197
Cylindrical cast 349
Cylindrical cord of nervous tissue 183
Cystometric capacity 311

D

Daily bladder diary 311
Daily living, activities of 35, 80, 154, 270,
        271, 303, 304, 375
Daycare rehabilitation 387
Daytime drowsiness 323
Deafness, mild 12
Decubitus ulcers 246
Deformity 99, 343, 349
    prevention of 343
Dejerine's syndrome 11, 23
Dementia 111, 138
Depression 32, 364
Descending tracts 185-187, 223
Desipramine 155
Detrusor
    areflexia 310, 311
    hyperreflexia 311
    instability 311
    overactivity 310, 313
    sphincter dyssynergia 310, 311, 314
Diabetes 390
    mellitus 172, 176, 331, 336
Diaphoresis 325
Diaphragm 286
Dietary
    fiber 178, 316
    management 337
    modification 149
Digital substraction angiography 34
Dipyridamole 329
Disability
    moderate 373
    rating scale 373
Discourse comprehension test 116
Distraction force 203
Dizziness 299, 364
Docosahexaenoic acid 177
Doppler sonography 34
Dorsal pontine syndrome
    lower 24
    upper 24
Dorsal root fibers, complete destruction
        of 197

Dorsolumbar lesions 290
Dressing apraxia 20
Drezotomy 299, 300
Drowsiness 299
Drug 327
    administration systems 258
Dry swallow 421
Dysarthria 114
    clumsy hand syndrome 21
Dyselectrolytemia 172
Dyslipidemia 172, 336
Dysphagia 138, 172, 321-323, 363
    management of 147
Dyspnea 322, 323
Dysreflexia 344
Dystonia 297, 372
Dysuria 311

E

Echocardiography 33, 51
Eicosapentaenoic acid 177
Elbow 289, 345, 348
    crutch gait, bilateral 294*f*
    flexing 347
    orthosis 351
    spastic 301
Electrical stimulation
    functional 70, 254, 317, 376
    system, functional 419
Electrically powered wheelchair 259
Electroencephalography 34
Electrolyte 175
    tests 47
Electromyographic
    evidence of clonus 230*f*
    recording 231*f*
Electromyography 224, 229
    biofeedback 376
Electrophrenic pacing 324, 325
Electrophysiological methods 229, 230
Electrophysiological tests 223*t*
Electrostimulus devices 419
Electrotherapy unit 390
Elemental diet 173
Emergency medical services 51, 56
Endocrine dysfunction 363
Energy 174
Enoxaparin 330
Epilepsy 364, 372
Erectile dysfunction 234
Erythrocytosis 323
Esophageal
    dysmotility 322
    stage 140, 143
European Cooperative Acute Stroke Study 40
European Stroke Scale 15
Evoked potential studies 234

Expressive disorders 110
Extrapyramidal tracts 188
Extremity
    dressing, lower 306
    flexor patterns, lower 271
    lower 102, 352
    upper 350
Eye forward 242

F

Face, flushing of 87
Fampridine 318
Fascia-lata 365
Fascicles innervating 301
Fasciculus
    cuneatus 186, 198
    gracilis 186
    interfascicularis 186
    medial longitudinal 22, 190
    septomarginalis 186
Fat
    excess 175
    low 176
Fatal pulmonary embolism 329
Fatigue 344
    central 228
    evaluation of 228
Fecal impaction 316
Fecal incontinence 316
Fesoterodine 313
Fiber 268
    foods, high 339
    of Clarke's column 193
    of corticospinal tract 187
    tracing of 192
Fiberoptic endoscopic evaluation of
        swallowing 145
Fibromuscular dysplasia 43
Fibrous foods 339
Fighting spirit 220
Finger
    flexion 289, 354
    nail loop 352
Flexion of knee, loss of 199
Flexor synergy of upper limb, spastic 102
Fluids 174
Food, types of 173, 340*t*
Foot, spastic 301
Footplates 346
Forearm flexor, spastic 351
Fourth sacral anterior nerve 318
Foville syndrome 24
Fractures of ribs 287
Frankel classification, modified 210
Frog breathing 287
Frontoparietal operculum 18
Fugl-Meyer assessment 32

Functional communication 115
Funiculus, posterior 186, 198

G

Gait 106
    analysis 228, 390
    facilitation of 107
    training 106, 292, 376
Gamma motor neurons 185
Gamma-amino butyric acid 276, 299
Gastostomy feeding 150
Gastric emptying 318
Gastrocolic reflex 316
Gastroesophageal reflux 150, 322
Gastrointestinal
    intolerance 172
    reflexes 316
    tract 316
Gastrostomy 173
    feeding 150
Gelatinosa 300
Genitalia 235
Genitourinary complications 93
Geriatric depression scale 32
Glasgow
    coma scale 36, 143, 364, 373
    outcome scale 373
Glossopharyngeal breathing 287, 324,
        326, 327
Glottic muscles 322
Glottis 287, 322, 327
Glucocorticoid 340
Glucose 175
    test 47
Glycerine 317
Glycopyrrolate 318
Gray horns, posterior 198
Grip strength training 288*f*
Gulps air bolus 327
Gutter splint 352

H

Habitual constipation 172
Haemophilus influenzae 329
Hamstring stretches 290
Hand 289
    dexterity, insufficient 312
    exercises 384*f*
    grip 346
    mouth functions 289
    orthosis 351
    rim projection 346
    spastic 301
    training of 304*f*
Head
    back, throw 347
    injury 372

Headache 299, 364
  pounding 87
Health locus of control scale 219
Healthcare system 408
Hematoma 362
Hemiparesis 20, 361, 365
Hemiplegia 104, 106
  contralateral 9
Hemiplegic
  hand 99
  lower limb 104
  shoulder 85
Hemisection of cord 197
Hemispheric stroke scale 36
Hemorrhagic stroke 16
Hemorrhoids 316
Hemothorax 319
Heparin 329
Heterotrophic ossification 82, 83, 372
Highfiber foods 339
Hip
  extension, selective 104
  joint 304
  knee-ankle-foot orthosis 354
  muscles 287
  spastic 301
Hoffman reflex 230
Homocysteine 176
  level, high 172
Horn
  cells, posterior 299
  dorsal 300
Horner's syndrome 198, 240
Hydrocephalus 363-365, 372
Hydrochloride 313
Hydrophilic catheters 312
Hydrotherapy 276
Hygiene, facilitate 306
Hyperbaric oxygen 327
Hypercholesterolemia 47
Hyperesthesia 198
Hyperexcitability
  contribution of segmental 229
  of alpha motor neuron 233
Hyperglycemia 52
Hyperinsulinemia 336
Hyperlipidemia 176
Hyperparathyroidism 336
Hyperpyrexia 9
Hyperreflexia 314
Hyperreflexic bowel 315
Hypersensitivity of skin 199
Hypertension 172, 176
  unit 390
Hypertonia 300
Hypertonicity 300, 372
Hyperviscosity 329

Hypocalcemia 330
Hypocholesterolemic agents 178
Hypoglycemia 52
Hypogonadism 363
Hypokalemia 330
Hypomagnesemia 330
Hyponatremic state 173
Hypothalamospinal tract 198
Hypothyroidism state 172
Hypotonia 199
Hypoventilation 320, 321
Hypoxic insults 363

I

Immobilization, complication of 329
Implantation
  of intrathecal catheter, technique of 280*f*
  technique of 278
Index muscle 210*t*, 212
Indoor team rehabilitation 388
Indwelling catheterization 312
Infection 130
  prevention of 324, 328
  treatment of 328
Inhalation, deep 287
Inhalational method 34
Inhibit motor activity 376
Injury 200, 287, 320, 364, 372
  basis of level of 348
  bilateral 12
  functional level of 286
  level of 87
  mechanism of 203
  nature of 203
  of local cord segments 198
  site of 320
  types of 348*t*
Inspiration
  cough, deep 227
  deeper 287
Integumentary system 92
Intensive care unit 328
Intercostal muscles 320
Intermittent abdominal pressure
    respirator 327
Intermittent catheterization 312
Intermittent positive pressure
    ventilation 328
International Continence Society 309, 310*t*
International Medical Society of Paraplegia
    209, 241
Internuclear ophthalmoplegia 23
Intestinal obstruction 316
Intracerebral hemorrhage 87
Intracranial pressure 48, 374
Intractable pain, chronic 300

Intrapulmonary percussive ventilation 328
Intrathecal baclofen 277, 314
   pump 277, 297, 299
   therapy 277
Ipratropium 323
Ischemic penumbra 42*f*
Ischemic stroke, mechanisms of 43
Ischial pressure sore 135
Isokinetic systems 230

J

Jaw 421
Joint Commission on Accreditation of Health
      Care Organizations 396
Joint range of motion 85

K

Kidneys, ultrasound of 253
Knee 199, 352
   ankle-foot orthosis 352, 353*f*
   instability 352
   jerk 199
Knife injury 197
Korsakoff's syndrome 6

L

Labial function 421
Labyrinthine reflex 98
Lacunar
   infarcts 15
   stroke 43
      syndrome 20
Laryngeal
   closure 143
   elevation 143
   function 421
   substage 140
Laryngitis 322
Laryngopharynx 140
Laryngoscope 325
Larynx 327
Left ventricular ejection fraction 34
Leg
   control of 103
   rests 345, 346
   stabilization of 346
Lesion of
   dorsal root 196
   motor area 12
   sensory area 12
   thalamus, severe 6
Levator scapulae 320
Limb
   contralateral 269
   kinetic apraxia 19
   lower 290, 350
   muscle strength assessment 323

   posterior 10
   upper 193, 289, 350
Limits range of motion 270
Linen, care of 134
Lingual function 421
Linolenic acid, alpha 177
Lipid abnormalities 336
Lipoprotein, low density 56
Liver synthesizes 178
Living skills 303
Locomotion 356
Locomotor ataxia 199
Loop handle 306
Loop splint 352
Lowenstein occupational therapy cognitive
      assessment 159
Lumbar enlargement 183
Lumbar puncture 51
Lumbar spinal cord 354
Lumbosacral
   brace 350*f*
   nerves 317
   region 299
   spine films 244
Lung 320
   airlessness of 322
   collapse 325
   restriction of 321

M

Macular vision 5
Magnetic stimulation, functional 317
Malone antegrade continence enema 318
Mania 365
Manipulate bolus 422
Manofluorography 145
Manometry 145
Medical Rehabilitation Center 382
Medical Research Council 32, 36
   Muscle Grading 36
Medulla oblongata 11
Medullary syndrome
   lateral 11
   medial 11
Melodic intonation therapy 120
Memory deficit 377
Meningitis 138, 365
Mental
   barriers 154
   confusion 87
   well-being, care of 331
Mesenteric artery syndrome, superior 316
Metabolic
   and endocrine changes 336
   disorder unit 390
Metaproterenol 323
Methylprednisolone 242

Metoclopramide 318
Micturition 309
  reflex 313
Midbrain
  cross-section of 7*f*
  syndrome
    dorsal 25
    ventral 24
  vascular supply of 6
Middle cerebral artery 3, 5, 10, 43, 17
  clot 49*f*
  stroke syndrome 17
Millard-Gubler syndrome 24
Minerals supplementation 174
Mini-mental status examination 31, 36, 159
Minnesota test 115
Mobilization, continuous passive 80
Molecular weight heparin, low 90
Morbidity 44, 309
Motor assessment scale 32
Motor functional performance 161
Motor imagery 167
Motor neuron 223
  bowel syndrome, lower 315
Motor paralysis 363
Motor paralytic bladder 310
Motor stroke, pure 20
Moving paralyzed limbs 304
Mucus plugging 320
Muscle
  belly of quadriceps 236
  bulk 337
  function evaluation system 256*f*
  major involved 271
  sense, loss of unconscious 197
  spastic 269
  spindle, bypasses 232
  strength
    quantification of 228
    testing 227
  tone 33, 229, 268
    and mass, maintain 270
  weakness and atrophy 81
Muscular disinsertion 301
Musculocutaneous nerve 301
Musculoskeletal complications 249
Myelotomy 298, 299, l299
  midline posterior 300
Myocardial failure 87
Myotatic reflex, segmental 268
Myotomes 210*t*

N

Nasal
  drip, posterior 362
  intermittent positive pressure
    ventilation 324
  stuffiness 87

Nasopharyngeal leak 362
National acute spinal cord injury study 209, 242, 417
National Institute of Health Stroke Scale 46
National Institute of Neurologic Disorders and Stroke 40
National Spinal Cord Injury Statistical Center 248
Natural liquid foods 173
Nausea 299
Neck
  accessory 286
  bending of 203
  rests 345
Neocortex 365
Neostigmine 318
Nerve 327
  injuries 363
  root 198, 223
Nervous system 3, 223*t*
  central 138, 359
  part of 223*t*
Neural
  circuits 299, 300
  plasticity 60
  precursor cells 418
  stem cells 416
Neuroablative procedures 297, 299
Neurobehavioral
  cognitive status examination 31
  sequelae 361, 364
Neurodevelopmental rehabilitation 68
Neurogenic bladder 309, 310
  classification of 309, 310*t*
  dysfunction 309
  management of 309
Neurogenic bowel
  dysfunction 314
  management 316
Neurogenic hypomotile intestine 339
Neurogenic pain 297
Neurologic disease 309
Neurologic dysfunction 309
Neurological
  deficit 14, 361
  disease 314
    progressive 150
  disorders, progressive 138
  examination scales 210
Neurolysis of peripheral nerve 277
Neuromuscular
  function, quantification of 227
  weakness 324
Neurons, alpha 185
Neuropathology, nature of 117
Neuropeptide 313
Neurophysical sequelae 361, 362

Neurosyphilis 197
Neurotomies 301
Nocturnal desaturation 323
Nonfunctional cough 287
Noninvasive ventilation 325
Nonmechanical ventilatory
    assistance 326
Nonreacting pupil 364
Non-reflux stoma 318
Nonskid mat 306
Nortriptyline 155
Nosocomial
  infection 324
  pneumonia 328, 329
Noxious stimuli 88
Nucleus
  ambiguous 141
  tractus solitarius 141
Nutrition 132
  enteral 173
Nutritional management of stroke 172

O

Obesity 172, 175
Obstructive sleep apnea 323
Ocular plethysmography 34
Oculomotor nucleus 7
Odontoid 243*f*
Odynophagia 322
Olfactory ensheathing cells 418
Olivospinal tract 189
Onabotulinum toxin 313
One-and-a-half syndrome 24
Ophthalmic artery 21
Oral
  motor evaluation 421
  transport stage 139
Organum vasculosum lamina
    terminalis 4
Orthosis 349, 350, 355, 390
Osmolar fluid 374
Osteoporosis 81, 340, 354
  prevention of 340
Osteotomies 301
Oxfordshire Community Stroke
    Project 15
Oxybutynin 313
Oxygen, supplemental 52

P

Pain 191*f*, 240
  biochemical theory of 194
  control mechanism 193
  felt, sharp 196
  loss of 199
  management unit, interventional 389
  stabbing 198

syndrome 93
  central 86, 87
Palm oil, low levels of 178
Paradoxical motion 321
Paralysis 286, 320
  bilateral 9, 240
  contralateral 4, 8
  of eye muscles 7
  of levator palpebrae superioris 7
  of lower limb 4
  spastic 198
  total 211
  types of 200
Paramedian branches 6
Paranasal sinuses 362, 368*f*
Paraplegia, spastic 300
Paraplegics 291
  walk again 419
Parenchyma 325
Parenteral nutrition 175
  total 175
Parinaud's syndrome 7
Parkinson's disease 138
Pectoralis 320
  major 306
  minor 306
Pelvic 343
  floor 315
    muscles 234
  girdle 105
  rotation, functional 69*f*
Pelvis 106
Pendulum test 229, 233
Penile tip erosion 312
Penoscrotal fistula 312
Pentadecapeptide 313
Penumbra system 41*f*
Percutaneous
  endoscopic gastrostomy 54
  gastrostomy 150
Perianal abscess 316
Peripheral
  nerves 223, 299, 301
  neurotomies 299, 301
  pain 240
Peristalsis 315, 339
Perisylvian cortex, destruction of left 158
Persistent vegetative state 373
Pharmacotherapy 122, 377
Pharyngeal
  muscles 143, 287
  paralysis 143
  stage 139, 143
  tongue 139, 140
Pharyngolaryngeal sensation 143
Pharynx 327
Phenoxybenzamine 314

Philadelphia geriatric center 35
Phonetic paraphasia 110
Phosphodiesterase-5 inhibitors 314
Phrenic nerves 320, 327
Physical medicine 54
Physical therapy sessions 290*f*
Physiotherapy 285, 297
Pillows, positioning of 100*f*
Placing hemiplegic leg 103
Plan implementation 406
Plantar flexion of foot 231*f*
Plantar withdrawal reflex 233
Pneumococcal vaccination 329
Pneumoencephalocele 367
Pneumonia 319, 322, 323, 325, 326, 328
Pneumothorax 319
Pollicis brevis muscle, abductor 232*f*
Polyethylene glycol 317
Polymeric mixtures, commercially
    supplied 173
Polyphenolic antioxidants 176
Polyunsaturated 177
Pontine hemorrhage 9
Pontine paramedian reticular formation 22
Pontine syndrome, ventral 24
Porch index of communication ability 115
Poststroke
    anxiety 155
    rehabilitation 64
    subluxation 85
Post-traumatic
    amnesia 373, 374
    epilepsy 362
    glioma 364
    seizures 361
    syndrome 364
Postural drainage 324, 328
Postural hypotension 89
Potassium 174
    chloride 173
Pragmatic therapy 120
Premorbid
    language skills 117
    personality 154
Pressure
    management 343
    palsies 226
    reducing support surface 92
    relief 133
    sore 128, 131*f*, 132*f*
        distribution of 131
        grading 130
        management of 132
        multiple 136
    ulcers sore 92
    ventilation, negative 325
Presynaptic inhibition, reflex indicates 233

Primitive oral reflex 142
Prophylaxis 330
Proprioceptive neuromuscular
    facilitation 273
Prosthesis unit 390
Protein 174
Prothrombin time 47, 90
Proximal key points 104, 105
Prucalopride 318
Pseudomonas aeruginosa 130, 329
Psychological deficit 374
Psychosis 155, 365
Ptosis 363
Pudendal motor nerve latency 234
Pudendal nerve latency 235
Pulmonary
    edema 87
    embolism 89, 90, 319, 329
    function 323
    muscles, function of 286
Pulse 33
    oximetry 323
Pump catheter 279*f*
Pyogenic meningitis 365
Pyramidal tract 7, 187, 188, 197

Q

Quadrantanopsia 18
Quadrigeminal artery emerging 7
Quadriplegia index of function 216

R

Radial wrist extensor 305
Radicular arteries, quarter of anterior 195
Radionuclide angiography 34
Rancho los amigos scale 373
Range of motion 80, 100
Ratchet-W-H orthosis 354
Raymond-Céstan syndrome 24
Recreational therapists 396
Recreational therapy 392, 393, 402
    benefits of 407
Rectal placement 317
Rectal prolapsed 316
Reflex 315, 343
    bradycardia 87
    functions, loss of 197
    inhibiting movement patterns 100, 102
    neurogenic bladder 310
    sympathetic dystrophy 83
    voiding 312
Refractory period 226
Rehabilitation 54, 60, 63, 392, 412
    active 375
    acute 167
        care 250*f*
    goals, long-term 161

long-term 72, 251
main goals of 375
models of 381
of oral feeding 149
of spinal cord injury 264
systems of 387
Relaxation techniques 273
Relaxes 287
Renal failure 331
Residual function 235
Residual spasticity 365
Resiniferatoxin 313
Respiration 242
electrophonic 326, 327
Respiratory
care 319, 324, 331
complications 319
function 251, 286
optimal 343
insufficiency 322
muscle conditioning 327
Restrict radial deviation 354
Restrictive defect 321
derives 321
Reticulospinal tracts 189
Retrolentiform part 10
Reversible syndromes 241
Rhizotomies, posterior 299, 301
Rhizotomy 258, 301
posterior 300*f*
Rhomboid 305
stretches 289
Rim projections 346
Road traffic accidents 372
Root
dorsal 198, 300
entry zone, dorsal 299
posterior 299
Rotational force 203
Rotator cuff injury 100
Rubber band 349
traction 352
Rubrospinal tract 188

S

Sacral anterior root stimulator 318
Sacral nerve 313
Sacral pressure sore 135
Sacral reflex 234
Sacral rhizotomy, dorsal 313
Safflower oil 177
Saturated fatty acid ratio 177
Scandinavian neurological stroke scale 15
Scapula 289
Scapular elevation 100
Sensation, loss of 199
Sensorimotor stroke, mixed 21

Sensory
assessment 287
cortical areas 5
disturbances 200
examination 33
integration of 228
loss 4
mild 4
nerve action potential 226
neurogenic bladder 310
perception 315
score 212
stroke, pure 21
tract 198
Sepsis 319
Serotonin reuptake inhibitors 155
Serratus anterior 306, 320
Sexual dysfunction 372
Sexuality rehabilitation 377
Shockwave therapy 275
Shoulder 289
air 331
flexion 289
girdle 105
orthosis 350
rotators 305
subluxation 67*f*
Sickle cell disease 43
Sigmoid
colon 315
volvulus 316
Skeletal models 295*f*
Skim milk 173
powder 174
Skin
care of 128, 330, 341
protectors 92
Sleep
abnormalities 364
apnea 327
Smooth muscle 235, 313
Social reliance 220
Social stimulation and benefit 304
Social worker 381
Sodium 174, 179
low 173
Soft tissue elements 203
Soleus muscle 231*f*
Soluble fiber 316
Somatosensory
evoked potential 224, 373
pathways 235
Sound stimuli 227
Spasm, relief of 132
Spasticity 93, 269, 270, 297, 301, 306, 350
assessment of 271
management of 297

medical management of 268, 276
quantification of 229
reduce 247
surgical management of 298
treatment of 277
   planning 272
Speech
   and language
      pathologist 384
      therapist 381
   communication therapy 386*f*
   therapist 366, 377
Sphincter 315
   constriction 315
   control 217
   electromyography 234
   muscles 312
   pupillae 7
Spinal
   and stroke rehabilitation clinic 389
   artery
      distribution, anterior 195*f*
      distribution, posterior 195*f*
      joins 194
      posterior 195
   canal 297, 300
   column injury 202-204
   column, biomechanics of injured 202
   cord 183, 191*f*, 194, 196, 264, 299, 327, 338
      anatomy of 183
      certain zones of 195
      comprehensive evaluation of 208
      disorders of 222, 237
      independence measure 215
      repair research 417
      stimulation 258, 297, 298
      white matter of 185
   cord injury 78, 128, 205, 215, 222, 226,
      244*f*, 245, 247, 248, 258, 264, 269, 285,
      291, 297, 303, 305, 309, 311, 312, 314,
      319-321, 321*t*, 323, 324, 336, 338, 342,
      349, 353, 381, 387, 389, 412, 416
      chronic 336
      classification of 213*f*
      evaluation of 207
      functional ambulation inventory 215
      functional restoration of 303
      nature of 416
      rehabilitation 248, 254
   gray matter 184
   injury 218, 239, 311, 348, 361, 364, 402,
      418
      mechanism of 203
      pathophysiology of 202
   instability 286
   model 269

shock 320
surgery clinic 389
Spine 286
Spinocerebellar tract 192
   anterior 192, 197
   lateral 197, 198
   lesion 197
   posterior 193
Spirometer 286
Splint 350
   classification system 350
   types of 349
Splitting spinal cord 299
Squint, internal 8
Staphylococcus aureus 329
State trait anxiety inventory 219
Static lung 321
Static progressive 350
Static splint 349
Stercoral perforation 316
Stimulate peristalsis 317
Stimulation of nerves, electrical 376
Stomach 173
Stools, hard 339
Strabismus, external 7
Streptococcus pneumoniae 329
Striate, posterolateral 5
Stroke 28-31, 44, 47, 53*t*, 60, 68, 71, 74, 109,
      128, 138, 152, 158, 175, 232*f*, 269, 349,
      381, 382, 387, 409
   acute 47, 48, 50*f*, 52*t*
   causes of 43
   evaluation of 28
   management, acute 40, 51
   medical care 51
   mimics, common 47
   prevention, secondary 73
   recovery predictors 62
   rehabilitation 1, 62, 222, 402, 411
      programs 62
   syndromes 14
   treatment of 165
      acute 14
   victim 172
Subarachnoid hemorrhage 12
Subcutaneous adipose 337
Subglottic stenosis 323
Substantia gelatinosa 184
   cells 194
Sudden acute hypertension 87
Sugars, excess 175
Sulcus, posterolateral 301
Sunflower oil 177
Supine 286, 287, 289
   lying position 99
Supramarginal gyri 12

Suprapubic
catheter 312
tapping 312
Swallow saliva 421
Swallowing 323
assessment of 145, 422
care of 324
central control of 141
disorders 142
problems 138
Swivel spoon 306
Sympathetic
nervous system 321
skin response 226, 235
Syringomyelia 197
Systemic infection 172
Systemic measures 132

T

Tabes dorsalis 198
Tachycardia 325
Tachypnea 323
T-cells 194
Tectospinal tract 189
Temperature fibers 191
Tendo achilles 199, 290
Tendon
jerk 230
electrical equivalent of 230
exaggerated 268
lengthening 301
loss of 199
reflexes 198, 236
transfers 301
Tenodesis grasp 306
Tenodesis grip 289
Tenotomy 301
Terazosin 314
Tetraplegics 216
Thalamus 6
Theophylline 327
Therapeutic
exercise program 97
massage 274
nerve blocks 257
recreation 393, 398, 402
rehabilitation 268
Thoracic
cage 319
region 286
spinal cord injury 320
spine films 244
Thoracic/lumbar instability, low 287
Thoracolumbar spine stabilization 246f
Throat clearing 421
Thrombolysis candidates, potential 52t
Thrombolytic therapy 49f

Thromboplastin time, activated partial 47
Thrombosis of anterior spinal artery 197
Tibial nerve 301
posterior 317
Tibialis anterior 230f, 231f
Tissue plasminogen activator 40
Tolterodine 313
Tone normalization 343
Tongue 287
driving force 140
Tonic stretch reflexes 297
Toothbrush 306
Top of basilar syndrome 23
Torsional force 203
Toxin therapy 313
Tracheal stenosis 322
Tracheobronchial secretions 326
Tracheostomy 323
tube 421
Tracheotomy 325
tube 327
Tract cells 191, 194
Tract of Lissauer, posterolateral 191
Traction immobilization 244
Tractotomy 199
Tracts
arrangements of 185
ascending 186, 190, 223
of posterior column 198
Transanal irrigation 317
Transcortical aphasia 19
Transcranial Doppler 50
ultrasonography 160
Transcutaneous electrical nerve stimulation
84, 257, 274
Transesophageal echocardiography 51
Transient ischemic attacks 47
Transthoracic echocardiography 51
Transurethral sphincterotomy 314
Trapezius 320
stretch 289
Trauma 289, 372, 377
centers 372
external 309
Traumatic brain injury 138, 359, 361, 369,
372-374
consequences of 361
Traumatic fat embolism 330
Traumatic hypospadias 312
Trigeminal nerve 142
Trochanteric pressure sore 135
Trophic ulcers 197
Trospium chloride 313
Trunk
bending of 203
mobilization 104
stability 343

Tube feeding 174*t*
Tube, flexible 312
Two-dimensional interpretation 159

U

Ulcer
    complicated 130
    long standing 130
Ulnar deviation 289
Ultimately pneumonia 321
Upper extremity, movements of 102
Upper motor syndrome 268
Ureters, ultrasound of 253
Urethra 312
Urethral
    function 309
    sphincter 234
Urinary
    bladder 309
        and rectum, emptying of 200
    incontinence 310, 372
    rehabilitation unit 390
    sepsis 250
    tract infection 88, 312, 338, 419
Urogenital dysfunction 234

V

Vaccination 324
Vasculitis 43
Vegetarian diet, advantage of 178
Vein thrombosis, deep 89, 285
Velcro fastening facilitate dressing 306
Vena cava filter placement 330
Ventilation 242
Ventilator-associated pneumonia 328
Ventilatory management, chronic 326
Ventilatory support, chronic 324
Ventral root produce, destruction of 198
Verbal paraphasia 110
Vertebral canal 183
Vertebrobasilar
    artery thrombosis 22
    insufficiency 22
        syndromes 22
Vestibulospinal tract 189
Videoendoscopic swallowing study 145
Videofluoroscopic swallowing study 145
Viral infection 197
Vision 32, 258

Visual
    action therapy 120
    deficits 18
    evoked potential 223
Vital capacity 286, 287, 321, 327
Vitamin 174, 175
    A, supplement of 179
    B$_{12}$ neuropathy 198
Vocal quality 421
Vocational counselor 381, 386
Voiding dysfunction
    evaluation of 311
    management of 311
Voluntary contraction of tibialis 233
Voluntary cough 421

W

Walker, types of 355*f*
Walking index 215, 216
Wallenberg syndrome 22
Warfarin aspirin recurrent stroke 56
Watsu approach 276
Weakness 299
    of movement 198
Weber's syndrome 8, 24
Weight shift techniques 133
Western aphasia battery 115
Wheelchair
    maneuvers 347
    selection 342
    types 343
World Health Organization 393
World Recreational Therapy 393
Wound
    care 250
    resurfacing, methods of 135
Wriggle right buttock 347
Wrist 289, 351
    extended 347
    extension 289
    extension grip 347
    flexion 100, 289
    tightness of 100

X

Xiphoid 286, 287

Y

Yawning 322